"With this book, you can design a customized healing plan to take your health as far as it needs to go. Whether your focus is mental health or physical health, whether you want chronic symptom relief or you'd like to prevent frightening diagnoses, whether you want to make big changes or take small steps, these tools are yours.

This is not one size fits all. Each individual has their own signature blend of poisons, toxins, pathogens, exposures, and emotional experiences. No person has the exact same health situation as another. This is why the information here can be tailored so you have every opportunity to heal. I've always said that there is no single 'Medical Medium protocol.' There are countless Medical Medium protocols because these tools are endlessly personalizable for your unique needs. You're welcome to dip your toe into the waters of just one or explore them all."

— Anthony William, Medical Medium

"Even if you lack the faith that what you're doing will heal you, you can still heal when you give your body what it needs, remove from your body what it doesn't need, know why you got sick to begin with, and know what to do to recover. These steps will still allow you to heal, even if you don't believe you can heal or believe you ever will heal."

— Anthony William, Medical Medium

PRAISE FOR ANTHONY WILLIAM

"Anthony William has a powerful gift that our family has now experienced firsthand. After years of doctors being unable to diagnose, identify, or pinpoint our child's gastrointestinal issues, Anthony's expertise and intuition led us to not only identifying the issue, but more importantly, Anthony's precise protocols have been the invaluable catalyst in our daughter's healing, recovery, and her happiness. As parents, there is no greater gift you can pray for than the health of your children, and we are eternally grateful to you, Anthony, for your powerful gifts. Thank you for your time, energy, guidance, and comfort on a journey that wasn't overnight, and for restoring our daughter's and many of our family members' health, Anthony."
— Dwayne "The Rock" Johnson and Lauren Hashian

"Celery juice is sweeping the globe. It's impressive how Anthony has created this movement and restored superior health in countless people around the world."
— Sylvester Stallone

"Anthony William has been there for my wife at all times to make sure she is as healthy as she could possibly be. I will always thank him and love him for that."
— Adam Sandler, writer, filmmaker, actor, comedian

"Anthony's understanding of foods, their vibrations, and how they interact with the body never ceases to amaze. Effortlessly he explains the potential harmony or disharmony in our choices in a way anyone can understand. He has a gift. Do your body a favor and treat yourself."
— Pharrell Williams, 13-time Grammy-winning artist and producer

"Anthony is a healing encounter."
— Diane von Furstenberg, iconic fashion designer

"Anthony is a trusted source for our family. His work in the world is a light that has guided many to safety. He means so much to us."
— Robert De Niro and Grace Hightower De Niro

"Anthony doesn't offer gimmicks or fads to finding ultimate health. His recommended foods and cleansing programs are simple and delicious and THEY WORK! If you're done living with pain, fatigue, brain fog, intestinal disorders, and a myriad of other nasty ailments, drop everything and read this (and his other) books. He will quickly bring health and hope back into your life."
— Hilary Swank, Oscar-winning actress and film producer

"For over 40 years I have been teaching the principles of vital health and alkalinity in my books and seminars. Sage and I are passionate about the cleanse-to-heal approach to nutrition and wellness that naturally supports the body and fortifies our immune system to keep it functioning at its prime. We are so grateful for the dear friendship, guidance, alignment, and insights of Anthony William, not only in his teaching and best practices, but also for the way he has personally ushered us through our own health challenges. He is a brother on this path and a gift to this world. His routines have proven results to all who seek to optimize their inner terrain."

— Tony Robbins

"While there is most definitely an element of otherworldly mystery to the work he does, much of what Anthony William shines a spotlight on—particularly around autoimmune disease—feels inherently right and true. What's better is that the protocols he recommends are natural, accessible, and easy to do."

— Gwyneth Paltrow, Oscar-winning actress, #1 *New York Times* best-selling author, founder and CEO of GOOP.com

"Anthony William's philosophy on food and health protocols has profoundly changed my life and health for the better. I am forever grateful for him."

— Miranda Kerr, international supermodel, founder and CEO of KORA Organics

"Anthony has turned numerous lives around for the better with the healing powers of celery juice."

— Novak Djokovic, #1-ranked tennis champion in the world

"All great gifts are bestowed with humility. Anthony is humble. And like all the right remedies, his are intuitive, natural, and balanced. These two make for a powerful and effective combination."

— John Donovan, CEO of AT&T Communications

"Anthony William is truly dedicated to sharing his knowledge and experience to spread the word of healing to all. His compassion and desire to reach as many people as he can to help them heal themselves is inspiring and empowering. Today, in a world of obsession with prescription medication, it is so refreshing to know that there are alternative options that truly work and can open a new door to health."

— Liv Tyler, star of *9-1-1: Lone Star*, *Harlots*, the *Lord of the Rings* trilogy, *Empire Records*

"Anthony is a magician for all my label's recording artists, and if he were a record album, he would far surpass Thriller. His ability is nothing short of profound, remarkable, extraordinary, and mind-blowing. He is a luminary whose books are filled with prophecies. This is the future of medicine."

— Craig Kallman, Chairman and CEO, Atlantic Records

"Anthony's knowledge on the food we consume, the impact it has on our body, and our overall well-being has been a game changer for me!"
— Jenna Dewan, star of *The Rookie, Soundtrack, World of Dance, Step Up*

"Anthony is a wonderful person. He identified some long-term health issues for me, he knew what supplements I needed, and I felt better immediately."
— Rashida Jones, Grammy-winning director of *Quincy*,
star of *Parks and Recreation* and *The Office*

"My family and friends have been the recipients of Anthony's inspired gift of healing, and we've benefited more than I can express with rejuvenated physical and mental health."
— Scott Bakula, executive producer and star of *NCIS: New Orleans*; Golden Globe–
winning star of *Quantum Leap* and *Star Trek: Enterprise*

"I rely on Anthony William for my and my family's health. Even when doctors are stumped, Anthony always knows what the problem is and the pathway for healing."
— Chelsea Field, *NCIS: New Orleans, Andre, The Last Boy Scout*

"I refer to Anthony William's books constantly for the most insightful wisdom and recipes to restore energy and good health. Interested in the unique and powerful qualities of each food he describes, I'm inspired to consider how I can enhance the ritual of cooking and eating for the sake of wellness each day."
— Alexis Bledel, Emmy-winning star of *The Handmaid's Tale, Gilmore Girls,
Sisterhood of the Traveling Pants*

"I was diagnosed with a serious autoimmune disorder two years ago. The disease compromised my liver and resulted in debilitating, episodic flare-ups, often resulting in hospitalizations. I went through a battery of consultations with world-renowned experts, as well as tried numerous prescribed medicines such as steroids and immunosuppressants, all of which were challenging. I was intent on exploring alternative treatments to exhaust all possible cures, which is when I spoke with Anthony William. Anthony's compassion, combined with his extensive knowledge and understanding on dietary solutions to heal chronic diseases, resulted in a true miracle. Based on my liver disease and gastroparesis, Anthony customized a daily regimen my body and mind could handle. Within six weeks, my blood work showcased a 50 percent improvement in my liver function, and within three months, my blood work was the best it had been since the onset of my disease. My weight stabilized, my chronic symptoms were eradicated, and I literally got my life back. I cannot thank Anthony William enough for his expertise, patience, compassion, and for helping me to get my healthy life back. I am forever grateful."
— Dana Gerson Unger, Friends Board Member, Dana-Farber Cancer Institute

"Anthony's discovery and analysis of the values of celery juice is a game changer in our family. Both in my wife's work and in our regular routines. I firmly believe our ease with recovery on all three bouts of COVID we were dealt was largely due to our strict regimen of the Medical Medium virus protection packet."
— Corey Feldman, artist, creator, actor, musician, philanthropist

"Thank God for Anthony's gift, because it has not only inspired thousands of people to recover their health, but it has also helped my personal journey to recovery, as well as guiding my work with my own clients as a health coach as I help to teach the ways of plant-based whole foods nutrition."
— Courtney Feldman, health coach, model, singer, dancer, influencer

"Anthony's books are revolutionary yet practical. For anybody frustrated by the current limits of Western medicine, this is definitely worth your time and consideration."
— James Van Der Beek, creator, executive producer, and star of *What Would Diplo Do?* and star of *Pose* and *Dawson's Creek*, and Kimberly Van Der Beek, public speaker and activist

"Anthony's advanced understanding of the Epstein-Barr virus (medical science is just catching up with what he has been saying for years) has helped many people, including myself, reclaim their lives. When your health has been challenged, you appreciate what an incredible gift this is. I am so impressed with Anthony's compassion, kindness, and his dedication to helping people heal. His extensive and undeniable understanding of the true causes of illness is remarkable. And his solutions are simple and easy to apply, and most importantly, accessible to all. He has not only given hope to those of us who have struggled with mystery pain, autoimmune disease, depression, confusion, and the after-effects of COVID, but he has given us the maps we need to reclaim our lives. He is, in my opinion, a gift to humanity. And I recommend that anyone who has been struggling with their health to stop the struggle and immediately pick up his books and follow along."
— Carrie Ann Inaba, *Dancing with the Stars*, Emmy-nominated television host, executive producer, and founder of Carrie Ann Conversations

"Anthony is a great man. His knowledge is fascinating and has been very helpful for me. The celery juice alone is a game changer!"
— Calvin Harris, producer, DJ, and Grammy-winning artist

"I am so grateful to Anthony. After introducing his celery juice protocol into my daily routine, I have seen a marked improvement in every aspect of my health."
— Debra Messing, Emmy-winning star of *The Dark Divide*, *Will & Grace*, *Ned and Stacey*

"Anthony has dedicated his life to helping others find the answers that we need to live our healthiest lives. And celery juice is the most accessible way to start!"
— Courteney Cox, star of *Shining Vale*, *Cougar Town*, *Friends*

"Anthony is not only a warm, compassionate healer, he is also authentic and accurate, with God-given skills. He has been a total blessing in my life."
— Naomi Campbell, model, actress, activist

"Anthony has created global awareness about how to heal ourselves naturally. So thankful for his books. They are truly changing lives."
— Kelly Rutherford, star of *Gossip Girl* and *Melrose Place*

"Anthony's extensive knowledge and deep intuition have demystified even the most confounding health issues. He has provided a clear path for me to feel my very best— I find his guidance indispensable."
— Taylor Schilling, star of *Pam & Tommy* and *Orange Is the New Black*

"Anthony William is a gift to humanity. His incredible work has helped millions of people heal when conventional medicine had no answers for them. His genuine passion and commitment for helping people is unsurpassed, and I am grateful to have been able to share a small part of his powerful message in Heal."
— Kelly Noonan Gores, writer, director, and producer of the *Heal* documentary

"Anthony William's God-given gift for healing is nothing short of miraculous."
— David James Elliott, *Heart of Champions*, *Trumbo*, *Mad Men*, *CSI: NY*; star for 10 years of *JAG*

"We are incredibly grateful for Anthony and his passionate dedication to spreading the word about healing through food. Anthony has a truly special gift. His practices have entirely reshaped our perspectives about food and ultimately our lifestyle. Celery juice alone has completely transformed the way we feel and it will always be a part of our morning routine."
— Hunter Mahan, six-time PGA Tour–winning golfer

"Anthony is a truly generous person with keen intuition and knowledge about health. I have seen firsthand the transformation he's made in people's quality of life."
— Carla Gugino, star of *The Haunting of Bly Manor*, *Jett*, *Watchmen*, *Entourage*, *Spy Kids*

"A pathfinder. Truly ahead of his time. A vision of hope."
— Steve Harris, Iron Maiden

"I've been following Anthony for a while now and am always floored (but not surprised) at the success stories from people following his protocols . . . I have been on my own path of healing for many years, jumping from doctor to doctor and specialist to specialist. He's the real deal, and I trust him and his vast knowledge of how the thyroid works and the true effects food has on our body. I have directed countless friends, family, and followers to Anthony because I truly believe he possesses knowledge that no doctor out there has. I am a believer and on a true path to healing now and am honored to know him and blessed to know his work. Every endocrinologist needs to read his book on the thyroid!"
— Marcela Valladolid, chef, author, television host

"What if someone could simply touch you and tell you what it is that ails you? Welcome to the healing hands of Anthony William—a modern-day alchemist who very well may hold the key to longevity. His lifesaving advice blew into my world like a healing hurricane, and he has left a path of love and light in his wake. He is hands down the ninth wonder of the world."
— Lisa Gregorisch-Dempsey, senior executive producer of *Extra*

"Anthony William is changing and saving the lives of people all over the world with his one-of-a-kind gift. His constant dedication and vast amount of highly advanced information have broken the barriers that block so many in the world from receiving desperately needed truths that science and research have not yet discovered. On a personal level, he has helped both my daughters and me, giving us tools to support our health that actually work. Celery juice is now a part of our regular routine!"
— Lisa Rinna, star of *The Real Housewives of Beverly Hills* and *Days of Our Lives*, *New York Times* best-selling author, designer of the Lisa Rinna Collection

"I am a doctor's daughter who has always relied on Western medicine to ameliorate even the smallest of woes. Anthony's insights opened my eyes to the healing benefits of food and how a more holistic approach to health can change your life."
— Jenny Mollen, actress and *New York Times* best-selling author of *I Like You Just the Way I Am*

"I had the pleasure of working with Anthony William when he came to Los Angeles and shared his story on Extra. What a fascinating interview as he left the audience wanting to hear more . . . people went crazy for him! His warm personality and big heart are obvious. Anthony has dedicated his life to helping people through the knowledge he receives from Spirit, and he shares all of that information through his Medical Medium books, which are life changing. Anthony William is one of a kind!"
— Sharon Levin, senior producer of *Extra*

"Anthony William is one of those rare individuals who uses his gifts to help people rise up to meet their full potential by becoming their own best health advocates . . . I witnessed Anthony's greatness in action firsthand when I attended one of his thrilling live events. I equate how spot-on his readings were with a singer hitting all the high notes. But beyond the high notes, Anthony's truly compassionate soul is what left the audience captivated. Anthony William is someone I am now proud to call a friend, and I can tell you that the person you hear on the podcasts and whose words fill the pages of best-selling books is the same person who reaches out to loved ones simply to lend support. This is not an act! Anthony William is the real deal, and the gravity of the information he shares through Spirit is priceless and empowering and much needed in this day and age!"
— Debbie Gibson, Broadway star, iconic singer-songwriter

"Anthony William has a remarkable gift! I will always be grateful to him for discovering an underlying cause of several health issues that had bothered me for years. With his kind support, I see improvements every day. I think he is a fabulous resource!"
— Morgan Fairchild, actress, author, speaker

"Within the first three minutes of speaking with me, Anthony precisely identified my medical issue! This healer really knows what he's talking about. Anthony's abilities as the Medical Medium are unique and fascinating."
— Alejandro Junger, M.D., *New York Times* best-selling author of *Clean, Clean Eats, Clean Gut,* and *CLEAN 7* and founder of the acclaimed Clean Program

"Since reading Medical Medium Thyroid Healing, *I have expanded my approach and treatments of thyroid disease and am seeing enormous value for patients. The results are rewarding and gratifying."*
— Prudence Hall, M.D., founder and medical director of The Hall Center

"How very much we have been moved and benefited from the discovery of Anthony and the Compassion Spirit, who can reach us with healing wisdom through Anthony's sensitive genius and caring mediumship. His book is truly 'wisdom of the future,' so already now, miraculously, we have the clear, accurate explanation of the many mysterious illnesses that the ancient Buddhist medical texts predicted would afflict us in this era when over-clever people have tampered with the elements of life in the pursuit of profit."
— Robert Thurman, Jey Tsong Khapa Professor Emeritus of Indo-Tibetan Buddhist Studies, Columbia University; President, Tibet House US; best-selling author of *Wisdom Is Bliss*; host of *Bob Thurman Podcast*

"Anthony William is the gifted Medical Medium who has very real and not-so-radical solutions to the mysterious conditions that affect us all in our modern world. I am beyond thrilled to know him personally and count him as a most valuable resource for my health protocols and those for my entire family."
— Annabeth Gish, *The Haunting of Hill House*, *The X-Files*, *The West Wing*, *Mystic Pizza*

"Whenever Anthony William recommends a natural way of improving your health, it works. I've seen this with my daughter, and the improvement was impressive. His approach of using natural ingredients is a more effective way of healing."
— Martin D. Shafiroff, financial advisor, past recipient of #1 Broker in America ranking by WealthManagement.com, and #1 Wealth Advisor ranking by Barron's

"Anthony William has devoted his life to helping people with information that has truly made a substantial difference in the lives of many."
— Amanda de Cadenet, founder and CEO of The Conversation and the Girlgaze Project; author of *It's Messy* and *#girlgaze*

"I love Anthony William! My daughters Sophia and Laura gave me his book for my birthday, and I couldn't put it down. The Medical Medium has helped me connect all the dots on my quest to achieve optimal health. Through Anthony's work, I realized the residual Epstein-Barr left over from a childhood illness was sabotaging my health years later. *Medical Medium* has transformed my life."
— Catherine Bach, *The Young and the Restless*, *The Dukes of Hazzard*

"My recovery from a traumatic spinal crisis several years ago had been steady, but I was still experiencing muscle weakness, a tapped-out nervous system, as well as extra weight. A dear friend called me one evening and strongly recommended I read the book *Medical Medium* by Anthony William. So much of the information in the book resonated with me that I began incorporating some of the ideas, then I sought and was lucky enough to get a consultation. The reading was so spot-on, it has taken my healing to an unimagined, deeper, and richer level of health. My weight has dropped healthily, I can enjoy bike riding and yoga, I'm back in the gym, I have steady energy, and I sleep deeply. Every morning when following my protocols, I smile and say, 'Whoa, Anthony William! I thank you for your restorative gift . . . Yes!'"
— Robert Wisdom, *A Journal for Jordan*, *Ballers*, *The Wire*, *Ray*

"As a Hollywood businesswoman, I know value. Some of Anthony's clients spent over $1 million seeking help for their 'mystery illness' until they finally discovered him."
— Nanci Chambers, co-star of *JAG*; Hollywood producer and entrepreneur

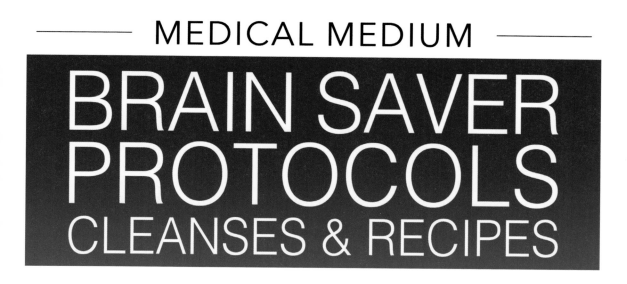

MEDICAL MEDIUM

BRAIN SAVER PROTOCOLS
CLEANSES & RECIPES

ALSO BY ANTHONY WILLIAM

Medical Medium: Secrets Behind Chronic and Mystery Illness and How to Finally Heal
(Revised and Expanded Edition)

Medical Medium Life-Changing Foods: Save Yourself and the Ones You Love
with the Hidden Healing Powers of Fruits & Vegetables

Medical Medium Thyroid Healing: The Truth behind Hashimoto's, Graves',
Insomnia, Hypothyroidism, Thyroid Nodules & Epstein-Barr

Medical Medium Liver Rescue: Answers to Eczema, Psoriasis, Diabetes,
Strep, Acne, Gout, Bloating, Gallstones, Adrenal Stress, Fatigue,
Fatty Liver, Weight Issues, SIBO & Autoimmune Disease

Medical Medium Celery Juice: The Most Powerful Medicine
of Our Time Healing Millions Worldwide

Medical Medium Cleanse to Heal: Healing Plans for Sufferers of Anxiety, Depression,
Acne, Eczema, Lyme, Gut Problems, Brain Fog, Weight Issues, Migraines, Bloating,
Vertigo, Psoriasis, Cysts, Fatigue, PCOS, Fibroids, UTI, Endometriosis & Autoimmune

Medical Medium Brain Saver: Answers to Brain Inflammation, Mental Health, OCD, Brain Fog,
Neurological Symptoms, Addiction, Anxiety, Depression, Heavy Metals, Epstein-Barr Virus,
Seizures, Lyme, ADHD, Alzheimer's, Autoimmune & Eating Disorders

All of the above are available at your local bookstore, or may be ordered by visiting:

Hay House USA: www.hayhouse.com®
Hay House Australia: www.hayhouse.com.au
Hay House UK: www.hayhouse.co.uk
Hay House India: www.hayhouse.co.in

***

MEDICAL MEDIUM

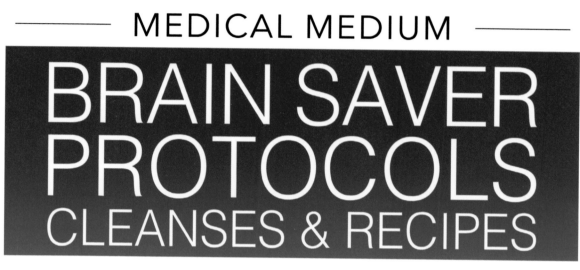

BRAIN SAVER
PROTOCOLS
CLEANSES & RECIPES

FOR NEUROLOGICAL, AUTOIMMUNE & MENTAL HEALTH

ANTHONY WILLIAM

HAY
HOUSE

HAY HOUSE, INC.
Carlsbad, California • New York City
London • Sydney • New Delhi

Copyright © 2022 by Anthony William

Published in the United States by: Hay House, Inc.: www.hayhouse.com®
Published in Australia by: Hay House Australia Pty. Ltd.: www.hayhouse.com.au
Published in the United Kingdom by: Hay House UK, Ltd.: www.hayhouse.co.uk
Published in India by: Hay House Publishers India: www.hayhouse.co.in

Cover design: Vibodha Clark
Interior design: Julie Davison
Interior illustrations: Vibodha Clark
Indexer: J S Editorial, LLC

Cataloging-in-Publication Data is on file at the Library of Congress

Hardcover ISBN: 978-1-4019-7133-5
E-book ISBN: 978-1-4019-7134-2
Audiobook ISBN: 978-1-4019-7139-7

10 9 8 7 6 5 4 3 2 1
1st edition, October 2022

Printed in the United States of America

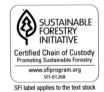

SUSTAINABLE FORESTRY INITIATIVE
Certified Chain of Custody
Promoting Sustainable Forestry
www.sfiprogram.org
SFI-01268
SFI label applies to the text stock

For the people of the future who will run
into challenges with their health.

If you have lost hope along the way of your journey,
know that as you open the pages of this book,
you open a window into healing. Remember these
words, for they shall enter your soul, take root,
blossom, and bear fruit. Take solace from the many
who have come before you over the years and have
healed. You can be one of them. Your time has come.

— Anthony William, Medical Medium

CONTENTS

FOREWORD

Anthony is a combination of brother from another mother with shades of guru, guardian angel, and gifted healer. Anthony is a truly good man and an outstanding friend. I love Anthony. We have been there for each other. Anthony is always there for me. If you pay close attention, you will understand that I am not just blowing smoke up to the Spirit of Compassion. My high opinion of Anthony stems from my experience of meeting many gurus and healers, some real, some fake.

We have in our generation a true seer (and listener), the Medical Medium.

In 1990 I graduated from medical school in Uruguay and moved to New York to specialize in internal medicine and then cardiovascular diseases. The change in lifestyle was so drastic that I did not even see it coming. Four years into my training I was overweight, suffering from irritable bowel syndrome and severe allergies. But the worse part was that I was severely depressed. I couldn't function.

A visit to a gastroenterologist, an allergist, and a psychiatrist left me with seven prescription medications for three diagnoses. I kept staring at my prescriptions and something inside of me kept screaming, "Find another way." And so I took off and searched. I've spent time in monasteries in India and met the most influential gurus of our time. I've met more healers, therapists, doctors, practitioners, coaches, shamans, mediums, and witches than I could ever remember. I found the way to heal myself through detox and gut repair. I have become a known functional-medicine doctor. I wrote four books. I've helped thousands of people in their healing processes, bringing what I know and finding the team that brings whatever I don't know into the healing journey of so many. I often go with them to consultations with other specialists or healers. I want to learn, to see, and to understand what works. I've learned a thing or two in the world of healing.

But nothing makes my head spin more than what Anthony speaks about. Mostly because of its success rate.

When I met Anthony over 10 years ago, the Medical Medium books had not been published yet. At my first book launch we were introduced. He had come with a mutual friend. Our friend had pulled me aside and told me that Anthony hears a voice that tells him about health and disease, in general and specific to certain people. I was immediately interested in meeting him. I kept thinking, *Is it real? Is he just psychotic and should be on psych meds? Or does he make any sense?* When we started talking, I critically observed Anthony, not only listening to what he was saying. *Is he lying or is he telling the truth? Does he actually hear a voice? Where is that coming from? Does the voice tell him things that are accurate? Does what the voice says help at all?*

The first minute of our conversation, I thought he was shy. After five minutes I realized he was far from shy, in fact, incredibly alive and outgoing. His style of communicating is amusing and honest, and he chooses his words very precisely when talking about health and disease. He is very organized in his mind. He was talking about diseases with conviction and somehow a deep understanding, as if he were a medical doctor. But his information was to me, at that time, as if out of a *Star Wars* movie. I was convinced. He hears a voice. So the question that remained was, *Does this voice know what it is talking about?* One way of measuring that was for me to search publications of research and trials that prove that what he was saying was scientifically correct, medically proven. Another way was to judge by the results. I started doing both.

On the research and publications front, I did not accomplish much for a long time. It turned out that the voice of his information was advanced, ahead of many publications. One of the pillars of Anthony's understanding is that most chronic diseases, and many acute ones, are caused by viruses. Some of the viruses can stay dormant for years and only cause trouble when your defenses go down. Some old, some mutated, and some undiscovered viruses. Some of the ones that we've known about for a long time, and that are so ubiquitous we barely even test for them in routine check-ups. Such an example is the herpes virus that causes a lip sore every once in a while. We live with these viruses and we are not scared of them. Another prime example of a virus Anthony has always said is at the root of many symptoms and diseases is the Epstein-Barr virus. Anthony teaches that almost everyone is exposed to EBV and that it either lives dormant or low-grade active in our organs and glands, eventually affecting our central nervous system. He has always said that many of us got it as a baby from our parents, who got it from their parents. What has been well known is that EBV is transmitted commonly through saliva when someone has infectious mononucleosis, also known as the "kissing disease" because that's how some people get it.

In the research, I found theoretical understandings here and there that some diseases such as cancer could be linked to viruses. After the Medical Medium books started to come out, there was chatter among the autoimmune practitioner community that autoimmune disease could be triggered by common viruses. Almost a decade after I wrote the foreword for the first Medical Medium book, they are now saying the Epstein-Barr virus causes multiple sclerosis, which is exactly what Anthony originally said in that first book, that the true cause of MS is EBV. Anthony provided the intricate details of how the Epstein-Barr virus actually causes the physical and neurological symptoms involved with multiple sclerosis. The research is mounting in an accelerated way and things that Anthony was telling me more than a decade ago, that sometimes made me doubt what he spoke about, are now front page in the media. Articles are now pointing out clues that link long COVID with the reactivation of EBV, something that Anthony had already published before long COVID was connected to EBV.

These are just a couple of examples of how Anthony, I believe, gets his information from a source that knows what it is talking about, often preceding scientific evidence for decades.

As a functional-medicine doctor and a cardiologist, I see and help people with many chronic diseases. I use Anthony's teachings in one way or another with most of my patients. It has made me a better doctor. I can help people I couldn't help before.

That is why I was so happy to read *Brain Saver* and *Brain Saver Protocols, Cleanses & Recipes*, Anthony's latest books. The brain is the organ that we understand the least, but has the most impact in our experience of life. That is why we can keep people alive with artificial and transplanted hearts, kidneys, livers, lungs, and other organs, but when you are diagnosed as brain-dead, they recommend to pull the plug.

I can't wait for you to read these books, too, and for them to bring you the solution to your healing that you've been looking for.

With much love and respect,
Alejandro Junger, M.D.,
New York Times best-selling author of
Clean, Clean Eats, Clean Gut, and *CLEAN 7*

AUTHOR'S PERSONAL NOTE

How *Brain Saver* Became Two Books

"Anthony, the book is going to be well over a thousand pages. It's too big to print." That was the call I got from my publisher the week after handing in the *Brain Saver* manuscript.

I can't say it came as a surprise. Over the months and then years it took to write "the brain book," I had watched the pages pile up and up and up on my desk. Anyone who knew what I was working on would ask, "Don't you think you're close to wrapping up by now?"

"People need answers," I would say and then get back to work.

I hadn't set out to write such a voluminous book, and I realized I would have to wrap it up someday if the material was ever going to reach people. Yet the material just kept coming. The world was changing faster. People were getting sicker. And Spirit of Compassion was forewarning me of what's to come in the next 5 to 10 years and beyond.

There were many times when I would push a 20-hour day, sometimes a 22-hour day, because I was devoting so much time to receiving information from Spirit of Compassion. Periodically, I'd fall asleep on my office floor with the lights on and then wake up a few hours later to start the day all over again. If there's anything you pick up from my work, it's that I believe people should take care of themselves whenever possible. They should eat well, get plenty of sleep, get sun, take walks, and so forth when they can. Still, I'm guilty of ignoring my personal needs while listening to the voice of Spirit and doing what God intended me to do. I'd often remind others that life goes by quickly, and if I disappear and leave this earth, it was from burning the candle at four ends under enormous pressure and outside forces of darkness trying to die this light out so the world doesn't receive Spirit's prophecies. Many times, I joked that I would burn a hole in my seat with the amount of time I spent sitting down to work on this material with Spirit. The joke has now come pretty close to reality. This might be the moment when I do finally throw away my office chair—the seat cushion is torn up pretty badly.

I've always said that receiving information from Spirit of Compassion causes a whiteout, a foggy, glaring haze, a snow blindness—making it so that I feel surrounded by an energy source, making me feel that I'm somewhere else even though I'm aware that I haven't gone anywhere because I'm still completely conscious in the moment. Most of the time that I was writing *Brain Saver*, I was in the white cloud. This is because Spirit wants me to not only visually see the images that the words represent as I'm hearing them but even to feel the essence of what people are feeling through their suffering. The white cloud is to remove me from my personal life, responsibilities, and experiences so my focus is only on the information given to me and the suffering of others. It's not just about receiving information and writing it down. It's about receiving the complete experience and connecting this to what others go through in their health struggles. The feeling is a roller coaster of sadness and happiness— sadness about what people have gone through and happiness that this could be that door of opportunity they could open to overcome the sickness. Once I've received and connected with the information, I have to learn this content that Spirit provides and study it just like anyone else does.

Each year that goes by, as I work on another book with Spirit of Compassion, I notice that the voice I hear stays the same while I, as a person, change. The changing comes from the continual realization that there are over eight billion people on this planet who will eventually become ill, and not all of them may ever get the chance to experience what Spirit has delivered here in front of me. It's one of the hard parts about this journey: to know that many will find their way to this information, these living words, yet so many won't. As a child, I thought surely everyone was going to be able to behold the wisdom from above when they became challenged by a health issue. Now the older me, who knows this may not be true, confronts the younger me, who had tremendous confidence that everyone on the planet would find this information. With each passing year, the dawning realization keeps changing me. It leads me to ask Spirit a lot of "Why"s and "How come"s and extra questions as I'm receiving Spirit's information and writing books about how hard this world really is to live in for all of us.

The writing process also gave me opportunities to identify firsthand with what people go through. As I struggled to sneak in a shower, wash my face, brush my teeth, change my clothes, I thought of what the chronically ill deal with as they try to accomplish these day-to-day tasks that those who aren't sick take for granted. My constraint was merely time as I fulfilled a mission. For people up against painful or limiting symptoms, these practices can be like mountains to climb. I always support wherever someone is in their capacity to take care of themselves during their healing process.

I could identify with the chronically ill, too, as I lost touch with important people in my life to write the brain book. I sacrificed time away from loved ones. I'm usually an avid studier of the seasons as they change before my eyes and ears. I like to listen to the peepers. I like to listen to the wind blow. I like to watch the leaves change and the grass turn color. I don't really remember partaking in or even registering any of that while putting together *Brain Saver*. Not that I'm complaining. These are little things to forego. Those who are chronically ill or suffering have much bigger bridges to cross, far more sacrifices and losses. I always keep them in mind as each hour passes that I spend getting the scripture needed to heal others from above. The joy comes later, when someone holds one of these books in their hands and starts their journey of rising out of the ashes.

Which brings us back to how *Brain Saver* became two books. Spirit of Compassion doesn't stop producing and could have me write continuously. I have to be the one to say uncle. There comes a point when I have to give in and get the information out to the ones who need it. I had wanted this material to fit in one book, so you could hold all the answers in your hands at once. When the publisher called to tell me just how big it would be, I had to face the reality: no one wants to hold a 10-pound book, least of all someone struggling with neurological symptoms.

I wrestled with whether there was any material I could take out. It was clear that any healing answers and protocols needed to stay. What about the parts where I explained Medical Medium information as the uncited source of many new medical understandings of chronic illness, such as that Epstein-Barr virus causes multiple sclerosis? After all, this isn't about me. I consulted with Spirit of Compassion. The determination was clear: showing readers that, for example, certain insights into long-haul COVID originated from Medical Medium material was itself a healing answer. When readers see that information circulating out in the world originally came from Medical Medium teachings, they get the opportunity to discover the full picture here, most notably the full picture of how to heal.

I kept thinking about how the book could be trimmed. Some of the material was going to be controversial. Was it worth it? Well, publishing truth about why the chronically ill are chronically ill is always controversial. I've already spoken and written about this for years. For the most part, the chronically ill have been disrespected and swept under the carpet. It's a hidden controversy, one you don't realize is out there until you stand up for the chronically ill and present the truth of why they're suffering. Darkness thrives on people who have symptoms being confused and lost about their direction, why they're sick. Darkness thrives on the chronically ill pursuing unproductive avenues, making their journey more difficult. So yes, it all needed to stay in the book.

That's when it was time to take the publisher's suggestion and turn "the brain book" into companion volumes: *Brain Saver* and *Brain Saver Protocols, Cleanses & Recipes*. We figured out the details: Both books would be published at the same time, so people could access the information all at once. Both books would have essential Medical Medium tools—Heavy Metal

Detox, Brain Shot Therapy, and fourteen customizable cleanses—printed in full. This way, if someone only had one book in hand, they wouldn't be missing out on critical healing resources.

You'll read more about what appears in this book and what material you can find in its companion book in "How This Book Works," which comes next. The books are designed to stand alone, each volume filled to the brim with information you can put to use now. As you can see from the story of how these books came together, you'll get the most protection out of reading both, whenever you can bring each into your life.

If I can give any advice about how to go about reading these two books, it's this: there is such comprehensive information, methodically and providentially placed, that once you're finished reading, you may benefit from giving it another go so that both your soul and physical brain get a chance to receive and store all that's here. Take your time. When you're ready, give each book another read-through. With every read, you may find powerful pieces of information and insight you never even noticed before.

Many blessings,
Anthony William, Medical Medium

"Spirit of Compassion has always said to me throughout the years of helping so many people heal that knowing the true cause of why you're sick is half the battle won. Knowing what to do, what to take, and how to apply those tools is the other half of the battle won."

— Anthony William, Medical Medium

HOW THIS BOOK WORKS

With this book, you can design a customized healing plan to take your health as far as it needs to go. Whether your focus is mental health or physical health, whether you want chronic symptom relief or you'd like to prevent frightening diagnoses, whether you want to make big changes or take small steps, these tools are yours.

This is not one size fits all. Each individual has their own signature blend of poisons, toxins, pathogens, exposures, and emotional experiences. No person has the exact same health situation as another. This is why the information here can be tailored so you have every opportunity to heal. I've always said that there is no single "Medical Medium protocol." There are countless Medical Medium protocols because these tools are endlessly personalizable for your unique needs. That's never been truer than here in *Brain Saver Protocols, Cleanses & Recipes*, which offers chapter after chapter of healing options. You're welcome to dip your toe into the waters of just one or

explore them all. Healing momentum builds on itself.

Part I, "Supplement Gospel," opens with a chapter dedicated to being your own health detective and avoiding the missteps it's easy to make when you're trying to heal. Next, find the vital "Golden Rules of Supplements" to guide you through the supplement lists with dosages that follow, as well as nine Medical Medium Shock Therapies for in-the-moment relief. With over 300 symptoms and conditions covered, "Supplement Gospel" can serve as a reference for you and your family to turn to over and over again, year after year, as life sends its challenges.

Part II, "Brain Betrayers," provides a deep dive into the foods, supplements, and additives that undermine our brain and nervous system health without our consent. Finding ways to limit or remove these items from your life can have a profound healing effect all its own. This isn't about condemning comfort food or associating what we eat with shame. It's about bringing you the ultimate comfort: freedom to make choices based on an understanding of what does and doesn't serve your health.

With Part III, "Brain Shot Therapy," you can find instant relief while you're working to fix problems at a deeper level in your brain, nervous system, and body. Using the recipes here, craft easy-to-make healing elixirs using combinations of ingredients specifically designed to address your needs. Choose from 30 different Brain Shots spread across three categories— Exposures, Shifters, and Stabilizers—to meet you wherever you are. This brand-new Medical Medium tool can be put to use as a flexible, stand-alone therapy, or you can try any of the seven Brain Shot Therapy cleanse options provided.

Part IV, "Heavy Metal Detox," takes the classic Medical Medium tool that has become a life-changing practice for people around the world to a whole new level. In addition to shining a light on how the Heavy Metal Detox Smoothie formula is able to make such a profound difference in brain health and why we need it, this section introduces new staples: the Advanced Heavy Metal Detox Smoothie plus an Extractor Smoothie and Advanced Extractor Smoothie that work together with the original smoothie to provide an even more effective brain detox. For maximum benefit, tailor any of the seven Heavy Metal Detox cleanses to your own individual needs.

The title of Part V, "Brain Saver Recipes," says it all. Over 100 delicious recipes will help you answer the question of how to nourish your brain. From fast, simple ideas

to impressive crowd pleasers, these recipes provide you with option after option in a world that can make decoding healthy eating feel impossible. With full-color photos to engage your whole family, choosing what to make for breakfast, lunch, dinner, or snacks can become a joyful experience.

Part VI, "Brain and Soul Rehabbing," is your refuge to revisit again and again. Life takes its toll. When you've struggled with persistent symptoms without answers, or you've watched a loved one suffer, or you've experienced emotional injuries, it's easy to lose faith that you could ever feel like yourself again. It's critical that you get a chance to tend to your frayed nerves and fractured soul. The healing meditations and techniques offered here, which are specifically geared to increase your ability to heal the symptoms and conditions listed in this book, offer that opportunity. You didn't bring your suffering upon yourself. It's far from your fault. With new insights and practices to add to your life, your truest self is always within reach.

By the way, if you'd like to learn more about the "why" of your symptoms or conditions, this book's companion, *Brain Saver*, offers extensive details about the causes of chronic physical and mental suffering. What does it mean to have a static brain, an alloy brain, a viral brain, an emotional brain, inflamed cranial nerves, a burnt out and deficient brain, an addicted brain, an acid brain? Find explanations of more than 100 symptoms and conditions, with special chapters dedicated to anxiety, depression, eating disorders, OCD, bipolar disorder,

Alzheimer's and dementia, addiction, burn-out, and cranial nerve problems, including vagus nerve inflammation. Also discover how to reduce your exposure to toxins and contaminants in your everyday life, how to protect yourself when getting blood drawn, why "everything in moderation" isn't as harmless as it sounds, and how to rethink brain fuel.

Whether you're using these companion books together or *Brain Saver Protocols, Cleanses & Recipes* is all you have in hand for now, consider it a lifelong reference.

Keep it in your kitchen, keep it by your bedside, keep it wherever it's within easy reach so you can continue to study the living words in these pages. Once you've gotten used to a favorite tool, you may decide to branch out and try more. Our needs and challenges change over time. Tools that don't seem relevant now may become your future go-to. Your brain has abilities to heal beyond what medical research and science are aware of today. Hold on to that knowledge, and you'll become a beacon of light for others who need answers.

"Medical Medium information is not one size fits all. You can customize what's right for you and your condition and take your healing as far as it needs to go. It's endlessly customizable. When you have a symptom that's not letting up, or multiple persistent symptoms, it's critical to learn the details. The details matter when you're chronically sick. The details matter when it comes to healing."

— Anthony William, Medical Medium

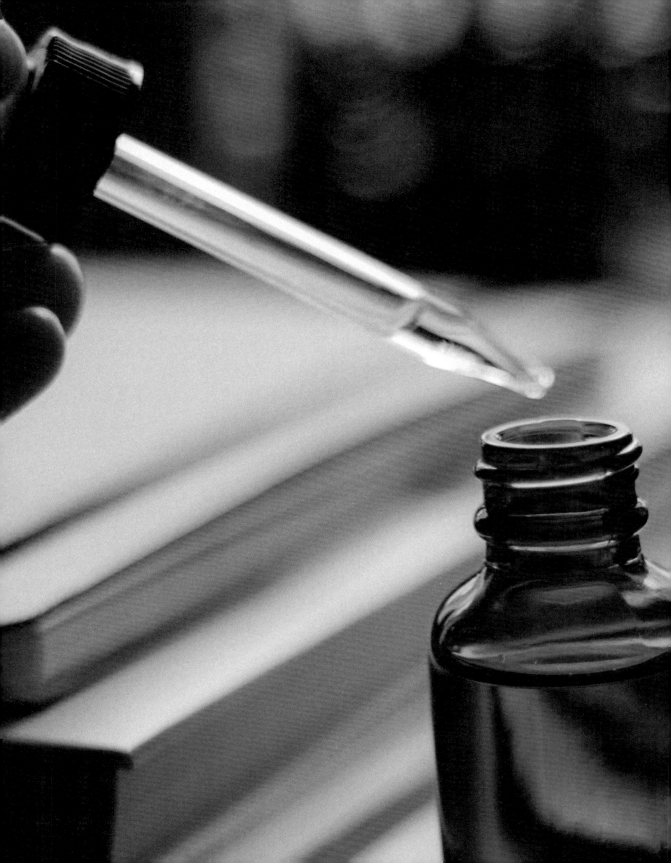

PART I

SUPPLEMENT GOSPEL

"There are ongoing exposures we can't always control, or new exposures of which we're not aware. For example, you could have been in a recent relationship and picked up a new virus. People have ongoing exposures all the time. It's not uncommon to heal a pathogen with Medical Medium information, feel like you're on top of your game, and then pick up a new virus or bacteria (or even multiple strains) from a new relationship—and start experiencing fatigue and brain fog again, thinking all your healing failed, when really, all the tools and knowledge you used to heal the first time will get you out of the jam you're in now too."

— Anthony William, Medical Medium

CHAPTER 1

Your Healing Process

Everyone is different. Not in the way we normally think. While our souls are different, our physical bodies, as humans, are meant to function in the same way. We eat food, drink water, urinate and defecate; our hearts beat and our blood pumps; we walk on our feet, we see with our eyes, we hear with our ears, our stomachs are meant to digest . . . until something goes wrong and we can't. We can't walk, we can't talk, we can't hear, we can't see; our blood gets clogged or our heart doesn't beat right. Different internal problems with our physical bodies can create endless differences. Our injuries, pathogens, stresses, metals, traumas, relationships, environmental surroundings, resources, support, pharmaceuticals, experiences, deficiencies, amounts of blood drawn, number of flus we've had, how many exposures we come into the world with— all these make us different. Our differences make our healing processes and their timelines different.

If you're reading this book, you most likely have a health problem. A health problem that's consistent in your life, while healing is less consistent. Maybe you have a serious condition, one that interferes with your life in some shape or form. In this book's companion title, *Brain Saver*, you can discover how you got sick to begin with and what's physically inside you that's interfering with your ability to heal. In both *Brain Saver* and this book, you can find out what to avoid and what tools to use to get your life back.

Your healing timeline will never be exactly the same as someone else's because someone else has a different compilation of problems within their body than you may have. If you're coming into this healing information with the intention of dabbling, you're welcome. Choosing 16 ounces of celery juice and some high-quality B$_{12}$ and staying away from gluten is dabbling. It's powerful. It's still dabbling. Another person who's struggling with difficult symptoms and conditions may need 32 ounces of celery juice, the Heavy Metal Detox Smoothie, a full protocol of supplements, a Medical Medium Mono Eating Cleanse, and to avoid eggs, dairy, and vinegar. Someone who has a very serious condition may even consider *that* dabbling, as they need additional Medical Medium tools. Still, if all you can do is one thing and one thing only, it's progress. Your body will receive it like it's heavenly light from above.

The healing process is not just the passive process of waiting for the body to heal. The healing process is the steps you take so your body can heal. Healing is an active combination of your free will, learning the information, your body's ability to heal on its own, the tools you're using, what you give your body so it can heal, and the details within it all.

Your healing process also depends on what was done in the past. The world of guessing games can set you back in your healing process. And that's okay. You're going in the other direction now. You're putting what you have tried in the past behind you.

Even if you lack the faith that what you're doing will heal you, you can still heal when you give your body what it needs, remove from your body what it doesn't need, know why you got sick to begin with, and know what to do to recover. These steps will still allow you to heal, even if you don't believe you can heal or believe you ever will heal. When people are on the journey of healing and they're not using the right tools, and they don't know why they became sick to begin with, they lose faith where they once had faith. It burns out. If you're someone who has tried everything, been through so much during your process of healing throughout the months or years, and you land here with

very little faith or no faith left at all because you lost it along the way through endless trial and error based on misinformation, you can still heal. Your faith will restore as you're healing and you see the light.

If you're a goal-setting person, it's good to set two types of goals: goals for what healing steps you're going to take, like accomplishing a cleanse or taking various supplements for your condition, and goals for where you see yourself in the future. If there was a time when you felt good or at least better in your life, keep that in mind. Don't lose touch with how you were feeling when you were living your life less compromised or even not sick at all. Hold on to those moments. You can add that feeling to your goal of getting better, getting back to where you once were.

Medical Medium information is not one size fits all. You can customize what's right for you and your condition and take your healing as far as it needs to go. It's endlessly customizable. When you have a symptom that's not letting up, or multiple persistent symptoms, it's critical to learn the details. The details matter when you're chronically sick. The details matter when it comes to healing.

BE YOUR OWN DETECTIVE

Many people who first embark on Medical Medium protocols find immediate relief from one to ten symptoms or more. Deeper healing and relief from additional symptoms may take a little more time. Complete healing doesn't happen right away. Everybody's on a different time clock, plus there are interruptions. No one can do everything "perfectly" without skipping a beat.

As you go through your healing process, be your own detective. If you're not getting the results you want, ask yourself about the details of what you're doing. Many people pick up a Medical Medium cleanse, try it once, get some results, and don't realize they could repeat the cleanse or venture into supplementation and other tools to keep going.

Also investigate where you might be consuming trendy products, supplementation, foods, and beverages that could be slowing down your healing process. Many people stick with old habits or fall back into old habits without even realizing it. As they're embarking on something new, they're continuing the old at the same time without an awareness of the effect that habit is having. Hanging on to old habits changes timelines. What is your caffeine intake like? How much chocolate are you doing? Coffee drinks? Matcha teas? Are you doing vinegars? Are you doing vegan cheeses? Nutritional yeast? How much coconut ice cream? Natural flavors? These habits could be tipping the scale in an unproductive direction when it comes to feeling better.

If you're not dealing with a symptom or condition, these habits may not be enough to put you out of balance yet. On the other hand, if you are sick and you have a symptom or condition, your scale has already tipped. It's not balanced. How much further that scale tips into poor health depends on

what unproductive things you may be doing that you don't even realize are unproductive.

If you feel like you need to hold on to your vices, know that this could slow down your healing. If you're anxious to heal something and you want to put it behind you as quickly as possible, the details are really going to matter to you.

GIVE YOURSELF TIME TO HEAL

Another reason that it can take some time to heal is if you have multiple viral infections, not just one, or if you have multiple varieties of toxic heavy metals, or larger deposits of metals.

Plus there are ongoing exposures we can't always control, or new exposures of which we're not aware. For example, you could have been in a recent relationship and picked up a new virus. People have ongoing exposures all the time. It's not uncommon to heal a pathogen with Medical Medium information, feel like you're on top of your game, and then pick up a new virus or bacteria (or even multiple strains) from a new relationship—and start experiencing fatigue and brain fog again, thinking all your healing failed, when really, all the tools and knowledge you used to heal the first time will get you out of the jam you're in now too.

Many people could see results quickly, with symptoms minimizing, as they get rid of their problems by killing off pathogens and removing toxic heavy metals, old pharmaceuticals, toxic chemicals, and toxic foods. It depends how much was there that needed to come out and heal. Some people take longer to feel results because the central nervous system and nerves all through the body need some restoration time.

(Some people take longer to feel results because excessive sexual activity or masturbation on a regular basis is depleting them of their zinc reserves, other trace mineral and vital nutrient reserves, and adrenaline reserves, lowering the immune system. When men's healing process takes longer than expected, this is a common reason why, especially if their immune system is battling a low-grade or high-grade viral infection.)

The brain itself may need time to physically repair itself too. When poisons, toxins, and even fatty deposits take up residence in the brain, they interfere with healthy brain tissue. These and other brain betrayers can slowly eat away at the brain, creating divots and hollows. When you remove what shouldn't be in the brain and feed the brain what it needs, brain cells develop, filling in these brain craters.

COMPARING YOURSELF

It's easy to judge yourself and your healing process against someone else's.

Many women compare their healing to the healing process of men in their life, whether partner, spouse, boyfriend, or friend. "Jeff is losing weight and healing faster. How come it's taking me longer?"

Traditionally, we're used to the image of men who get up and go, go, go, not having too many ups and downs with their health. If they catch a cold, they shake it off. Then they may die of a heart attack (meaning that something was going on all along, even if it didn't cause noticeable symptoms, or symptoms that anybody knew how to interpret). Traditionally, women tend to develop a myriad of mystery symptoms that often plague them on and off throughout their life. These roles can also be reversed, where a man seems to be healing more slowly, or what feels like not healing at all, while he compares himself to a woman who is recovering very quickly and getting back on track. Either way, it's easy to get caught up comparing yourself.

You never know, from person to person, who has more or less to heal. For example, if you've been through pregnancy and childbirth, your adrenals have gone under enormous strain. This can mean additional time is needed for the healing process. Caffeine use to power through the effects of adrenal strain can complicate the situation further.

If you don't seem to be getting better as fast as someone else, keep this in mind: it doesn't mean your body's healing more slowly than your partner, spouse, family member, friend, or person you follow on social media. It just means there's more to heal.

DEBUNKING TRENDS TO MAKE BRAIN SPACE FOR HEALING

I've witnessed many trends throughout the decades that have not restored people's health from the symptoms and conditions that are listed inside this book.

Or, when a very helpful trend starts, I've witnessed it eventually get twisted so that it's changed into something else and doesn't help people anymore. For example, flushing the body with fresh lemon water in the morning is a helpful practice. When it gets changed into drinking a cup of hot lemon water, that changes the effects. While lemon still has medicinal properties when it has been cooked, hot lemon water does not flush the bloodstream, liver, and body of poisons and toxins. That's only accomplished with lemon water made with water that is room temperature, lukewarm, cool, or even cold. The same twisting-a-practice-until-it's-not-helpful-anymore can happen with celery juice. Celery works on its own when it's freshly juiced with nothing added. Yet it becomes trendy to add lemon, ice, or water, which no longer allows celery juice to work.

It takes brain space to apply healing information, tools, and techniques. It takes brain space to gather what you need during the healing process. And it takes brain space to understand and learn the details so you can maximize your healing. When you have a life to live with lots of distractions and daily challenges, you can lose precious space in your brain. So if you're following a trend that doesn't work, or you're convinced it works when it isn't really doing what it promises, there's that much less capacity to keep up with what does work, to implement new tools and healing options that can really move the needle. You're taking up a lot of room in your head with trends that are wasting time.

There's mass confusion in the health world about the difference between someone who is chronically ill with neurological symptoms and someone who isn't chronically ill with neurological symptoms. You cannot apply the same health trends.

For example, if you aren't suffering from a neurological symptom or condition, and you dabble in cold plunging, you may believe you're succeeding in something that's wonderful for your health. In reality, cold plunging brings your body into a very quick state of near-hypothermia that shocks your nervous system, cardiovascular system, and endocrine system, prompting an adrenaline rush and high—because your brain is sending emergency messages to your adrenals that there is a physical crisis occurring that is becoming life-threatening. Lowering the body's temperature forcefully and abruptly for an extended period can also lower the immune system. All of this is disastrous for someone who has chronic neurological health problems, whose nerves are not working properly because of pathogens, metals, and other challenges inside the body. Cold plunging is not a great idea for someone who has tendonitis, neuropathy, migraines, or fatigue, to name just a few of the hundreds of symptoms and conditions that would not warrant a cold plunging party. (Note that a very quick cold shower, or a short cold bath to bring down a very high fever, is far different from lying in the snow or being out in the blistering cold wearing practically nothing or spending time submerged in icy cold water.)

This is how it works with all trends. Not enough consideration is being given to who can have fun dabbling with a trend and who doesn't have that room to play. The same goes for water fasting and even intermittent fasting. There are differences from one person to another in their symptoms and conditions when it comes to whether it's a good idea to partake or not. Certain trends get in the way, tip the scale, send healing in the opposite direction. Alkaline ionizer water machines are a prime example of a trend that's working against you while you're trying to apply healing tools that work for you.

One way to navigate through trends and know if they work or not is to follow the history. Back when people in the health movement were using alkaline ionizer water machines as their sole health investment, not only were they not seeing improvements—they saw a decline in health. Now the world has changed. People are eating better, playing hit-and-miss in the supplement world that can offer some benefits, choosing wisely, avoiding the basics of preservatives, fillers, processed food, and fast food, and these improvements work for them. Because they have these positives on their side, they can't clearly see the negative effects of following a trend such as alkaline ionizer water machines at the same time. Especially if they're using Medical Medium tools that advance them quickly and further in their healing process, overriding the negative effects of something like alkaline ionizer water machines, they don't realize

the decline they'd be experiencing if they weren't balancing out the water machine's effects. If you don't know the history, what happened in the past with alkaline ionizer water machines used on their own, you don't know that you would be that much further along in your healing without the machines.

WHAT MODERATION REALLY MEANS

Understanding what "moderation" means takes some next-level thinking. Your own personal approach to moderation will come down to whether you want to heal faster, more slowly, or even possibly not at all.

You may think you're living life in moderation. As you can read about in *Brain Saver*'s "The Moderation Trap" chapter, that's what we're taught: a little bit of this, a little bit of that. A little bit of espresso, say, or a little bit of wine—it all sounds very reasonable and balanced and levelheaded. Yet what really is moderation when you look at the bigger picture?

People are afraid of lemons, bananas, grapes, fruit sugars eroding their teeth . . . yet have they consumed 10,000 or even 1,000 lemons or bananas or grapes in their lifetime? No. They *have* had chocolate or coffee 10,000 times or more. Maybe you didn't start drinking coffee until the recent past, so you've only had 1,000 cups of it. Fifteen years in, will you have reached 11,000 doses of coffee? Will you be drinking coffee at night by then? Will you be eating chocolate regularly too? Say you regularly consume vinegar. You could have consumed well over 20 gallons of vinegar in 10 years.

People are drinking 10,000 cups of coffee, eating 10,000 servings of chocolate, 10,000 servings of vinegar, and they're *not* eating 10,000 bananas or lemons or grapes. And still, it's the bananas and lemons and grapes—the healing options we could all benefit from bringing into our lives in greater quantities—that we're warned away from, not the coffee, chocolate, or vinegar.

Maybe you're someone who doesn't know anything about how to heal, and you're learning that now. Everything in this book is here to move you forward, to get you past your illness, sickness, disease, or symptoms. That also means that most everything you'll see in this book is counter to what you've been taught is okay for your health—what you've been taught to do wrong.

I'm not saying you have to stop everything you've ever loved or are addicted to. Armed with the knowledge in this book, maybe you can pick and choose what to let go. When we're told to let go of past grievances, past traumas, past relationship hurt, or any kind of past hardship, we know that's not going to be easy. "Just let it go": that's what we're told sometimes. It's more difficult than that when it comes to our minds and emotions, which we can't see or touch. And while it is still difficult to let go of the physical items in front of us—the chocolate bar, the nutritional yeast, the vinegar we pour on our food, the egg we crack into a sizzling pan of butter—we have empowerment because we see them before us. We

can open our hands to physically let them go. When you learn that letting that egg go could move you forward, you have the choice to let it go. You have the power to do it. You can use your free will to keep some or all of these items out of your diet, out of your life.

I understand. Addictive impulses, cravings, and struggles with food are real. They don't make it easy to "let it go" when it comes to certain ingredients that we hold dear. What's different now is that you can understand why they happen and what to do about these challenges. With knowledge you can gain from *Brain Saver*'s "Your Addicted Brain," "The Moderation Trap," and "Eating Disorders" chapters, they're no longer unsolvable mysteries. You can understand the brain's needs that they reveal, and this book's protocols, cleanses, and recipes give you healing actions to take, all of which means you are not powerless in the face of cravings.

Many of the items I'm telling you to let go of in Part II of this book, "Brain Betrayers," are supposed to be good for you. Apple cider vinegar, nutritional yeast, coffee, chocolate, matcha tea, green tea: they're all supposed to be healthy. That's all part of the deception. No one really knows what's good for us or not. The people giving you the advice to consume them are only going by their own addictions, or what they heard was in a study or article somewhere. Science doesn't have all the answers. That's why everybody is sick.

Meanwhile, we're told to stay away from what will help us. These days we hear that certain fruits and vegetables have anti-nutrients in them. Again, there's no sound science behind that. People don't eat red bell peppers every day of their life. They do drink caffeine every single day, or they try to. People don't eat celery every day of their life, unless they're learning from Medical Medium information. They don't eat red cabbage or spinach every day of their life. They've been told to avoid spinach and cruciferous vegetables such as cabbage and make sure they drink their matcha tea every day for the rest of their life. People will, by habit, use vinegar every day for the rest of their life, or every other day, whether in the restaurant food they take out or a dish they make. They aren't told to eat mango or papaya every day for the rest of their life. They're told to stay away from fruit. "Too much sugar." Then there's chocolate. People are told that 70 to 90 percent cacao is better for you—"the more potency, the better"—when in reality, a higher cacao percentage means more caffeine, which is more damaging to the adrenals.

The concept of moderation is not going away. As long as there are human beings here on this planet, moderation will be here too. Human nature harbors human desire, which is partly conditioned toward instant gratification, vices, and addiction. The world is a hard place. Moderation is a friendly way of saying, "I need my vices to get through the day while in survival mode, while fighting my uphill battles, while trying to live my life." Healing is not about making moderation your enemy. It's about becoming friends with moderation so it doesn't sneak up behind you, kick your legs out, trip you up, and make you fall right on your face. Understanding moderation is a great way of understanding how to protect your brain.

"Understanding what 'moderation' means takes some next-level thinking. Your own personal approach to moderation will come down to whether you want to heal faster, more slowly, or even possibly not at all."

— Anthony William, Medical Medium

CHAPTER 2

Golden Rules of Supplements

Before you leap into the supplement protocols in the following chapters, first make sure you read this chapter fully so you can interpret the lists correctly.

If you're wondering about whether supplementation is right for you, know that the supplements recommended in this book are an optional step. If you prefer to focus on foods for healing (both adding helpful recipes and foods to your life and removing brain betrayer foods), you're more than welcome to do that. The cleanses in this book are also a powerful healing option. You don't have to play in Supplement Land yet if you don't want to.

Do stay open to supplements for the future if you're struggling with severe symptoms and conditions that are not dissipating as quickly as desired. You may be someone who started out with over 50 to 100 different symptoms, and perhaps you've conquered and healed many of these symptoms and yet still have some left that seem stubborn or need more time. In this case, too, you may want to be open to specific supplementation for your symptoms or conditions. Or

consider revolving through different Medical Medium cleanses, including the option to do the cleanses back-to-back to speed up healing, before you decide to embark on supplements.

The supplement protocols in this book are for people looking for something more, looking for options because their situations are perplexing to them. If that's you, then delve into the treasure trove of options in the form of specialized supplement lists for the individual symptoms and conditions in this book. These supplement protocols have a working, healing track record and history of recovering countless people from complicated health conditions.

It's important to know that our deficiencies are a big part of why we're sick. Zinc, for example, is practically nonexistent in food today, and a zinc deficiency lowers the immune system, so we're always in need of it. We also have a lot of toxic heavy metals and toxic chemicals in us, and spirulina is critical for removing those metals and newly manufactured toxic chemicals.

The supplements in each list throughout Chapter 4, "Medical Medium Protocols," are in alphabetical order, not necessarily in order of importance. Exceptions include celery juice, the Heavy Metal Detox Smoothie, Brain Shot Therapies, and Shock Therapies, which you'll see at the top of each list.

Keep in mind that the extent of what these supplements do for your body and brain remains undiscovered by medical research and science. While a few are on their radar for being beneficial, many of them are completely unknown as health rescuers, and the benefits go far beyond what anyone realizes. This is part of how and why results happen with Medical Medium supplement protocols.

Spirit of Compassion has always said to me throughout the years of helping so many people heal that knowing the true cause of why you're sick is half the battle won. Knowing what to do, what to take, and how to apply those tools is the other half of the battle won. Throughout this book's companion, *Brain Saver*, you can gain insights into the true causes of over 100 neurological symptoms and conditions. You can understand why the population is up against this epidemic of chronic illness and why you yourself may have been living with a symptom or even fighting for your life to get through each day. Here, you can discover what to do about it. The supplement options in this book are powerful tools to help you address the "why," take back control over your life, and win the *whole* battle.

For any questions on supplementation that this chapter doesn't address, see this book's other companion, *Cleanse to Heal*.

CRITICAL TIPS FOR INTERPRETING SUPPLEMENT LISTS

These critical tips will help you interpret the supplement protocols in the chapters that follow:

- When you see the term *dropperful*, that means as much liquid supplement as fills the bottle's eye dropper when you squeeze its rubber top. It may only fill up halfway or less; that's still considered a dropperful. The eye dropper does not have to be filled to the top.

- There are also some supplements where dosages are given in drops. Make sure to check carefully whether it says *drops* or *dropperfuls*.

- Most of the liquid and powder supplements are meant to be taken in water or juice. Check the directions on the supplement's label.

- When it comes to herbal tinctures, actively seek out alcohol-free versions (avoid the word *ethanol* too). If you have no other options and alcohol-based tincture is all you can find, try to look for the dried herb form and make a tea instead.

- When you see multiple herbal tinctures in a list, you're welcome to combine them into 1 ounce or more of water or juice and take them together.

- The same goes for teas. If multiple teas are listed for your symptom or condition, feel free to combine the herbs to make yourself a special tea blend or use a few different tea bags together.

- One cup of tea translates to either 1 tea bag or 1 to 2 teaspoons of loose leaf tea.

- For any supplement list that includes aloe vera, see the instructions under "Medical Medium Aloe Vera Shock Therapy" in Chapter 3 for how to prepare the fresh gel.

- Some of the dosages are listed in milligrams. If you can't find capsules that line up with the exact suggestions, try to get ones that are close.

- Most of the protocols in Chapter 4, "Medical Medium Protocols," list adult dosages. Talk to a physician about what's right for a child.

- When you see the term *daily*, that means to take the given dosage of the supplement over the course of the day, and it's your choice how you do that. You're welcome to take the whole dose once a day. If you're sensitive, you may want to break it up into multiple servings. For example, if it says to take 2 teaspoons of barley grass juice powder daily, you may decide either to put both teaspoons together into a smoothie or have 1 teaspoon in a morning smoothie and 1 teaspoon in some water at night.

- When you see *twice a day*, that means two installments taken at any time of day, as long as they're at least four hours apart. If you miss one of the installments on any given day, try to start fresh the next day.

- You're welcome to take your supplements with or without food.

WHERE TO START?

Once you've found your symptom or condition in Chapter 4, "Medical Medium Protocols," you don't need to take every supplement listed for it. If you're sensitive for any reason, you can try one supplement a day. If not, you can put them all together as your daily regimen. Or as a middle ground, you can choose a couple to start off with, and then take it from there.

Celery juice is always a good place to begin, or try a Brain Shot Therapy and/or Heavy Metal Detox Smoothie.

Beyond that, if vitamin B_{12}, zinc, vitamin C, and/or lemon balm are in your list, bring in those.

Then, if you're ready to move forward and your list contains spirulina, curcumin, cat's claw, and/or L-lysine, add those as your next step.

Later on, if you're not experiencing what you want from these supplements, you can add a few more from your list.

You can always take smaller amounts than the listed dosages if you feel you're sensitive.

You also have the option to intermix supplements from the different lists in this book. Any supplement from this book is an option to use, if your expert sense of what your body needs or your physician's recommendation tells you to do so. They're all helpful supplements for chronic health issues.

(When I mention tailoring a supplement protocol for yourself, I'm not talking about bringing in supplements other than what I recommend in this book or its companions, *Cleanse to Heal* and *Medical Medium*. More in a moment.)

If you're living with more than one symptom or condition at the same time and want one clear place to begin, pick the health struggle that looms largest in your life. For example, if you're plagued by fatigue and that feels most pressing, you can focus on the supplements for fatigue in Chapter 4. Over time, you may find that working on one issue takes care of another, or you can switch off after a little while and focus on a different supplement list in these pages.

If your condition is not named in Chapter 4, either try to find a symptom you experience that is named there and follow that supplement list, or find a supplement list for a condition in the chapter that's similar to yours. If your autoimmune disease isn't listed in this book, seek out the "Autoimmune Disorders and Diseases" supplement protocol in Chapter 4.

Some neurological symptoms and conditions may take longer healing time, because even after metals, toxins, chemicals, and viruses are removed, nerves still need time to heal. Supplementation can slowly repair longtime nerve damage, so you want to give your nerves some time to heal by sticking with the protocol.

DOSAGES

You're welcome to start at a much lower dose with any supplement listed in this book's protocols. For example, you could begin with a partial dropperful or partial capsule. Even with a smaller dose of one of these high-quality supplements, you will get more health benefits than from a large amount of ingredients in a lower-quality supplement. If you're sensitive, use your own experience or healing intuition or talk to your physician about what dosage your body can handle.

CHILDREN

The dosages listed in most of Chapter 4's supplement protocols are for adults. If you're considering supplements for a child, consult with their physician about what's safe and appropriate.

For celery juice amounts for children, see the table later in this chapter.

QUALITY MATTERS

I'm continually asked, What is the most effective form of a given supplement, and does it really matter? Yes, it matters greatly. There are subtle and sometimes critical differences among the different supplement types available that can affect how quickly your viral or bacterial load dies off, if at all; whether your central nervous system repairs itself and how fast; how quickly your inflammation reduces; how long it takes for your symptoms and conditions to heal; and whether or not you can safely remove toxic heavy metals and/or chemical toxins. The supplement variety you choose can make or break your progress. To speed up healing, you need the right kinds of supplements. For these very important reasons, I offer a directory on my website (www.medicalmedium.com) of the best forms of each supplement listed in this book.

You'll notice that almost every one of the supplements listed in this book's protocols is a single herb or nutrient. There's a reason for this—and you can learn more about why in *Cleanse to Heal*. Know that each one of the supplements in these lists holds God-given powers to help your body heal. Your liver, a processing center of your body, can understand each one of these herbs and nutrients and knows how to use it.

One powerful undiscovered tip is to consider taking your supplements with a piece of fruit such as a banana or even some potato, sweet potato, winter squash, raw honey, pure maple syrup, or coconut water (that's not pink or red). Natural sugar is what carries vitamins, minerals, and other nutrients through the bloodstream to help them find where they need to go, so taking your supplements with natural sugars ensures that your liver (the processing center) and other parts of your body can actually use them. (The exception to this tip is celery juice and Brain Shot Therapies, which you should drink by themselves.)

SUPPLEMENTS TO AVOID WHILE HEALING

Be very discerning about supplements not recommended in the Medical Medium book series. A lot of supplements have ingredients that work against you. As you can read in Chapter 6, "Brain Betrayer Supplements," some supplements such as fish oil and whey protein powder can work against your healing by feeding pathogens that create the symptoms and conditions in this book. That is, supplements other than what I recommend may be contributing to your problems in the first place, setting you back or setting you up for future problems. Something you have taken for years could finally catch up with you and set you back later in life, or create a new health problem that gets in the way of your healing. If you stay on a non-recommended supplement while working to cleanse and heal, you may not see the benefits you want to see.

HOW LONG?

The length of time to stay on these supplements depends on factors such as how deficient you are (in areas that blood work cannot even determine) and how viral you are (meaning what kind of low-grade, undetected, undiagnosed viral infections or viral loads you're dealing with). It also depends on how many toxic heavy metals and chemical toxins you may have in your brain and liver; how depleted your organs are of glucose and mineral salts; how much mystery inflammation you're experiencing from undiagnosed, low-grade viral and bacterial infections; how injured parts of your nervous system are; and how weakened your overall body systems may be—all of it occurring beyond detection at the doctor's office. You may be someone who says, "My doctor checked me. I'm not deficient. They didn't say anything about heavy metals. Why should I be on supplements?" The point is that a doctor isn't given the training or tools to see all the factors behind chronic illness. Heavy metal tests do not show how many metals are inside organs. Tests don't always see what our bodies are really up against in today's age of toxic exposure. Even if you

checked out at the doctor's office, are your symptoms and conditions still persisting? That's a sign to stick with supplementation to address the underlying issues.

The other measures you're taking to care for yourself—that is, regularly turning to Medical Medium cleanse options and supporting yourself at other times by incorporating healing foods, lowering fats, and avoiding brain betrayers and brain betrayer foods—will make a big difference to your healing timeline. How much your body was struggling and how long you'd been suffering when you started on your healing path will make a big difference too. Everyone has a different healing process and time frame. You may have been ill for a long time, in which case supplements are great for maintaining critical progress after you heal. Even as you're feeling better and recovering, with your specific symptoms fading away, continuing with supplements is important.

PREGNANCY AND BREASTFEEDING

Every woman who is pregnant should check with her doctor about any type of supplements she's considering.

If you're a mom struggling with symptoms or conditions while breastfeeding, you're welcome to partake in any of the supplementation listed here. If you have any questions about using supplements in your particular situation, talk to your doctor.

CELERY JUICE AS A MEDICINAL

In every supplement list in Chapter 4, "Medical Medium Protocols," you'll find a recommended amount of fresh celery juice. Celery juice is a powerful medicinal that elevates whatever you're doing right in your life. You can find the recipe for celery juice in Chapter 12, "Medical Medium Brain Saver Recipes."

The same guidelines apply for celery juice as always:

- Fresh, plain, unadulterated, straight celery juice. No added ice, water, lemon juice, apple cider vinegar, collagen, or other mix-ins. Also, as beneficial as green juice blends can be, they're not a substitute for pure celery juice.

- Juice means juice. Drinking blended celery without straining the pulp doesn't yield the same benefits. See "The Juicing versus Fiber Debate" in *Cleanse to Heal* for more on why.

- Fresh means fresh. Making a drink from reconstituted celery powder won't deliver the right benefits, nor will drinking pasteurized or HPP (high-pressure pasteurization) celery juice. Any kind of juicer is okay, although a cold press, masticating juicer is best. You can also choose to purchase your fresh celery juice from a juice bar rather than making your own. For best results, drink it freshly made. If you can't drink it immediately after juicing—for example, if you're having a second serving in the day—that's okay. Store it chilled in an airtight container.

- If you need to store your celery juice, it will stay strong and beneficial for 24 hours in the fridge. You can store it for as long as 48 to 72 hours in an airtight container in the refrigerator. After the 48-hour mark, celery juice does start losing some of its healing strength. Try your best not to exceed 24 hours. That period is when it's at its strongest.

- You can freeze celery juice, although that's not ideal either. If it's your only option, then go ahead and freeze it, and when you're ready, take it out and drink it as soon as it's thawed. Don't add water to the thawing celery juice. That will interfere with its benefits.

- Drink your fresh celery juice on an empty stomach. If you drank some water or lemon water beforehand, wait at least 15 to 20 and ideally 30 minutes before drinking your celery juice. After finishing your celery juice, wait at least 15 to 20 minutes and ideally 30 minutes before consuming anything else.

- If you're drinking celery juice later in the day, give any food you've eaten plenty of time to digest first. If your last snack or meal was high in fat/protein, it's best to wait a minimum of two hours and ideally three hours before having your celery juice. If you last ate something lighter such as fruit, leafy greens, vegetables, potatoes, or a fruit smoothie, you can drink your celery juice 60 minutes after eating.

- If you are on a doctor-prescribed medication, it's okay to take it either before or after your celery juice, depending on whether it's supposed to be taken on an empty stomach or with food. (Please note that if your medication is supposed to be taken with food, celery juice does not count as a food.) If you take the medication first, try to wait at least 15 to 20 minutes and ideally 30 minutes before you drink your celery juice. If you drink your celery

juice first, try to wait at least 15 to 20 minutes and ideally 30 minutes before you take your medication. For any further questions or concerns, consult your physician.

- When it comes to the other supplements in this book, please hold off on taking them with your celery juice. While the supplements will do fine with the celery juice, the celery juice is better without most supplements. It's best to wait to take your supplements until at least 15 to 20 minutes and ideally 30 minutes after you've finished your celery juice.

- If you have any further questions about bringing celery juice into your life, the Medical Medium title *Celery Juice* is an entire book of answers waiting for you.

Celery Juice Amounts for Children

When selecting celery juice amounts for children, you can refer to this table. These are recommended daily minimums. It can be less if that feels right for your child, or more. You don't need to worry that going over these minimums is harmful.

AGE	AMOUNT
6 months old	1 ounce or more
1 year old	2 ounces or more
18 months old	3 ounces or more
2 years old	4 ounces or more
3 years old	5 ounces or more
4 to 6 years old	6 to 7 ounces or more
7 to 10 years old	8 to 10 ounces or more
11 years old and up	12 to 16 ounces

HOW TO NAVIGATE THE HEAVY METAL DETOX SMOOTHIE, SPIRULINA, AND BARLEY GRASS JUICE POWDER IN PROTOCOLS

If you're doing the Medical Medium Heavy Metal Detox Smoothie daily and your supplement protocol also lists barley grass juice powder and/or spirulina, you don't need to take these supplements separately. You can take your barley grass juice powder and/or spirulina as part of your Heavy Metal Detox Smoothie, since they are already ingredients in it. If you're not on the Heavy Metal Detox Smoothie, you can choose to take barley grass juice powder and/or spirulina on their own.

CHAPTER 3

Medical Medium Shock Therapies

You'll find that some of the supplement protocols in the next chapter call for optional:

- Medical Medium Zinc Shock Therapy

- Medical Medium Vitamin C Shock Therapy

- Medical Medium Lemon Balm Shock Therapy

- Medical Medium Goldenseal Shock Therapy

- Medical Medium Thyme Tea Shock Therapy

- Medical Medium Propolis Shock Therapy

- Medical Medium Aloe Vera Shock Therapy

- Medical Medium B_{12} Shock Therapy

- Medical Medium California Poppy Shock Therapy

These are powerful healing tools to rebuild your immune system by fueling it with what it needs to fight an infection, support your brain and body through an emotional challenge, calm and restore your nervous system, strengthen and heal your digestive system, and/or purge, rebuild, and fortify your lymphatic system—whether you're dealing with a condition that's occurring for the first time or you're experiencing a relapse.

Medical Medium Shock Therapies have a profound record of helping people overcome health obstacles. These supplement therapies can be useful for almost anything you're ailing with. Medical Medium Shock Therapies are powerful whether you're up against intense stress or need a shift from a long-standing chronic illness roller coaster ride.

Medical Medium Shock Therapies are critical to this day and age. As darkness tries to destroy all that's good, we rise against darkness using light-created health weapons to regain empowerment. As the changing times bring additional stress upon us, humankind goes into a deeper health deficit than during previous decades. Sickness now dominates the lives of billions of people. Medical Medium Shock Therapies are

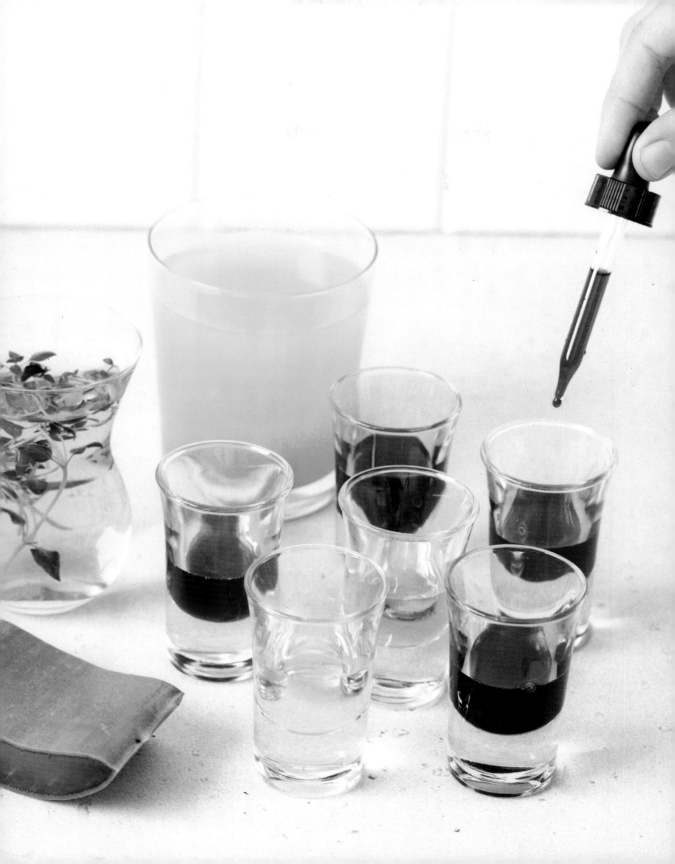

here to help level the playing field, where chemical and medical industries are playing dirty against humankind.

UNIVERSAL NOTES FOR ALL MEDICAL MEDIUM SHOCK THERAPIES

- You'll find suggestions for best applications for various ailments within each Shock Therapy protocol. These are examples and not exhaustive lists of symptoms and conditions. If you want to use a Medical Medium Shock Therapy for a symptom, condition, or circumstance not listed, you can still partake.

- If you feel a need to use more than one Shock Therapy on the same day(s), avoid mixing them directly together. Space the therapies apart by at least 15 minutes.

- You're welcome to lower the dosage of any Medical Medium Shock Therapy. Bring it down to whatever amount you'd like.

MEDICAL MEDIUM ZINC SHOCK THERAPY

Medical Medium Zinc Shock Therapy is a useful technique because most everyone is zinc deficient. It's a mineral that left our soils long ago due to a reaction that occurs when toxic heavy metals enter our soils, including our organic farm soils, and create dead soil over time by destroying the soil's immune system. Trace mineral zinc in foods at this point is minuscule and only becoming rarer as passing-by pollutants (such as herbicides, car exhaust, old asbestos from car brakes in decades past, DDT, toxic heavy metals falling from the sky, chem trails, worldwide mosquito spray, chemical fragrances, fungicides, burning plastic, burning in general, fireworks, and missile testing) continue to enter our soil and deplete the soil's immune system. Zinc is supposed to be our own immune system's number one defense, and because we're deficient, we're in dire need of it.

If we don't have enough zinc in the body, our immune system may overreact to an invader such as a flu strain or underreact to a chronic viral infection such as Epstein-Barr. Overreaction could mean higher fever and other more advanced, severe symptoms. Underreaction could mean prolonged low-grade symptoms that become chronic over time. When our immune system is well supplied with an abundant amount of zinc, this overreaction or underreaction doesn't take place. Zinc also slows down viruses and unproductive, aggressive bacteria on its own merits. Viruses and unproductive bacteria are allergic to zinc; the mineral repels and weakens them, even making pathogens docile, which allows the immune system to kill off and eliminate the pathogens more quickly.

Many cases of infertility are due to zinc deficiency, because procreation requires an optimum level of zinc. Excessive sexual activity can deplete zinc reserves.

Suggested Applications for Medical Medium Zinc Shock Therapy

Cold, flu, COVID, mononucleosis, tonsillitis, sore throat, strep throat, allergies, UTIs, bladder infections, kidney infections, yeast infections, bouts of neurological symptoms, Bell's palsy, acute nerve pain, body pain, herpes simplex 1, herpes simplex 2, bouts of brain inflammation, shingles flare-ups, acute shingles outbreaks, traumatic emotional events, exposure to a virus of any kind, after a plane flight or airport exposure, autoimmune flare-ups, acute tinnitus episodes, vertigo flare-ups

Medical Medium Zinc Shock Therapy Directions

- If you think you're coming down with a bug, you're already sick with the flu, or you have one of the infections or symptom flare-ups listed above, then for an adult, squirt 2 dropperfuls of high-quality liquid zinc sulfate into your mouth every three waking hours. If the taste is too strong, you can take the zinc in an ounce of water; it will still work the same. Let the zinc sit in your mouth for 10 seconds to one minute before swallowing, or spit out and don't swallow if your stomach is sensitive. You can follow this with a water or juice chaser to reduce the potent flavor.

- If the flu isn't making you nauseated and you can palate the zinc, you can do this up to five or six times a day (that is, two squirts of zinc every three hours for a total of 10 to 12 dropperfuls a day) for two days. You have the option to continue for a third or even fourth day if severe symptoms persist.

- If your palate is more sensitive, you're welcome to try a milder Medical Medium Zinc Shock Therapy: 1 dropperful every three waking hours up to five times a day or 2 dropperfuls three times a day.

- In any version of Medical Medium Zinc Shock Therapy, after the two to four days, bring the zinc dosage down to what your supplement list says.

- If you find, a week or more later, the need to apply Zinc Shock Therapy for a second round, you're welcome to do so.

For children, here are the adjusted amounts of liquid zinc sulfate for this supplement therapy:

- **Ages 1 to 2:** 2 tiny drops (not dropperfuls) in a teaspoon of juice or water every three waking hours

- **Ages 3 to 4:** 3 tiny drops (not dropperfuls) in juice, water, or directly in the mouth every three waking hours

- **Ages 5 to 8:** 4 tiny drops (not dropperfuls) in juice, water, or directly in the mouth every three waking hours

- **Ages 9 to 12:** 10 tiny drops (not dropperfuls) in juice, water, or directly in the mouth every three waking hours

- **Ages 13 and up:** 1 dropperful in juice, water, or directly in the mouth every four waking hours

Because of children's special sensitive nature, it's especially important to get the right kind of liquid zinc sulfate, which you can find on my directory online at www.medicalmedium.com. Almost all companies make zinc that's aggressive in taste and hard to palate, often with harsh additives too.

MEDICAL MEDIUM VITAMIN C SHOCK THERAPY

Why does Medical Medium Vitamin C Shock Therapy bring healing to a new level? Because it takes a specific type of glucose that you'll find mainly in raw honey, pure maple syrup, and fresh-squeezed citrus to bind on to the right type of non–ascorbic acid vitamin C to drive it into cells and organs. Vitamin C is an antioxidant that feeds your immune system. The raw honey and the squeezed orange combined attach themselves directly to the vitamin C, allowing this powerful antioxidant delivery of antiviral, antibacterial healing nutrients to occur within the body.

On top of which, the viruses and unproductive bacteria that are responsible for symptoms and conditions are highly allergic and sensitive to vitamin C. While protecting your own cells from oxidation, vitamin C has the ability to oxidize a pathogen, causing it to become injured, break down, and disperse.

As our bodies are bombarded by manufactured toxins, including manufactured medical treatments, we're in need of vitamin C more than ever before in our history. Our immune system needs extra strengthening to give us a fighting chance on this planet. Vitamin C is that nutrient our body craves to help keep us strong.

Suggested Applications for Medical Medium Vitamin C Shock Therapy

Bronchitis, pneumonia, cough, cold, flu, COVID, mononucleosis, tonsillitis, sore throat, strep throat, allergies, UTIs, bladder infections, kidney infections, yeast infections, bouts of neurological symptoms, Bell's palsy, acute nerve pain, body pain, herpes simplex 1, herpes simplex 2, bouts of brain inflammation, shingles flare-ups, acute shingles outbreaks, traumatic emotional events, exposure to a virus of any kind, after a plane flight or airport exposure, autoimmune flare-ups, acute tinnitus episodes, vertigo flare-ups, moments of high stress, relationship breakups, episodes of depression, episodes of anxiety, episodes of OCD, post-seizure, post-surgery, post–medical procedure, physical injuries, post–physical accident, emotional adrenaline surges, post–recreational drug and alcohol use, post-vacation, post–heavy workout, dental procedures

Medical Medium Vitamin C Shock Therapy Directions

- For Medical Medium Vitamin C Shock Therapy for adults, the ingredients are 2 500-milligram capsules of Micro-C or comparable buffered vitamin C, 1 cup of water (preferably warm), 2 teaspoons of raw honey, and the freshly squeezed juice from one orange.

- Here's how to prepare it: Open the Micro-C capsules and pour their powder into the warm water. Stir until dissolved. Add the raw honey and orange juice and stir well.

- Starting at the first sign of cold, flu, or any of the infections or symptom flare-ups listed, drink this tonic every two waking hours. You can do this for two days and then switch to the dosage in an individual

supplement list, or you can use this technique throughout the duration of a cold or flu.

- If you feel you need more vitamin C per drink, you can add more than 2 capsules of Micro-C to each. If you don't want to use raw honey, you can use 100 percent pure maple syrup (not maple-flavored syrup) in its place. If you don't like orange, you can substitute the juice of half a lemon.

For children, here are the adjusted amounts of vitamin C for this supplement therapy:

- **Ages 1 to 2:** 1 500-milligram capsule Micro-C emptied and mixed with ½ cup water, 1 teaspoon raw honey, and the freshly squeezed juice from half an orange, every six waking hours

- **Ages 3 to 4:** 1 500-milligram capsule Micro-C emptied and mixed with ½ cup water, 1 teaspoon raw honey, and the freshly squeezed juice from 1 orange, every five waking hours

- **Ages 5 to 8:** 1 500-milligram capsule Micro-C emptied and mixed with 1 cup water, 2 teaspoons raw honey, and the freshly squeezed juice from 1 orange, every four waking hours

- **Ages 9 to 12:** 1 500-milligram capsule Micro-C emptied and mixed with 1 cup water, 2 teaspoons raw honey, and the freshly squeezed juice from 1 orange, every two waking hours

- **Ages 13 and up:** 2 500-milligram capsules Micro-C emptied and mixed with 1 cup water, 2 teaspoons raw honey, and the freshly squeezed juice from 1 orange, every three waking hours

MEDICAL MEDIUM LEMON BALM SHOCK THERAPY

Lemon balm stabilizes nerve cells. Lemon balm does this by entering into nerve cells, recalibrating them, and reestablishing a balance after nerve cells have been triggered into high-intensity reaction. Lemon balm also protects nerve cells from corrosive adrenaline that is released during an emotional crisis—adrenaline that is otherwise antagonistic to nerve cells.

Suggested Applications for Medical Medium Lemon Balm Shock Therapy

Stress, emotional turmoil, emotional challenges, emotional trauma, emotional events, episodes of OCD, heightened ADHD, anxiety, depression, emotional confrontations, betrayal, emotional crisis, neurological episodes, pre- and post-seizure, incidents, physical accidents, nerve pain, outbreaks of shingles, post-shingles, bipolar episodes, mania, psychosis, nervousness, unease, anxiousness, nervous stomach, cranial nerve inflammation, body pain

Medical Medium Lemon Balm Shock Therapy can also be used as a backbone to come off psychiatric drugs, such as antidepressants, antianxiety medications, and benzodiazepines, with guidance and help from your doctor.

Medical Medium Lemon Balm Shock Therapy Directions

- For an adult, take 4 dropperfuls of alcohol-free lemon balm tincture in an ounce or more of water or juice (or directly in the mouth, with an optional juice or water chaser) every three waking hours.

- You can do this for three to five days, and then switch to the dosage in an individual supplement list.

- You're welcome to cycle through Lemon Balm Shock Therapy on a continual basis to steady the nervous system if an emotional event is ongoing. Here's how: Apply Lemon Balm Shock Therapy for a three-to-five-day period, and then dial back to the dosage listed in an individual supplement list for three days. Then you can repeat the Lemon Balm Shock

Therapy protocol for three to five days, and so on.

- You also have the option to lower the dosage of Lemon Balm Shock Therapy as you're navigating the terrain of your nervous system and emotional crisis.

For children, here are the adjusted amounts of alcohol-free lemon balm tincture for this supplement therapy:

- **Ages 1 to 2:** 12 tiny drops (not dropperfuls) in juice or water every three waking hours

- **Ages 3 to 4:** 20 tiny drops (not dropperfuls) in juice or water every three waking hours

- **Ages 5 to 8:** 1 dropperful in juice or water every three waking hours

- **Ages 9 to 12:** 2 dropperfuls in juice or water every three waking hours

- **Ages 13 and up:** 3 dropperfuls in juice or water every three waking hours

MEDICAL MEDIUM GOLDENSEAL SHOCK THERAPY

Goldenseal is antibacterial and antiviral, and as a result, goldenseal is anti-inflammatory because it reduces pathogens and aids in restoring weakened immune cells. White blood cells utilize goldenseal's antiviral, antibacterial compounds by carrying and then releasing these compounds into battle zones—areas of the body where white blood cells are at war with pathogens. Medical Medium Goldenseal Shock Therapy can be used with both acute conditions and ongoing chronic conditions.

Suggested Applications for Medical Medium Goldenseal Shock Therapy

Cold, flu, COVID, sinus congestion, allergies, bronchitis, pneumonia, lung infections, acute cough or chronic cough, earaches, ear infections, strep throat, sore throat, runny nose, postnasal drip, sties, conjunctivitis, UTIs, bladder infections, kidney infections, bacterial vaginosis (BV), pelvic inflammatory disease (PID), yeast infections, all varieties of acne, cold sores/fever blisters, herpes simplex 1, herpes simplex 2, shingles, acute neurological symptoms, difficult menstruation cycles, *H. pylori*, methicillin-resistant *Staphylococcus aureus* (MRSA), mononucleosis

Medical Medium Goldenseal Shock Therapy Directions

- For an adult, take 6 dropperfuls of alcohol-free goldenseal tincture in an ounce or more of water or juice (or directly in the mouth, with an optional juice or water chaser) every four waking hours.

- You can do this for three to five days, and then switch to the dosage in an individual supplement list.

- As with all the other Medical Medium Shock Therapies, you're also welcome to lower the amount to whatever dosage you're comfortable with, if you're sensitive.

- If a bout of illness, infection, or symptoms is still not subsiding a week or more after completing a round of Goldenseal Shock Therapy, you're welcome to apply Goldenseal Shock Therapy for another three to five days. Do wait a minimum of one week between rounds of this therapy.

For children, here are the adjusted amounts of alcohol-free goldenseal tincture for this supplement therapy:

- **Ages 1 to 2:** 10 tiny drops (not dropperfuls) in juice or water every four waking hours

- **Ages 3 to 4:** 20 tiny drops (not dropperfuls) in juice or water every four waking hours

- **Ages 5 to 8:** 1 dropperful in juice or water every four waking hours

- **Ages 9 to 12:** 2 dropperfuls in juice or water every four waking hours

- **Ages 13 and up:** 3 dropperfuls in juice or water every four waking hours

MEDICAL MEDIUM THYME TEA SHOCK THERAPY

Thyme contains a phytochemical compound that is antiviral, antibacterial, anti-mold, anti-yeast, and anti–unproductive fungus that stays circulating inside the bloodstream long after nutrients from other foods have either been utilized, dissipated, or eliminated out of the body. Thyme lingers, creating a time-released protective barrier against pathogens. Thyme's phytochemical compounds enter every organ inside the body, versus other herbs that only enter certain organs in the body.

Suggested Applications for Medical Medium Thyme Tea Shock Therapy

Flu, COVID, colds, lung infections, bronchitis, pneumonia, allergies, sinus congestion, coughs, sore throats, strep throat, scratchy throat, ear infections, UTIs, bladder infections, kidney infections, HPV, shingles, EBV-caused infections, SIBO, *H. pylori*, *E. coli*, *Streptococcus*, MRSA, *C. difficile*, acute jaw pain, tongue pain, mouth pain, gum pain, fever, body aches, cold sores/fever blisters, herpes simplex 1, parasite concerns, autoimmune flare-ups, episodes of neurological symptoms

Medical Medium Thyme Tea Shock Therapy Directions

- Make a special brew of Thyme Tea with 12 sprigs of fresh thyme per cup of hot water. (If you only have access to dried thyme, use 2 tablespoons dried herb per cup of hot water.) Let steep for at least 15 minutes. Remove the thyme sprigs or strain the tea, especially if you're using dried thyme.

- Drink 1 cup of this potent Thyme Tea every three waking hours.

- You can do this therapy for three to five days, and then switch to the dosage in an individual supplement list.

- After a week or more off Thyme Tea Shock Therapy, you're welcome to try another round of it.

- You can make your Thyme Tea with less thyme if you're sensitive.

- You have the option to sweeten your Thyme Tea with the juice of a half lemon and/or 1 teaspoon of raw honey per cup of tea.

- You're welcome to make more than one serving of Thyme Tea at a time, multiplying the ingredients accordingly, and then set aside the extra portions to drink throughout the day. You don't have to drink the tea hot or warm. It's fine to drink the tea lukewarm or cool.

For children, brew the same Thyme Tea as above, and then give your child these adjusted amounts for this therapy:

- **Ages 1 to 2:** 1 ounce of cool or warm (not hot) tea every three waking hours

- **Ages 3 to 4:** 2 ounces of cool or warm (not hot) tea every three waking hours

- **Ages 5 to 8:** 3 ounces of cool or warm (not hot) tea every three waking hours

- **Ages 9 to 12:** 4 ounces of cool or warm (not hot) tea every three waking hours

- **Ages 13 and up:** 6 ounces of cool, warm, or hot tea every three waking hours

MEDICAL MEDIUM PROPOLIS SHOCK THERAPY

Propolis is a powerful antiviral, antibacterial medicinal tool. If the propolis is high quality and used correctly, it has the ability to slow down, reverse, and even stop infections of many different varieties. Propolis doesn't just contain one antiviral agent compound. Propolis carries multiple antiviral agent compounds—sometimes even dozens.

You'll find two variations of Medical Medium Propolis Shock Therapy here. The first is for propolis tincture taken internally, and the second is for direct application of propolis tincture on mouth sores. These two variations can be used together or separately. Read on for more details.

Suggested Applications for Medical Medium Propolis Shock Therapy

Sore throat, strep throat, tonsillitis, sinus infections, allergies, lung infections, bronchitis, pneumonia, cough, postnasal drip, cold, flu, COVID, ear infections, UTIs, bladder infections, kidney infections, fever, chills, night sweats, trigeminal neuralgia, gum pain, mouth pain, tooth pain, tongue pain, migraines, headaches, shingles, bouts of neurological symptoms, cold sores/fever blisters, herpes simplex 1, canker sores, mouth ulcers

Medical Medium Propolis Shock Therapy Directions

- For an adult, take 4 dropperfuls of alcohol-free* propolis tincture in an ounce or more of water or juice every three waking hours.

- You can do this for three to five days, then switch to the dosage in an individual supplement list.

- You're welcome to continue cycling through Propolis Shock

Therapy. You can either take a week off and then apply it again, or you can repeat rounds of Propolis Shock Therapy back-to-back if you choose. If your supplement list doesn't include propolis, you can do 2 dropperfuls of propolis tincture daily in between rounds of Propolis Shock Therapy.

*Even propolis tincture labeled alcohol-free can contain traces of different forms of alcohol. Use propolis tincture with the least amount of alcohol you can find. Check the directory at www.medicalmedium.com for the only true alcohol-free propolis.

For children, here are the adjusted amounts of alcohol-free propolis tincture for this supplement therapy:

- **Ages 1 to 2:** 8 tiny drops (not dropperfuls) in juice or water every three waking hours

- **Ages 3 to 4:** 16 tiny drops (not dropperfuls) in juice or water every three waking hours

- **Ages 5 to 8:** 1 dropperful in juice or water every three waking hours

- **Ages 9 to 12:** 2 dropperfuls in juice or water every three waking hours

- **Ages 13 and up:** 3 dropperfuls in juice or water every three waking hours

Suggested Applications for Medical Medium Propolis Mouth Sore Shock Therapy

Cold sores/fever blisters, herpes simplex 1, canker sores, mouth ulcers

You can do external Propolis Mouth Sore Shock Therapy while also using internal Propolis Shock Therapy. If you're living with cold sores/fever blisters, it's ideal to do both versions of Propolis Shock Therapy. If, on the other hand, you're living with a canker sore, you're welcome to simply use the external Propolis Mouth Sore Shock Therapy.

Medical Medium Propolis Mouth Sore Shock Therapy Directions

- If the sore is in a spot where it's wet with saliva (for example, inner lip, gumline, side of the mouth, tongue) and you can reach it, first dry the sore quickly with a paper towel.

- Once the sore is dry, or if the sore is outside of the mouth and dry already, apply a few drops of propolis tincture directly onto the sore. Leave for 30 seconds to one minute.

- If the sore is in a spot where you had to dry it off first, then repeat the technique right away: quickly soak up the saliva again with a paper towel, and then place a few drops of propolis tincture directly onto the sore and let the propolis sit for another 30 seconds to one minute. Then dry and reapply one more time, for a total of three applications at a time. After the third application, don't dry it off. You can relax your mouth and let the propolis stay on the sore as you continue on with your day.

- If the sore was dry to begin with, you don't need to repeat the propolis application back-to-back like this—you only need to do one application at a time. Once you've applied the propolis droplets onto the sore, you can leave the propolis on and carry on with your day. (Or it's okay to wipe off the propolis after 30 seconds to one minute if needed.)

- Use this technique four to six times daily until the problem is gone.

- For quicker healing, make Propolis Mouth Sore Shock Therapy the last technique you use before bed.

MEDICAL MEDIUM ALOE VERA SHOCK THERAPY

Many people struggle with gastrointestinal pain that radiates all through the abdomen and torso without realizing that it originates from the stomach or intestinal tract. Aloe vera has chemical compounds that neutralize acid and calm nerves in the intestinal tract linings, slowing down and stopping intestinal spasms. Aloe neutralizes acids and inhibits bacterial and viral growth as well as yeast, unproductive fungus, and mold growth. Aloe vera also soothes the linings of the intestinal tract, calming inflamed intestinal tract nerves, inhibiting gastric nerve spasms, and alleviating pressure on the vagus nerves.

Suggested Applications for Medical Medium Aloe Vera Shock Therapy

Stomach pain, gastrointestinal pain, intestinal and stomach pain that rises into the chest or runs through the back and up to the neck and shoulders, colitis, IBS, Crohn's, celiac, acid reflux, ulcers, stomach burning, *H. pylori*, SIBO, stomach pain shortly after eating a meal, stomach and intestinal cramping, gastritis, severe bloating that's painful, constipation, acid attacks, gastroparesis

Medical Medium Aloe Vera Shock Therapy Directions

- For an adult, consume 2 to 4 inches of fresh aloe vera gel (skin removed) every two to four waking hours.

- Continue this therapy for one to seven days.

- After three or more days off Aloe Vera Shock Therapy, you're welcome to cycle through one to seven days of the therapy again. In between rounds of Aloe Vera Shock Therapy, you can do 2 or more inches of fresh aloe vera gel daily or twice a day.

- To prepare the aloe gel, carefully slice open your 2- to 4-inch piece of aloe vera leaf, filleting it as if it were a fish and trimming away the green skin and spikes. Scoop out the clear gel.

- Make sure you do not use the skin. As you're scooping out the aloe gel, try not to scrape the skin. The chemical compound in the green skin can be irritating for some people.

- Also cut off 1 inch from the very end of the base of the aloe leaf and discard; it's too bitter.

- Eat the gel straight if possible for best results. If you have trouble eating the aloe gel, it's okay to blend it with water. (Still make sure not to use the green skin.)

- This recipe is based on using a large, store-bought aloe vera leaf, which you can find in the produce section of many grocery stores. If you're using a homegrown aloe vera plant, make sure it's an edible source.

- You're welcome to prepare all of your aloe gel for the day at once. Store your aloe gel portions for later in the day in an airtight container in the refrigerator.

- If you're storing a partial leaf, wrap the cut end in a damp towel or plastic wrap and place it in the refrigerator.

- Avoid aloe leaves where the gel is very red inside and extra watery. These leaves aren't fresh and are starting to decay.

- As with the other Medical Medium Shock Therapies, you can always choose to use less than the amount listed. Use the amount of aloe gel you're comfortable with.

For children, here are the adjusted amounts of fresh aloe vera gel for this therapy:

- **Ages 1 to 2:** 1 teaspoon fresh gel every two to four waking hours

- **Ages 3 to 4:** 2 teaspoons fresh gel every two to four waking hours

- **Ages 5 to 8:** 1 tablespoon fresh gel every two to four waking hours

- **Ages 9 to 12:** 2 tablespoons fresh gel every two to four waking hours

- **Ages 13 and up:** 2 inches fresh gel every two to four waking hours

MEDICAL MEDIUM B_{12} SHOCK THERAPY

When we go through difficult physical or mental events, including long-term chronic illness, we lose B_{12} reserves. B_{12} depletion can be rapid in the moment of a crisis and then show up years later as additional health problems. For more insights into B_{12}, see the chapter "Your Burnt Out, Deficient Brain" in this book's companion, *Brain Saver*.

Suggested Applications for Medical Medium B_{12} Shock Therapy

Stress, accidents where the physical body has been injured, accidents where the emotional body has been injured, emotional events, emotional trauma, loss, acute bouts of anxiety, acute bouts of depression, heightened episodes of OCD, anger episodes, neurological episodes, seizures, post-fever (after an infection or after COVID or flu), post-surgery, post–medical procedure, after recreational drug or alcohol use, difficult caffeine withdrawal, post-vacation, acute attacks of body pain, following overuse of the brain for work, creativity, school studies, exams, or intense play

Medical Medium B$_{12}$ Shock Therapy Directions

- For an adult, take 2 dropperfuls of vitamin B$_{12}$ (as adenosylcobalamin with methylcobalamin) directly in the mouth (with an optional juice or water chaser) or mixed in an ounce or more of juice or water every three waking hours.

- Continue this therapy for one to two days. You have the option to continue for a third or even fourth day if needed.

- After the one to four days, bring your vitamin B$_{12}$ dosage down to what your supplement list says. Wait a minimum of one week between rounds of B$_{12}$ Shock Therapy.

For children, here are the adjusted amounts of vitamin B$_{12}$ (as adenosylcobalamin with methylcobalamin) for this supplement therapy:

- **Ages 1 to 2:** 2 tiny drops (not dropperfuls) in juice or water every three waking hours

- **Ages 3 to 4:** 3 tiny drops (not dropperfuls) in juice or water every three waking hours

- **Ages 5 to 8:** 5 tiny drops (not dropperfuls) in juice or water every three waking hours

- **Ages 9 to 12:** 10 tiny drops (not dropperfuls) in juice or water every three waking hours

- **Ages 13 and up:** 1 dropperful in juice or water every three waking hours

MEDICAL MEDIUM CALIFORNIA POPPY SHOCK THERAPY

California poppy contains specific alkaloids that soothe and calm pain receptor cells, specifically around cranial nerves and the brain stem. California poppy can be used to take the edge off or minimize heightened pain.

Suggested Applications for Medical Medium California Poppy Shock Therapy

Nerve pain, neuralgia, trigeminal neuralgia, neck pain, back pain, sciatic pain, tooth pain, mouth pain, tongue pain, jaw pain, body pain, head pain, shoulder pain, hip pain, knee pain, vagus nerve symptoms, emotional hardship, trauma, loss, emotional pain, anxiety, emotional suffering, intense stress

California poppy can be used to help wean off recreational drugs or prescription drugs, including pain medications, with guidance from your doctor.

Medical Medium California Poppy Shock Therapy Directions

- For an adult, take 3 dropperfuls of alcohol-free California poppy tincture in an ounce or more of water or juice, or 3 capsules, every four waking hours.

- For acute pain, use this therapy for one to three days. If still needed, you can repeat another back-to-back cycle of this therapy, for a total of up to six days. Then cut back to 3 dropperfuls twice a day for three days, if still needed. If pain continues to persist, you can follow the chronic pain relief cycle described next.

- For chronic pain, use this therapy when needed for up to seven days at a time. Cut back to 3 dropperfuls twice a day (if still needed) for three days before venturing into another seven-day cycle.

- If you're someone who gets sleepy using California poppy, then choose to use it wisely. Use it with caution when operating equipment or machinery, or on long car drives.

For children, here are the adjusted amounts of alcohol-free California poppy tincture for this therapy. For any questions about California poppy, check with your child's physician:

- **Ages 5 to 8:** 10 tiny drops (not dropperfuls) in juice or water every four waking hours

- **Ages 9 to 12:** 15 tiny drops (not dropperfuls) in juice or water every four waking hours

- **Ages 13 and up:** 1 dropperful in juice or water or 1 capsule every four waking hours

"This is how it works with all trends: not enough consideration is being given to who can have fun dabbling with a trend and who doesn't have that room to play."

— Anthony William, Medical Medium

CHAPTER 4

Medical Medium Protocols

These supplement protocols have a working, healing track record and history of recovering countless people from complicated health conditions. To interpret these lists and figure out where to start, please read Chapter 2, "Golden Rules of Supplements." You'll find critical guidance there. For example:

You have many options within these supplement protocols. You can apply one of the recommended supplements, or you can apply multiple supplements. These full lists of supplements are offered to give you options to take your health as far as you would like to go.

You have the option to take it slowly as you monitor your progress, and you have the option of a quicker pace. You don't need to take the full dosages you see listed here. You have the option to minimize dosages. A lot of people find their healing through Medical Medium cleanses, the Heavy Metal Detox Smoothie, and many other Medical Medium tools.

The supplements in each protocol are, for the most part, in alphabetical order, not necessarily order of importance. Check "Where to Start?" in Chapter 2 for guidance about the most important supplements.

Read much more in Chapter 2.

Feel free to check with your health care provider when partaking in supplementation.

WHAT'S THE CAUSE?

The lists to come feature protocols only, without explanations of cause, to allow space for as many protocols as possible. If you'd like to know what's behind your health struggle, you can find detailed explanations of over 100 brain- and nervous system–related symptoms, conditions, diseases, and disorders in this book's companion title, *Brain Saver*.

EVERYDAY BRAIN AND HEALTH MAINTENANCE

Before applying these, be sure to read Chapter 2, "Golden Rules of Supplements."

- **Fresh celery juice:** work up to 32 ounces daily
- **Heavy Metal Detox Smoothie:** 1 serving daily (see Chapter 10)
- **5-MTHF:** 1 capsule daily
- **Aloe vera:** 2 or more inches of fresh gel (skin removed) daily
- **Barley grass juice powder:** 1 teaspoon or 3 capsules daily
- **B-complex:** 1 capsule daily
- **Celeryforce:** 1 capsule twice a day
- **Chaga mushroom powder:** 2 teaspoons or 6 capsules daily
- **Curcumin:** 2 capsules daily
- **EPA and DHA (fish-free):** 1 capsule daily (taken with dinner)
- **Glutathione:** 1 capsule daily
- **Lemon balm:** 3 dropperfuls daily
- **L-lysine:** 3 500-milligram capsules daily
- **Magnesium glycinate:** 2 capsules daily
- **Melatonin:** 1 5-milligram capsule at bedtime daily
- **Nascent iodine:** 4 small drops (not dropperfuls) daily
- **Nettle leaf:** 2 cups of tea or 3 dropperfuls daily
- **Raspberry leaf:** 1 cup of tea daily

- **Spirulina:** 1 teaspoon or 3 capsules daily
- **Vitamin B$_{12}$ (as adenosylcobalamin with methylcobalamin):** 1 dropperful daily
- **Vitamin C (as Micro-C or comparable buffered vitamin C):** 4 500-milligram capsules twice a day
- **Wild blueberry:** 1 teaspoon powder to 1 ounce juice daily
- **Zinc (as liquid zinc sulfate):** up to 1 dropperful daily

ACHES AND PAINS

Refer to Cranial Nerve Inflammation protocol.

ACUTE DISSEMINATED ENCEPHALOMYELITIS (ADEM)

Refer to Autoimmune Disorders and Diseases protocol and/or ALS protocol.

ADDICTION

Before applying these, be sure to read Chapter 2, "Golden Rules of Supplements."

- **Fresh celery juice:** work up to at least 16 ounces daily
- **Heavy Metal Detox Smoothie:** 1 serving daily (see Chapter 10)

- **Cravings Shifter:** 1 Brain Shot daily (see Chapter 8)

- **Adrenal Fight or Flight Stabilizer:** 1 Brain Shot daily (see Chapter 8)

- **Pharmaceutical Exposure:** 1 Brain Shot daily (see Chapter 8)

- **Energy Shifter:** 1 Brain Shot daily (see Chapter 8)

- **California Poppy Shock Therapy:** if needed (see Chapter 3)

- **Lemon Balm Shock Therapy:** if needed (see Chapter 3)

- **5-MTHF:** 1 capsule daily

- **Ashwagandha:** 1 dropperful twice a day

- **Barley grass juice powder:** 1 tablespoon or 9 capsules daily

- **Celeryforce:** 2 capsules three times a day

- **Chaga mushroom powder:** 2 teaspoons or 6 capsules daily

- **Curcumin:** 2 capsules twice a day

- **EPA and DHA (fish-free):** 2 capsules daily (taken with dinner)

- **GABA:** 1 250-milligram capsule daily

- **Lemon balm:** 4 dropperfuls three times a day

- **L-glutamine:** 2 capsules twice a day

- **Licorice root:** 1 dropperful daily (two weeks on, two weeks off)

- **Melatonin:** 1 5-milligram capsule twice a day

- **Peppermint:** 1 cup of tea daily

- **Raw honey:** 1 tablespoon daily

- **Spirulina:** 1 tablespoon or 9 capsules daily

- **Vitamin B$_{12}$ (as adenosylcobalamin with methylcobalamin):** 3 dropperfuls twice a day

- **Vitamin C (as Micro-C or comparable buffered vitamin C):** 4 500-milligram capsules daily

- **Wild blueberry:** 2 tablespoons powder or 2 to 4 ounces juice daily

- **Zinc (as liquid zinc sulfate):** 1 dropperful twice a day

ADDISON'S DISEASE

Refer to Autoimmune Disorders and Diseases protocol.

ADHD (ATTENTION-DEFICIT/ HYPERACTIVITY DISORDER)

Before applying these, be sure to read Chapter 2, "Golden Rules of Supplements."

Remember that you can take these adult dosages to your pediatrician to see what dosages are right for your child. Also see Chapter 8, "Brain Shot Therapy," Chapter 10, "Heavy Metal Detox," and Chapter 2, "Golden Rules of Supplements," for adjusted amounts of celery juice, Heavy Metal Detox Smoothie, and Brain Shot Therapies for children.

- **Fresh celery juice:** work up to 16 ounces daily

- **Heavy Metal Detox Smoothie:** 1 serving daily (see Chapter 10)

- **Burnout Stabilizer:** 1 Brain Shot daily (see Chapter 8)

- **Adrenal Fight or Flight Stabilizer:** 1 Brain Shot daily (see Chapter 8)

- **Barley grass juice powder:** 1 teaspoon or 3 capsules daily

- **B-complex:** 1 capsule daily

- **Celeryforce:** 2 capsules daily

- **Elderberry syrup:** 1 teaspoon daily

- **EPA and DHA (fish-free):** 1 capsule daily (taken with dinner)

- **GABA:** 1 250-milligram capsule daily

- **Goldenseal:** 1 dropperful daily (one week per month)

- **Lemon balm:** 3 dropperfuls daily

- **Licorice root:** 1 dropperful daily (two weeks on, two weeks off)

- **Magnesium glycinate:** 2 capsules daily

- **Melatonin:** 1 to 5 milligrams daily (preferably at night)

- **Mullein leaf:** 1 dropperful daily (one week per month)

- **Spirulina:** 1 teaspoon or 3 capsules daily

- **Vitamin B$_{12}$ (as adenosylcobalamin with methylcobalamin):** 1 dropperful daily

- **Vitamin C (as Micro-C or comparable buffered vitamin C):** 2 500-milligram capsules daily

- **Zinc (as liquid zinc sulfate):** 1 dropperful daily

AGE SPOTS

Refer to Hyperpigmentation protocol.

ALCOHOL WITHDRAWAL

Refer to Addiction protocol.

ALS (AMYOTROPHIC LATERAL SCLEROSIS, LOU GEHRIG'S DISEASE, MOTOR NEURON DISEASE)

Before applying these, be sure to read Chapter 2, "Golden Rules of Supplements."

- **Fresh celery juice:** work up to 32 ounces daily; then you have the option to work up to 32 ounces twice a day

- **Heavy Metal Detox Smoothie:** 1 serving daily (see Chapter 10)

- **Extractor Smoothie:** 1 serving daily (see Chapter 10)

- **Nerve Shifter:** 1 Brain Shot daily (see Chapter 8)

- **Any Shock Therapies from Chapter 3 can be used if needed**

- **5-HTP:** 1 capsule at bedtime daily

- **5-MTHF:** 1 capsule daily

- **Aloe vera:** 2 or more inches of fresh gel (skin removed) daily

- **Ashwagandha:** 1 dropperful daily

- **Barley grass juice powder:** 1 teaspoon or 3 capsules daily

- **B-complex:** 1 capsule daily

- **Cat's claw:** 2 dropperfuls twice a day

- **Celeryforce:** 2 capsules twice a day

- **CoQ10:** 1 capsule daily

- **Curcumin:** 2 capsules twice a day

- **Elderberry syrup:** 1 teaspoon daily

- **EPA and DHA (fish-free):** 2 capsules daily (taken with dinner)

- **GABA:** 1 250-milligram capsule twice a day

- **Glutathione:** 2 capsules twice a day

- **Goldenseal:** 4 dropperfuls twice a day (two weeks on, two weeks off)

- **Lemon balm:** 4 dropperfuls twice a day

- **Licorice root:** 1 dropperful twice a day (two weeks on, two weeks off)

- **L-lysine:** 2 500-milligram capsules twice a day

- **Magnesium glycinate:** 3 capsules twice a day

- **Melatonin:** 1 5-milligram capsule at bedtime daily

- **Milk thistle:** 1 dropperful daily

- **MSM:** 1 capsule daily

- **Nettle leaf:** 2 dropperfuls twice a day

- **Olive leaf:** 1 dropperful twice a day

- **Propolis:** 2 dropperfuls twice a day
- **Raw honey:** 1 tablespoon daily
- **Spirulina:** 1 teaspoon or 3 capsules daily
- **Vitamin B$_{12}$ (as adenosylcobalamin with methylcobalamin):** 3 dropperfuls twice a day
- **Vitamin C (as Micro-C or comparable buffered vitamin C):** 8 500-milligram capsules twice a day
- **Vitamin D$_3$:** 1,000 to 5,000 IU daily
- **Wild blueberry:** 1 tablespoon powder or 2 ounces juice daily
- **Zinc (as liquid zinc sulfate):** 2 dropperfuls twice a day

ALZHEIMER'S DISEASE

Before applying these, be sure to read Chapter 2, "Golden Rules of Supplements."

- **Fresh celery juice:** work up to 32 ounces daily
- **Freshly squeezed orange juice:** 16 ounces daily
- **Heavy Metal Detox Smoothie:** 1 serving daily (see Chapter 10)
- **Extractor Smoothie:** 1 serving daily (see Chapter 10)

- **Burnout Stabilizer:** 1 Brain Shot daily (see Chapter 8)
- **Mood Shifter:** 1 Brain Shot daily (see Chapter 8)
- **5-MTHF:** 1 capsule twice a day
- **Barley grass juice powder:** 1 tablespoon or 9 capsules daily
- **B-complex:** 1 capsule daily
- **Cat's claw:** 1 dropperful twice a day
- **Celeryforce:** 3 capsules three times a day
- **CoQ10:** 1 capsule twice a day
- **Curcumin:** 3 capsules twice a day
- **EPA and DHA (fish-free):** 2 capsules daily (taken with dinner)
- **GABA:** 1 250-milligram capsule twice a day
- **Glutathione:** 1 capsule daily
- **Lemon balm:** 3 dropperfuls twice a day
- **L-glutamine:** 2 capsules twice a day
- **L-lysine:** 1 500-milligram capsule twice a day
- **Magnesium glycinate:** 1 capsule twice a day
- **Melatonin:** 1 5-milligram capsule up to six times a day

- **Nettle leaf:** 3 dropperfuls twice a day
- **Spirulina:** 1 tablespoon or 9 capsules daily
- **Vitamin B$_{12}$ (as adenosylcobalamin with methylcobalamin):** 3 dropperfuls twice a day
- **Vitamin C (as Micro-C or comparable buffered vitamin C):** 2 500-milligram capsules twice a day
- **Wild blueberry:** 1 tablespoon powder or 2 ounces juice daily
- **Zinc (as liquid zinc sulfate):** 1 dropperful daily

AMNESIA

Refer to Concussion Recovery Side Effects protocol.

ANEMIA

Refer to Autoimmune Disorders and Diseases protocol.

ANEURYSM

Refer to Strokes protocol.

ANKYLOSING SPONDYLITIS

Refer to Autoimmune Disorders and Diseases protocol.

ANOREXIA

Refer to Eating Disorders protocol.

ANXIETY

Before applying these, be sure to read Chapter 2, "Golden Rules of Supplements."

- **Fresh celery juice:** work up to 32 ounces daily
- **Heavy Metal Detox Smoothie:** 1 serving daily (see Chapter 10)
- **Adrenal Fight or Flight Stabilizer:** 1 Brain Shot daily (see Chapter 8)
- **Nerve Shifter:** 1 Brain Shot daily (see Chapter 8)
- **Lemon Balm Shock Therapy:** if needed (see Chapter 3)
- **5-HTP:** 1 capsule at bedtime daily
- **5-MTHF:** 1 capsule daily
- **Aloe vera:** 2 or more inches of fresh gel (skin removed) daily
- **Ashwagandha:** 1 dropperful twice a day
- **Barley grass juice powder:** 2 teaspoons or 6 capsules daily

- **B-complex:** 1 capsule daily
- **Celeryforce:** 3 capsules three times a day
- **Curcumin:** 2 capsules daily
- **EPA and DHA (fish-free):** 1 capsule daily (taken with dinner)
- **GABA:** 1 250-milligram capsule daily
- **Ginger:** 2 cups of tea or freshly grated to taste daily
- **Hops:** 1 cup of tea daily
- **Lemon balm:** 4 dropperfuls four times a day
- **L-lysine:** 2 500-milligram capsules daily
- **Magnesium glycinate:** 3 capsules daily
- **Melatonin:** 1 5-milligram capsule at bedtime daily
- **Spirulina:** 2 teaspoons or 6 capsules daily
- **Vitamin B$_{12}$ (as adenosylcobalamin with methylcobalamin):** 3 dropperfuls twice a day
- **Vitamin C (as Micro-C or comparable buffered vitamin C):** 4 500-milligram capsules twice a day
- **Vitamin D$_3$:** 1,000 IU daily
- **Wild blueberry:** 2 teaspoons powder or 2 ounces juice daily

- **Zinc (as liquid zinc sulfate):** 1 dropperful daily

ANXIOUSNESS

Before applying these, be sure to read Chapter 2, "Golden Rules of Supplements."

- **Fresh celery juice:** work up to 32 ounces daily
- **Heavy Metal Detox Smoothie:** 1 serving daily (see Chapter 10)
- **Adrenal Fight or Flight Stabilizer:** 1 Brain Shot daily (see Chapter 8)
- **Nerve Shifter:** 1 Brain Shot daily (see Chapter 8)
- **Ashwagandha:** 1 dropperful daily
- **Barley grass juice powder:** 1 teaspoon or 3 capsules daily
- **B-complex:** 1 capsule daily
- **Celeryforce:** 2 capsules twice a day
- **Chaga mushroom powder:** 2 teaspoons or 6 capsules daily
- **Curcumin:** 1 capsule twice a day
- **EPA and DHA (fish-free):** 1 capsule daily (taken with dinner)
- **GABA:** 1 250-milligram capsule daily
- **Hibiscus:** 1 cup of tea twice a day

- **Lemon balm:** 3 dropperfuls twice a day
- **L-lysine:** 2 500-milligram capsules twice a day
- **Magnesium glycinate:** 1 capsule twice a day
- **Melatonin:** 1 5-milligram capsule at bedtime daily
- **Spirulina:** 1 teaspoon or 3 capsules daily
- **Vitamin B$_{12}$ (as adenosylcobalamin with methylcobalamin):** 2 dropperfuls twice a day
- **Vitamin C (as Micro-C or comparable buffered vitamin C):** 4 500-milligram capsules twice a day
- **Vitamin D$_3$:** 1,000 IU daily
- **Wild blueberry:** 2 teaspoons powder or 2 ounces juice daily
- **Zinc (as liquid zinc sulfate):** 1 dropperful daily

APHASIA

Refer to Encephalopathy protocol.

APRAXIA

Refer to Encephalopathy protocol.

ARRHYTHMIA

Refer to Cranial Nerve Inflammation protocol and/or Heart Palpitations (Non-neurological) protocol.

ARTERIOSCLEROSIS

Before applying these, be sure to read Chapter 2, "Golden Rules of Supplements."

- **Fresh celery juice:** work up to 32 ounces daily
- **Barley grass juice powder:** 1 teaspoon or 3 capsules daily
- **Chaga mushroom powder:** 1 teaspoon or 3 capsules daily
- **CoQ10:** 1 capsule twice a day
- **Curcumin:** 3 capsules twice a day
- **EPA and DHA (fish-free):** 1 capsule daily (taken with dinner)
- **Glutathione:** 2 capsules twice a day
- **Hawthorn berry:** 1 dropperful twice a day
- **Magnesium glycinate:** 3 capsules twice a day
- **Melatonin:** 1 5-milligram capsule at bedtime daily
- **Milk thistle:** 2 dropperfuls twice a day
- **Nettle leaf:** 2 dropperfuls twice a day

- **Spirulina:** 1 teaspoon or 3 capsules daily
- **Vitamin B$_{12}$ (as adenosylcobalamin with methylcobalamin):** 2 dropperfuls twice a day
- **Vitamin C (as Micro-C or comparable buffered vitamin C):** 8 500-milligram capsules twice a day
- **Wild blueberry:** 1 tablespoon powder or 2 to 4 ounces juice daily
- **Zinc (as liquid zinc sulfate):** 1 dropperful daily

ARTHRITIS (REACTIVE)

Refer to Autoimmune Disorders and Diseases protocol.

ARTHRITIS (RHEUMATOID)

Refer to Autoimmune Disorders and Diseases protocol.

ATHEROMA

Refer to Arteriosclerosis protocol.

ATHEROSCLEROSIS

Refer to Arteriosclerosis protocol.

ATRIAL FIBRILLATION (AFIB)

Refer to Cranial Nerve Inflammation protocol and/or Heart Palpitations (Non-neurological) protocol.

AUDITORY PROCESSING DISORDER (APD)

Before applying these, be sure to read Chapter 2, "Golden Rules of Supplements."

Remember that you can take these adult dosages to your pediatrician to see what dosages are right for your child. Also see Chapter 8, "Brain Shot Therapy," Chapter 10, "Heavy Metal Detox," and Chapter 2, "Golden Rules of Supplements," for adjusted amounts of celery juice, Heavy Metal Detox Smoothie, and Brain Shot Therapies for children.

- **Fresh celery juice:** work up to at least 16 ounces daily
- **Heavy Metal Detox Smoothie:** 1 serving daily (see Chapter 10)
- **Nerve Shifter:** 1 Brain Shot daily (see Chapter 8)
- **5-MTHF:** 1 capsule daily
- **Barley grass juice powder:** 1 teaspoon or 3 capsules daily
- **Celeryforce:** 1 capsule twice a day
- **Curcumin:** 1 capsule daily
- **EPA and DHA (fish-free):** 1 capsule daily (taken with dinner)

- **GABA:** 1 250-milligram capsule daily
- **Glutathione:** 1 capsule daily
- **Lemon balm:** 1 dropperful twice a day
- **Magnesium glycinate:** 1 capsule twice a day
- **Melatonin:** 1 5-milligram capsule at bedtime daily
- **Spirulina:** 1 teaspoon or 3 capsules daily
- **Vitamin B$_{12}$ (as adenosylcobalamin with methylcobalamin):** 1 dropperful twice a day
- **Vitamin C (as Micro-C or comparable buffered vitamin C):** 2 500-milligram capsules twice a day
- **Wild blueberry:** 2 teaspoons powder or 2 ounces juice daily
- **Zinc (as liquid zinc sulfate):** 1 dropperful daily

AUTISM

Refer to ADHD protocol.

AUTOIMMUNE DISORDERS AND DISEASES

Before applying these, be sure to read Chapter 2, "Golden Rules of Supplements."

If your individual autoimmune issue does not appear with its own supplement list in the coming pages, turn back to this list for support.

- **Fresh celery juice:** work up to 32 ounces daily; then you have the option to work up to 32 ounces twice a day
- **Heavy Metal Detox Smoothie:** 1 serving daily (see Chapter 10)
- **Pathogen Exposure:** 1 Brain Shot daily (see Chapter 8)
- **Any Shock Therapies from Chapter 3 can be used if needed, especially for flare-ups**
- **5-MTHF:** 1 capsule twice a day
- **ALA (alpha lipoic acid):** 1 500-milligram capsule twice a week
- **Aloe vera:** 2 or more inches of fresh gel (skin removed) daily
- **Barley grass juice powder:** 2 teaspoons or 6 capsules twice a day
- **Cat's claw:** 2 dropperfuls twice a day
- **Celeryforce:** 3 capsules twice a day
- **Chaga mushroom powder:** 2 teaspoons or 6 capsules twice a day
- **Curcumin:** 2 capsules twice a day

- **Glutathione:** 1 capsule daily
- **Goldenseal:** 2 dropperfuls twice a day (two weeks on, two weeks off)
- **Hibiscus:** 1 cup of tea daily
- **Lemon balm:** 2 dropperfuls twice a day
- **Licorice root:** 1 dropperful daily (two weeks on, two weeks off)
- **L-lysine:** 4 500-milligram capsules twice a day
- **Lomatium root:** 1 dropperful daily
- **MSM:** 1 capsule twice a day
- **Mullein leaf:** 2 dropperfuls twice a day
- **Nascent iodine:** 3 small drops (not dropperfuls) twice a day
- **Nettle leaf:** 2 dropperfuls twice a day
- **Oregon grape root:** 1 dropperful twice a day (two weeks on, two weeks off)
- **Propolis:** 2 dropperfuls twice a day
- **Raw honey:** 1 to 3 teaspoons daily
- **Selenium:** 1 capsule daily
- **Spirulina:** 2 teaspoons or 6 capsules daily
- **Thyme:** 2 sprigs of fresh thyme in hot water as tea or 4 sprigs in room temperature water daily

- **Turmeric:** 1 capsule twice a day
- **Vitamin B$_{12}$ (as adenosylcobalamin with methylcobalamin):** 2 dropperfuls twice a day
- **Vitamin C (as Micro-C or comparable buffered vitamin C):** 6 500-milligram capsules twice a day
- **Wild blueberry:** 1 tablespoon powder or 2 ounces juice daily
- **Zinc (as liquid zinc sulfate):** up to 2 dropperfuls twice a day

AVOIDANT RESTRICTIVE FOOD INTAKE DISORDER (ARFID)

Refer to Eating Disorders protocol.

AYAHUASCA RECOVERY

Refer to Addiction protocol.

BALANCE ISSUES

Refer to Vertigo protocol.

BALO DISEASE

Refer to Multiple Sclerosis protocol.

BELL'S PALSY

Refer to Shingles protocol.

BINGE EATING DISORDER

Refer to Eating Disorders protocol and/or Mystery Hunger protocol.

BIPOLAR DISORDER

Before applying these, be sure to read Chapter 2, "Golden Rules of Supplements."

- **Fresh celery juice:** work up to 32 ounces daily

- **Fresh cucumber juice:** work up to 16 ounces daily

- **Heavy Metal Detox Smoothie:** 1 serving daily (see Chapter 10)

- **Mood Shifter:** 1 Brain Shot daily (see Chapter 8)

- **Adrenal Fight or Flight Stabilizer:** 1 Brain Shot daily (see Chapter 8)

- **Lemon Balm Shock Therapy:** if needed (see Chapter 3)

- **California Poppy Shock Therapy:** if needed for mania episode (see Chapter 3)

- **5-HTP:** 1 capsule at bedtime daily

- **5-MTHF:** 1 capsule daily

- **Ashwagandha:** 1 dropperful daily

- **Barley grass juice powder:** 1 teaspoon or 3 capsules daily

- **B-complex:** 1 capsule daily

- **Celeryforce:** 2 capsules twice a day

- **Curcumin:** 1 capsule twice a day

- **GABA:** 1 250-milligram capsule twice a day

- **Glutathione:** 1 capsule daily

- **Lemon balm:** 4 dropperfuls twice a day

- **Magnesium glycinate:** 2 capsules twice a day

- **Melatonin:** 1 5-milligram capsule at bedtime daily

- **Spirulina:** 1 teaspoon or 3 capsules daily

- **Vitamin B$_{12}$ (as adenosylcobalamin with methylcobalamin):** 2 dropperfuls twice a day

- **Vitamin C (as Micro-C or comparable buffered vitamin C):** 4 500-milligram capsules twice a day

- **Vitamin D$_3$:** 1,000 IU daily

- **Wild blueberry:** 2 teaspoons powder or 2 ounces juice daily

- **Zinc (as liquid zinc sulfate):** 1 dropperful daily

BLOATING (SEVERE)

Refer to Stomach Problems protocol.

BLOOD CLOTS

Before applying these, be sure to read Chapter 2, "Golden Rules of Supplements."

- **Fresh celery juice:** work up to 32 ounces daily

- **Fresh cucumber juice:** work up to 32 ounces daily

- **Lower fats in diet by eating Brain Saver Recipes**

- **Pharmaceutical Exposure:** 1 Brain Shot daily (see Chapter 8)

- **Thyme Tea Shock Therapy:** if needed (see Chapter 3)

- **CoQ10:** 1 capsule twice a day

- **Curcumin:** 2 capsules twice a day

- **EPA and DHA (fish-free):** 1 capsule daily (taken with dinner)

- **Glutathione:** 1 capsule daily

- **Goldenseal:** 2 dropperfuls twice a day (2 weeks on, two weeks off)

- **Hawthorn berry:** 1 dropperful daily

- **Magnesium glycinate:** 2 capsules twice a day

- **Milk thistle:** 1 dropperful twice a day

- **Thyme:** 2 sprigs of fresh thyme in hot water as tea or 4 sprigs in room temperature water twice a day

- **Vitamin B$_{12}$ (as adenosylcobalamin with methylcobalamin):** 2 dropperfuls twice a day

- **Vitamin C (as Micro-C or comparable buffered vitamin C):** 4 500-milligram capsules twice a day

BLOOD DRAW (FOR ONE WEEK DIRECTLY BEFORE)

This protocol shows options to strengthen your blood and prepare your brain and body for the week leading up to getting blood drawn. If you're on higher dosages of any of these supplements due to another protocol you're following in this chapter, it's fine to stay with those higher dosages. If you're on additional supplements from a protocol in this chapter, it's also fine to stay on them.

Read more critical tips about blood draw in the chapter "Blood Draining Agenda" in this book's companion title, *Brain Saver*.

Before applying these, be sure to read Chapter 2, "Golden Rules of Supplements."

- **Fresh celery juice:** 16 to 32 ounces daily

- **Lemon or lime water:** 32 ounces twice a day

- **Coconut water:** 20 to 40 ounces daily (not pink or red)

- **Try to incorporate as many Brain Saver Recipes from Chapter 12 as desired throughout the week**

- **Magnesium glycinate:** 2 capsules daily

- **Vitamin B$_{12}$ (as adenosylcobalamin with methylcobalamin):** 2 dropperfuls daily

- **Vitamin C (as Micro-C or comparable buffered vitamin C):** 4 500-milligram capsules daily

- **Zinc (as liquid zinc sulfate):** 2 dropperfuls daily

BLOOD DRAW (FOR ONE WEEK DIRECTLY FOLLOWING)

This protocol shows options to help rebuild your blood, lessen shock, and strengthen your immune system for the week directly following getting blood drawn. If you're on higher dosages of any of these supplements due to another protocol you're following in this chapter, it's fine to stay with those higher dosages. If you're on additional supplements from a protocol in this chapter, it's also fine to stay on them.

Read more critical tips about blood draw in the chapter "Blood Draining Agenda" in this book's companion title, *Brain Saver*.

Before applying these, be sure to read Chapter 2, "Golden Rules of Supplements."

- **Fresh celery juice:** 16 to 32 ounces daily

- **Fresh cucumber juice:** optional 16 to 32 ounces daily

- **Lemon or lime water:** 32 ounces twice a day

- **Coconut water:** 20 to 40 ounces daily (not pink or red)

- **Brain Builder:** optional 1 serving daily (see Chapter 12)

- **Brain Soother Juice:** optional 1 serving daily (see Chapter 12)

- **Melon:** half a melon such as honeydew or cantaloupe, or 2 to 3 cups watermelon, daily

- **Spinach Soup or Brain Saver Salad:** 1 serving daily (see Chapter 12)

- **Try to incorporate as many other Brain Saver Recipes from Chapter 12 as desired throughout the week**

- **Magnesium glycinate:** 2 capsules daily

- **Vitamin B$_{12}$ (as adenosylcobalamin with methylcobalamin):** 2 dropperfuls daily

- **Vitamin C (as Micro-C or comparable buffered vitamin C):** 4 500-milligram capsules daily

- Zinc (as liquid zinc sulfate): 2 dropperfuls daily

BLURRED VISION

Refer to Cranial Nerve Inflammation protocol.

BODY BUZZING AND HUMMING

Refer to Cranial Nerve Inflammation protocol.

BODY DYSMORPHIC DISORDER (BDD)

Refer to Obsessive-Compulsive Disorder (OCD) protocol and/or Eating Disorders protocol.

BRAIN ABSCESS

Before applying these, be sure to read Chapter 2, "Golden Rules of Supplements."

- Fresh celery juice: work up to 32 ounces daily; then you have the option to work up to 32 ounces twice a day
- Pathogen Exposure: 1 Brain Shot daily (see Chapter 8)
- Radiation Exposure: 1 Brain Shot daily (see Chapter 8)
- Goldenseal Shock Therapy: if needed (see Chapter 3)
- Zinc Shock Therapy: if needed (see Chapter 3)
- Vitamin C Shock Therapy: if needed (see Chapter 3)
- Barley grass juice powder: 2 teaspoons or 6 capsules daily
- Cat's claw: 2 dropperfuls twice a day
- Curcumin: 2 capsules twice a day
- Goldenseal: 3 dropperfuls twice a day (two weeks on, two weeks off)
- Lemon balm: 4 dropperfuls twice a day
- Mullein leaf: 3 dropperfuls twice a day
- Olive leaf: 2 dropperfuls twice a day
- Oregon grape root: 2 dropperfuls twice a day (two weeks on, two weeks off)
- Propolis: 2 dropperfuls twice a day
- Raw honey: 1 tablespoon daily
- Spirulina: 2 teaspoons or 6 capsules daily
- Vitamin B$_{12}$ (as adenosylcobalamin with methylcobalamin): 1 dropperful twice a day
- Vitamin C (as Micro-C or comparable buffered vitamin

C): 6 500-milligram capsules twice a day

- **Wild blueberry:** 2 tablespoons powder or 4 ounces juice daily
- **Zinc (as liquid zinc sulfate):** up to 2 dropperfuls twice a day

BRAIN AGING

Refer to Everyday Brain and Health Maintenance protocol.

BRAIN CANCER

Refer to Brain Tumors and Cysts protocol.

BRAIN FOG

Before applying these, be sure to read Chapter 2, "Golden Rules of Supplements."

- **Fresh celery juice:** work up to 32 ounces every morning
- **Fresh cucumber juice:** work up to 32 ounces daily
- **Freshly squeezed orange juice:** 16 to 32 ounces daily
- **Heavy Metal Detox Smoothie:** 1 serving daily (see Chapter 10)
- **Extractor Smoothie:** 1 serving daily (see Chapter 10)
- **Nerve Shifter:** 1 Brain Shot daily (see Chapter 8)

- **Burnout Stabilizer:** 1 Brain Shot daily (see Chapter 8)
- **5-MTHF:** 1 capsule twice a day
- **Ashwagandha:** 1 dropperful twice a day
- **Barley grass juice powder:** 1 teaspoon or 3 capsules twice a day
- **B-complex:** 1 capsule daily
- **Cat's claw:** 1 dropperful twice a day
- **Celeryforce:** 3 capsules three times a day
- **Chaga mushroom powder:** 1 teaspoon or 3 capsules twice a day
- **Dulse liquid:** 1 dropperful daily
- **Lemon balm:** 1 dropperful twice a day
- **Licorice root:** 1 dropperful daily (two weeks on, two weeks off)
- **L-lysine:** 2 500-milligram capsules twice a day
- **Nettle leaf:** 1 dropperful twice a day
- **Spirulina:** 1 teaspoon or 3 capsules twice a day
- **Vitamin B$_{12}$ (as adenosylcobalamin with methylcobalamin):** 1 dropperful twice a day
- **Vitamin C (as Micro-C or comparable buffered vitamin

C): 2 500-milligram capsules twice a day

- Wild blueberry: 1 tablespoon powder or 2 ounces juice daily
- Zinc (as liquid zinc sulfate): up to 1 dropperful twice a day

BRAIN INFLAMMATION

Before applying these, be sure to read Chapter 2, "Golden Rules of Supplements."

- Fresh celery juice: work up to 32 ounces daily; then you have the option to work up to 32 ounces twice a day
- Fresh cucumber juice: work up to 32 ounces daily
- Heavy Metal Detox Smoothie: 1 serving daily (see Chapter 10)
- Pathogen Exposure: 1 Brain Shot daily (see Chapter 8)
- Nerve Shifter: 1 Brain Shot daily (see Chapter 8)
- Radiation Exposure: 1 Brain Shot daily (see Chapter 8)
- Pharmaceutical Exposure: 1 Brain Shot daily (see Chapter 8)
- Goldenseal Shock Therapy: if needed (see Chapter 3)
- Zinc Shock Therapy: if needed (see Chapter 3)
- Vitamin C Shock Therapy: if needed (see Chapter 3)

- Thyme Tea Shock Therapy: if needed (see Chapter 3)
- 5-MTHF: 1 capsule daily
- Aloe vera: 2 or more inches of fresh gel (skin removed) daily
- Barley grass juice powder: 1 teaspoon or 3 capsules daily
- Cat's claw: 4 dropperfuls twice a day
- Celeryforce: 2 capsules twice a day
- Curcumin: 3 capsules twice a day
- Goldenseal: 4 dropperfuls twice a day (three weeks on, one week off)
- Lemon balm: 3 dropperfuls twice a day
- Licorice root: 2 dropperfuls twice a day (three weeks on, one week off)
- L-lysine: 4 500-milligram capsules twice a day
- Magnesium glycinate: 2 capsules twice a day
- Mullein leaf: 4 dropperfuls twice a day
- Nascent iodine: 6 small drops (not dropperfuls) daily
- Nettle leaf: 2 dropperfuls twice a day
- Olive leaf: 2 dropperfuls twice a day

- **Propolis:** 3 dropperfuls twice a day

- **Spirulina:** 1 teaspoon or 3 capsules daily

- **Vitamin B$_{12}$ (as adenosylcobalamin with methylcobalamin):** 3 dropperfuls twice a day

- **Vitamin C (as Micro-C or comparable buffered vitamin C):** 8 500-milligram capsules twice a day

- **Wild blueberry:** 2 tablespoons powder or 4 ounces juice daily

- **Zinc (as liquid zinc sulfate):** 2 dropperfuls twice a day

BRAIN LESIONS

Before applying these, be sure to read Chapter 2, "Golden Rules of Supplements."

- **Fresh celery juice:** work up to 32 ounces daily

- **Heavy Metal Detox Smoothie:** 1 serving daily (see Chapter 10)

- **Extractor Smoothie:** 1 serving daily (see Chapter 10)

- **Pharmaceutical Exposure:** 1 Brain Shot daily (see Chapter 8)

- **Radiation Exposure:** 1 Brain Shot daily (see Chapter 8)

- **Burnout Stabilizer:** 1 Brain Shot daily (see Chapter 8)

- **5-MTHF:** 1 capsule daily

- **ALA (alpha lipoic acid):** 1 capsule daily

- **Aloe vera:** 2 or more inches of fresh gel (skin removed) daily

- **Barley grass juice powder:** 1 teaspoon or 3 capsules daily

- **B-complex:** 1 capsule daily

- **Cat's claw:** 3 dropperfuls twice a day

- **Celeryforce:** 2 capsules twice a day

- **Chaga mushroom powder:** 1 teaspoon or 3 capsules daily

- **Curcumin:** 3 capsules twice a day

- **Dandelion root:** 1 cup of tea twice a week

- **EPA and DHA (fish-free):** 1 capsule daily (taken with dinner)

- **GABA:** 1 250-milligram capsule daily

- **Glutathione:** 2 capsules twice a day

- **Goldenseal:** 1 dropperful twice a day (three weeks on, one week off)

- **Lemon balm:** 2 dropperfuls twice a day

- **L-glutamine:** 2 500-milligram capsules twice a day

- **Licorice root:** 1 dropperful twice a day (three weeks on, one week off)

- **L-lysine:** 2 500-milligram capsules twice a day
- **Magnesium glycinate:** 2 capsules twice a day
- **Melatonin:** work up to 20 milligrams at bedtime daily
- **MSM:** 1 capsule daily
- **Nettle leaf:** 2 dropperfuls twice a day
- **Propolis:** 2 dropperfuls twice a day
- **Raw honey:** 1 tablespoon daily
- **Selenium:** 1 capsule once a week
- **Silica:** 1 teaspoon daily
- **Spirulina:** 1 teaspoon or 3 capsules daily
- **Vitamin B$_{12}$ (as adenosylcobalamin with methylcobalamin):** 3 dropperfuls twice a day
- **Vitamin C (as Micro-C or comparable buffered vitamin C):** 8 500-milligram capsules twice a day
- **Wild blueberry:** 2 teaspoons powder or 2 ounces juice daily
- **Zinc (as liquid zinc sulfate):** 1 dropperful twice a day

BRAIN TUMORS AND CYSTS

Before applying these, be sure to read Chapter 2, "Golden Rules of Supplements."

- **Fresh celery juice:** work up to 32 ounces daily; then you have the option to work up to 32 ounces twice a day
- **Advanced Heavy Metal Detox Smoothie:** 1 serving daily (see Chapter 10)
- **Advanced Extractor Smoothie:** 1 serving daily (see Chapter 10)
- **Radiation Exposure:** 1 Brain Shot daily (see Chapter 8)
- **Pharmaceutical Exposure:** 1 Brain Shot daily (see Chapter 8)
- **California Poppy Shock Therapy:** if needed (see Chapter 3)
- **Lemon Balm Shock Therapy:** if needed (see Chapter 3)
- **Aloe Vera Shock Therapy:** if needed (see Chapter 3)
- **5-HTP:** 1 capsule at bedtime daily
- **ALA (alpha lipoic acid):** 1 capsule twice a day
- **Aloe vera:** 2 or more inches of fresh gel (skin removed) daily
- **Amla berry:** 2 teaspoons daily
- **Barley grass juice powder:** 1 teaspoon or 3 capsules daily

- **Burdock root:** 1 cup of tea or 1 root freshly juiced daily
- **California poppy:** 1 dropperful daily
- **Cat's claw:** 5 dropperfuls twice a day
- **Celeryforce:** 2 capsules twice a day
- **Chaga mushroom powder:** 1 teaspoon or 3 capsules daily
- **Chrysanthemum:** 1 cup of tea three times a week
- **Curcumin:** 3 capsules twice a day
- **Elderberry syrup:** 2 teaspoons daily
- **EPA and DHA (fish-free):** 1 capsule daily (taken with dinner)
- **GABA:** 1 250-milligram capsule daily
- **Glutathione:** 2 capsules twice a day
- **Lemon balm:** 4 dropperfuls twice a day
- **L-lysine:** 2 500-milligram capsules twice a day
- **Magnesium glycinate:** 2 capsules twice a day
- **Melatonin:** work up to 80 milligrams at bedtime daily
- **Nascent iodine:** 1 dropperful daily (one week on, one week off)

- **Nettle leaf:** 3 dropperfuls twice a day
- **Raspberry leaf:** 1 cup of tea with 2 tea bags daily
- **Raw honey:** 1 tablespoon daily
- **Reishi mushroom powder:** 1 teaspoon or 3 capsules daily
- **Spirulina:** 1 teaspoon or 3 capsules daily
- **Vitamin B$_{12}$ (as adenosylcobalamin with methylcobalamin):** 2 dropperfuls twice a day
- **Vitamin C (as Micro-C or comparable buffered vitamin C):** 8 500-milligram capsules 3 times a day
- **Wild blueberry:** 2 teaspoons powder or 2 ounces juice daily
- **Zinc (as liquid zinc sulfate):** 1 dropperful twice a day

BREAST IMPLANT ILLNESS

Before applying these, be sure to read Chapter 2, "Golden Rules of Supplements."

- **Fresh celery juice:** work up to 32 ounces daily
- **Heavy Metal Detox Smoothie:** 1 serving daily (see Chapter 10)
- **Pharmaceutical Exposure:** 1 Brain Shot daily (see Chapter 8)

- **Mold Exposure:** 1 Brain Shot daily (see Chapter 8)
- **Radiation Exposure:** 1 Brain Shot daily (see Chapter 8)
- **5-MTHF:** 1 capsule daily
- **Aloe vera:** 2 or more inches of fresh gel (skin removed) daily
- **Ashwagandha:** 1 dropperful twice a day
- **Barley grass juice powder:** 1 teaspoon or 3 capsules daily
- **Cat's claw:** 2 dropperfuls twice a day
- **Celeryforce:** 2 capsules twice a day
- **Dandelion root:** 1 cup of tea daily
- **Glutathione:** 2 capsules twice a day
- **Goldenseal:** 3 dropperfuls twice a day (three weeks on, one week off)
- **Lemon balm:** 2 dropperfuls twice a day
- **Licorice root:** 1 dropperful twice a day (two weeks on, two weeks off)
- **Magnesium glycinate:** 2 capsules twice a day
- **Nettle leaf:** 2 dropperfuls twice a day
- **Spirulina:** 1 teaspoon or 3 capsules daily

- **Vitamin B_{12} (as adenosylcobalamin with methylcobalamin):** 2 dropperfuls twice a day
- **Vitamin C (as Micro-C or comparable buffered vitamin C):** 6 500-milligram capsules twice a day
- **Zinc (as liquid zinc sulfate):** 2 dropperfuls twice a day

BULIMIA

Refer to Eating Disorders protocol.

BURNING HOT FEELING WITH NO FEVER

Refer to Shingles protocol and/or Herpes Simplex 1 and 2 protocol.

BURNING SENSATIONS INSIDE MOUTH

Refer to Shingles protocol and/or Herpes Simplex 1 and 2 protocol.

BURNING SENSATIONS ON SKIN

Refer to Shingles protocol and/or Herpes Simplex 1 and 2 protocol.

BURNOUT

Before applying these, be sure to read Chapter 2, "Golden Rules of Supplements."

- **Fresh celery juice:** work up to 32 ounces daily
- **Heavy Metal Detox Smoothie:** 1 serving daily (see Chapter 10)
- **Burnout Stabilizer:** 1 Brain Shot daily (see Chapter 8)
- **5-MTHF:** 1 capsule twice a day
- **Aloe vera:** 2 or more inches of fresh gel (skin removed) daily
- **Ashwagandha:** 3 dropperfuls twice a day
- **Barley grass juice powder:** 1 tablespoon or 9 capsules daily
- **B-complex:** 1 capsule daily
- **California poppy:** 1 dropperful twice a day
- **Cat's claw:** 1 dropperful daily
- **Celeryforce:** 4 capsules three times a day
- **Chaga mushroom powder:** 1 tablespoon or 9 capsules daily
- **CoQ10:** 1 capsule daily
- **Curcumin:** 2 capsules twice a day
- **EPA and DHA (fish-free):** 1 capsule daily (taken with dinner)
- **Goldenseal:** 1 dropperful daily (two weeks on, two weeks off)
- **Lemon balm:** 3 dropperfuls four times a day
- **Licorice root:** 1 dropperful daily (two weeks on, two weeks off)
- **L-lysine:** 4 500-milligram capsules twice a day
- **Magnesium glycinate:** 2 capsules twice a day
- **Melatonin:** 1 5-milligram capsule at bedtime daily
- **Nettle leaf:** 2 dropperfuls twice a day
- **Selenium:** 1 capsule once a week
- **Spirulina:** 2 teaspoons or 6 capsules daily
- **Vitamin B$_{12}$ (as adenosylcobalamin with methylcobalamin):** 4 dropperfuls twice a day
- **Vitamin C (as Micro-C or comparable buffered vitamin C):** 5 500-milligram capsules twice a day
- **Wild blueberry:** 2 tablespoons powder or 4 ounces juice daily
- **Zinc (as liquid zinc sulfate):** 2 dropperfuls twice a day

BURSITIS

Refer to Fibromyalgia protocol.

BUZZING IN EARS

Refer to Tinnitus protocol.

CAFFEINE WITHDRAWAL

Refer to Addiction protocol.

CALCIFICATIONS ON BRAIN

Refer to Brain Lesions protocol.

CANKER SORES

Before applying these, be sure to read Chapter 2, "Golden Rules of Supplements."

- **Fresh celery juice:** work up to 32 ounces daily
- **Propolis Shock Therapy and Propolis Mouth Sore Shock Therapy:** if needed (see Chapter 3)
- **Cat's claw:** 2 dropperfuls daily
- **Curcumin:** 2 capsules daily
- **Goldenseal:** 3 dropperfuls twice a day (two weeks on, two weeks off)
- **Lemon balm:** 3 dropperfuls twice a day
- **Licorice root:** 2 dropperfuls daily (two weeks on, two weeks off)
- **L-lysine:** 4 500-milligram capsules twice a day

- **Propolis:** 3 dropperfuls twice a day; also try to dry off the canker sore with a paper towel, and then dab straight propolis drops onto the sore periodically throughout the day
- **Raw honey:** 1 tablespoon daily
- **Spirulina:** 2 teaspoons or 6 capsules daily
- **Vitamin B$_{12}$ (as adenosylcobalamin with methylcobalamin):** 2 dropperfuls daily
- **Vitamin C (as Micro-C or comparable buffered vitamin C):** 6 500-milligram capsules twice a day
- **Zinc (as liquid zinc sulfate):** 2 dropperfuls daily

CARPAL TUNNEL SYNDROME

Refer to Fibromyalgia protocol.

CASTLEMAN DISEASE

Refer to Autoimmune Disorders and Diseases protocol.

CELIAC DISEASE

Refer to Autoimmune Disorders and Diseases protocol.

CEREBRAL ATROPHY

Before applying these, be sure to read Chapter 2, "Golden Rules of Supplements."

- **Fresh celery juice:** work up to 32 ounces daily
- **Heavy Metal Detox Smoothie:** 1 serving daily (see Chapter 10)
- **Radiation Exposure:** 1 Brain Shot daily (see Chapter 8)
- **Pharmaceutical Exposure:** 1 Brain Shot daily (see Chapter 8)
- **Nerve Shifter:** 1 Brain Shot daily (see Chapter 8)
- **Burnout Stabilizer:** 1 Brain Shot daily (see Chapter 8)
- **5-HTP:** 1 capsule at bedtime daily
- **Barley grass juice powder:** 1 teaspoon or 3 capsules daily
- **B-complex:** 1 capsule daily
- **Celeryforce:** 3 capsules twice a day
- **EPA and DHA (fish-free):** 1 capsule daily (taken with dinner)
- **GABA:** 2 250-milligram capsules twice a day
- **Glutathione:** 1 capsule twice a day
- **L-glutamine:** 2 500-milligram capsules twice a day
- **Magnesium glycinate:** 2 capsules twice a day
- **Melatonin:** work up to 40 milligrams at bedtime daily
- **Nettle leaf:** 2 dropperfuls twice a day
- **Raw honey:** 1 tablespoon daily
- **Silica:** 1 teaspoon daily
- **Spirulina:** 1 teaspoon or 3 capsules daily
- **Vitamin B$_{12}$ (as adenosylcobalamin with methylcobalamin):** 2 dropperfuls twice a day
- **Vitamin C (as Micro-C or comparable buffered vitamin C):** 8 500-milligram capsules twice a day
- **Vitamin D$_3$:** 1,000 IU daily
- **Wild blueberry:** 2 tablespoons powder or 4 ounces juice daily
- **Zinc (as liquid zinc sulfate):** 1 dropperful daily

CEREBRAL HYPOXIA

Before applying these, be sure to read Chapter 2, "Golden Rules of Supplements."

- **Fresh celery juice:** work up to 32 ounces daily
- **Heavy Metal Detox Smoothie:** 1 serving daily (see Chapter 10)
- **Barley grass juice powder:** 1 teaspoon or 3 capsules daily

- **Celeryforce:** 4 capsules twice a day
- **GABA:** 1 250-milligram capsule twice a day
- **Lemon balm:** 4 dropperfuls twice a day
- **Magnesium glycinate:** 4 capsules twice a day
- **Raspberry leaf:** 1 cup of tea with 2 tea bags twice a day
- **Raw honey:** 1 tablespoon daily
- **Spirulina:** 1 teaspoon or 3 capsules daily
- **Vitamin B$_{12}$ (as adenosylcobalamin with methylcobalamin):** 3 dropperfuls twice a day
- **Vitamin C (as Micro-C or comparable buffered vitamin C):** 8 500-milligram capsules twice a day
- **Wild blueberry:** 2 tablespoons powder or 4 ounces juice

CEREBRAL PALSY

Before applying these, be sure to read Chapter 2, "Golden Rules of Supplements."

- **Fresh celery juice:** work up to 32 ounces daily
- **Heavy Metal Detox Smoothie:** 1 serving daily (see Chapter 10)
- **Extractor Smoothie:** 1 serving daily (see Chapter 10)
- **Pharmaceutical Exposure:** 1 Brain Shot daily (see Chapter 8)
- **Barley grass juice powder:** 1 teaspoon or 3 capsules daily
- **Celeryforce:** 3 capsules twice a day
- **Glutathione:** 1 capsule twice a day
- **Lemon balm:** 3 dropperfuls twice a day
- **Magnesium glycinate:** 3 capsules twice a day
- **Raw honey:** 1 tablespoon daily
- **Skullcap:** 1 dropperful twice a day
- **Spirulina:** 1 teaspoon or 3 capsules daily
- **Vitamin B$_{12}$ (as adenosylcobalamin with methylcobalamin):** 2 dropperfuls twice a day
- **Vitamin C (as Micro-C or comparable buffered vitamin C):** 6 500-milligram capsules twice a day
- **Wild blueberry:** 1 tablespoon powder or 2 ounces juice daily

CEREBROVASCULAR DISEASE

Before applying these, be sure to read Chapter 2, "Golden Rules of Supplements."

- **Fresh celery juice:** work up to 32 ounces daily
- **Heavy Metal Detox Smoothie:** 1 serving daily (see Chapter 10)
- **Extractor Smoothie:** 1 serving daily (see Chapter 10)
- **Pharmaceutical Exposure:** 1 Brain Shot daily (see Chapter 8)
- **Barley grass juice powder:** 1 teaspoon or 3 capsules daily
- **Burdock root:** 1 cup of tea or 1 root freshly juiced daily
- **Celeryforce:** 2 capsules twice a day
- **Chaga mushroom powder:** 2 teaspoons or 6 capsules daily
- **CoQ10:** 1 capsule twice a day
- **Curcumin:** 3 capsules twice a day
- **EPA and DHA (fish-free):** 1 capsule daily (taken with dinner)
- **Hawthorn berry:** 2 dropperfuls twice a day
- **Magnesium glycinate:** 3 capsules twice a day
- **Milk thistle:** 2 dropperfuls twice a day
- **Nettle leaf:** 2 dropperfuls twice a day
- **Raw honey:** 1 tablespoon daily
- **Spirulina:** 1 teaspoon or 3 capsules daily
- **Vitamin B$_{12}$ (as adenosylcobalamin with methylcobalamin):** 2 dropperfuls twice a day
- **Vitamin C (as Micro-C or comparable buffered vitamin C):** 6 500-milligram capsules twice a day
- **Wild blueberry:** 2 teaspoons powder or 2 ounces juice daily
- **Zinc (as liquid zinc sulfate):** 1 dropperful daily

CHEMICAL AND FOOD SENSITIVITIES

Before applying these, be sure to read Chapter 2, "Golden Rules of Supplements."

Daily:

- **Fresh celery juice:** try to work up to 16 ounces daily
- **Fresh cucumber juice:** try to work up to 16 ounces daily
- **Nerve-Gut Acid Stabilizer:** 1 Brain Shot daily (see Chapter 8)
- **Aloe vera:** 2 or more inches of fresh gel (skin removed) daily
- **Celeryforce:** 1 capsule daily
- **Raw honey:** 1 teaspoon or more daily

Cycle through, with one per day:

- 5-MTHF: 1 capsule
- Barley grass juice powder: ½ teaspoon or 1 capsule
- Lemon balm: 1 dropperful
- L-lysine: 500 milligrams
- Peppermint: 1 cup of tea
- Vitamin B$_{12}$ (as adenosylcobalamin with methylcobalamin): 1 dropperful
- Vitamin C (as Micro-C or comparable buffered vitamin C): 2 500-milligram capsules
- Vitamin D$_3$: 1,000 IU

Additional options:

- Aloe Vera Shock Therapy: if needed (see Chapter 3)
- Mono Eating Cleanse: consider one of the options from *Cleanse to Heal*

CHEST TIGHTNESS (MYSTERY)

Refer to Vagus Nerve Problems protocol.

CHEWING DIFFICULTY

Refer to Shingles protocol and/or Herpes Simplex 1 and 2 protocol.

CHOCOLATE AND CACAO WITHDRAWAL

Refer to Addiction protocol.

CHRONIC ANGER DISORDER

Before applying these, be sure to read Chapter 2, "Golden Rules of Supplements."

- Fresh celery juice: work up to 32 ounces daily
- Fresh cucumber juice: work up to 32 ounces daily
- Heavy Metal Detox Smoothie: 1 serving daily (see Chapter 10)
- Anger Shifter: 1 Brain Shot daily (see Chapter 8)
- Mood Shifter: 1 Brain Shot daily (see Chapter 8)
- Negative Energy Exposure: 1 Brain Shot daily (see Chapter 8)
- Lemon Balm Shock Therapy: if needed (see Chapter 3)
- California Poppy Shock Therapy: if needed (see Chapter 3)
- 5-HTP: 1 capsule at bedtime daily
- Barley grass juice powder: 1 teaspoon or 3 capsules daily
- Celeryforce: 3 capsules twice a day
- GABA: 1 250-milligram capsule twice a day

- **Lemon balm:** 4 dropperfuls twice a day
- **Magnesium glycinate:** 3 capsules twice a day
- **Raw honey:** 2 tablespoons daily
- **Spirulina:** 1 teaspoon or 3 capsules daily
- **Vitamin B$_{12}$ (as adenosylcobalamin with methylcobalamin):** 2 dropperfuls twice a day
- **Wild blueberry:** 1 tablespoon powder or 2 ounces juice daily

CHRONIC FATIGUE IMMUNE DYSFUNCTION SYNDROME (CFIDS)

Refer to ME/CFS protocol.

CHRONIC FATIGUE SYNDROME (CFS)

Refer to ME/CFS protocol.

CHRONIC INFLAMMATORY DEMYELINATING POLYNEUROPATHY (CIDP)

Refer to Cranial Nerve Inflammation protocol.

CHRONIC MYSTERY GUILT

Before applying these, be sure to read Chapter 2, "Golden Rules of Supplements."

- **Fresh celery juice:** work up to 16 ounces daily
- **Mood Shifter:** 1 Brain Shot daily (see Chapter 8)
- **Guilt and Shame Shifter:** 1 Brain Shot daily (see Chapter 8)
- **Lemon Balm Shock Therapy:** if needed (see Chapter 3)
- **5-MTHF:** 1 capsule twice a day
- **Ashwagandha:** 1 dropperful twice a daily
- **Barley grass juice powder:** 2 teaspoons or 6 capsules daily
- **B-complex:** 1 capsule daily
- **Celeryforce:** 2 capsules three times a day
- **CoQ10:** 1 capsule daily
- **Curcumin:** 2 capsules daily
- **EPA and DHA (fish-free):** 1 capsule daily (taken with dinner)
- **GABA:** 1 250-milligram capsule twice a day
- **Ginger:** 1 cup of tea or freshly grated or juiced to taste daily
- **Hibiscus:** 3 cups of tea daily
- **Lemon balm:** 3 dropperfuls three times a day
- **Licorice root:** 1 dropperful daily (two weeks on, two weeks off)

- **Magnesium glycinate:** 2 capsules daily

- **Melatonin:** 1 5-milligram capsule at bedtime daily

- **Nascent iodine:** 3 small drops (not dropperfuls) daily

- **Rose hips:** 1 cup of tea daily

- **Spirulina:** 2 teaspoons or 6 capsules daily

- **Vitamin B$_{12}$ (as adenosylcobalamin with methylcobalamin):** 2 dropperfuls twice a day

- **Zinc (as liquid zinc sulfate):** 1 dropperful daily

COFFEE WITHDRAWAL

Refer to Addiction protocol.

COLD, FLU, AND COVID

Supplements for Cold, Flu, and COVID in Adults

Before applying these, be sure to read Chapter 2, "Golden Rules of Supplements."

- **Fresh celery juice:** work up to at least 16 ounces daily

- **Pathogen Exposure Shot:** 1 Brain Shot daily (see Chapter 8)

- **Zinc Shock Therapy:** if needed (see Chapter 3)

- **Vitamin C Shock Therapy:** if needed (see Chapter 3)

- **Lemon Balm Shock Therapy:** if needed (see Chapter 3)

- **Goldenseal Shock Therapy:** if needed (see Chapter 3)

- **Thyme Tea Shock Therapy:** if needed (see Chapter 3)

- **Propolis Shock Therapy:** if needed (see Chapter 3)

- **Aloe Vera Shock Therapy:** if needed (see Chapter 3)

- **B$_{12}$ Shock Therapy:** if needed (see Chapter 3)

- **Cat's claw:** 2 dropperfuls four times a day

- **Elderberry syrup:** 1 tablespoon four times a day

- **Eyebright:** 3 dropperfuls four times a day

- **Ginger:** 1 cup of tea or freshly grated in water twice a day

- **Goldenseal:** 6 dropperfuls four times a day

- **Lemon balm:** 4 dropperfuls four times a day

- **Lomatium root:** 3 dropperfuls four times a day

- **Mullein leaf:** 6 dropperfuls four times a day

- **Olive leaf:** 3 dropperfuls four times a day

- **Oregano oil:** 1 capsule twice a day

- **Osha:** 3 dropperfuls four times a day

- **Propolis:** 4 dropperfuls four times a day

- **Thyme:** 2 sprigs of fresh thyme in hot water as tea or 4 sprigs in room temperature water twice a day

- **Vitamin B$_{12}$ (as adenosylcobalamin with methylcobalamin):** 2 dropperfuls twice a day

- **Vitamin C (as Micro-C or comparable buffered vitamin C):** 6 500-milligram capsules three times a day

- **Zinc (as liquid zinc sulfate):** 2 dropperfuls three times a day

Supplements for Cold, Flu, and COVID in Children Ages 1 to 2

Before applying these, be sure to read Chapter 2, "Golden Rules of Supplements."

- **Fresh celery juice:** refer to the table in Chapter 2 for children's amounts

- **Zinc Shock Therapy:** if needed (see children's dosages in Chapter 3)

- **Vitamin C Shock Therapy:** if needed (see children's dosages in Chapter 3)

- **Lemon Balm Shock Therapy:** if needed (see children's dosages in Chapter 3)

- **Goldenseal Shock Therapy:** if needed (see children's dosages in Chapter 3)

- **Thyme Tea Shock Therapy:** if needed (see children's dosages in Chapter 3)

- **Propolis Shock Therapy:** if needed (see children's dosages in Chapter 3)

- **Aloe Vera Shock Therapy:** if needed (see children's dosages in Chapter 3)

- **B$_{12}$ Shock Therapy:** if needed (see children's dosages in Chapter 3)

- **Elderberry syrup:** 1 teaspoon three times a day

- **Goldenseal:** 4 tiny drops (not dropperfuls) four times a day

- **Lemon balm:** 6 tiny drops (not dropperfuls) four times a day

- **Lomatium root:** 3 tiny drops (not dropperfuls) four times a day

- **Mullein leaf:** 6 tiny drops (not dropperfuls) four times a day

- **Olive leaf:** 4 tiny drops (not dropperfuls) four times a day

- **Propolis:** 6 tiny drops (not dropperfuls) four times a day

- Vitamin B$_{12}$ (as adenosylcobalamin with methylcobalamin): 4 tiny drops (not dropperfuls) twice a day

- Vitamin C (as Micro-C or comparable buffered vitamin C): open 1 500-milligram capsule and mix half (250 milligrams) into juice or smoothie twice a day

- Zinc (as liquid zinc sulfate): 3 tiny drops (not dropperfuls) in juice or water twice a day

Supplements for Cold, Flu, and COVID in Children Ages 3 to 4

Before applying these, be sure to read Chapter 2, "Golden Rules of Supplements."

- Fresh celery juice: refer to table in Chapter 2 for children's amounts

- Zinc Shock Therapy: if needed (see children's dosages in Chapter 3)

- Vitamin C Shock Therapy: if needed (see children's dosages in Chapter 3)

- Lemon Balm Shock Therapy: if needed (see children's dosages in Chapter 3)

- Goldenseal Shock Therapy: if needed (see children's dosages in Chapter 3)

- Thyme Tea Shock Therapy: if needed (see children's dosages in Chapter 3)

- Propolis Shock Therapy: if needed (see children's dosages in Chapter 3)

- Aloe Vera Shock Therapy: if needed (see children's dosages in Chapter 3)

- B$_{12}$ Shock Therapy: if needed (see children's dosages in Chapter 3)

- Elderberry syrup: 2 teaspoons three times a day

- Eyebright: 10 tiny drops (not dropperfuls) four times a day

- Ginger: freshly grated to taste in juice daily

- Goldenseal: 6 tiny drops (not dropperfuls) four times a day

- Lemon balm: 6 tiny drops (not dropperfuls) four times a day

- Lomatium root: 3 tiny drops (not dropperfuls) four times a day

- Mullein leaf: 6 tiny drops (not dropperfuls) four times a day

- Olive leaf: 10 tiny drops (not dropperfuls) four times a day

- Propolis: 15 tiny drops (not dropperfuls) four times a day

- Vitamin B$_{12}$ (as adenosylcobalamin with

methylcobalamin): 4 tiny drops (not dropperfuls) twice a day

- **Vitamin C (as Micro-C or comparable buffered vitamin C):** open 1 500-milligram capsule and mix half (250 milligrams) into juice or smoothie three times a day

- **Zinc (as liquid zinc sulfate):** 4 tiny drops (not dropperfuls) in juice, water, or directly in mouth (with optional water or juice chaser) three times a day

Supplements for Cold, Flu, and COVID in Children Ages 5 to 8

Before applying these, be sure to read Chapter 2, "Golden Rules of Supplements."

- **Fresh celery juice:** refer to table in Chapter 2 for children's amounts

- **Zinc Shock Therapy:** if needed (see children's dosages in Chapter 3)

- **Vitamin C Shock Therapy:** if needed (see children's dosages in Chapter 3)

- **Lemon Balm Shock Therapy:** if needed (see children's dosages in Chapter 3)

- **Goldenseal Shock Therapy:** if needed (see children's dosages in Chapter 3)

- **Thyme Tea Shock Therapy:** if needed (see children's dosages in Chapter 3)

- **Propolis Shock Therapy:** if needed (see children's dosages in Chapter 3)

- **Aloe Vera Shock Therapy:** if needed (see children's dosages in Chapter 3)

- **B$_{12}$ Shock Therapy:** if needed (see children's dosages in Chapter 3)

- **Elderberry syrup:** 1 tablespoon three times a day

- **Eyebright:** 1 dropperful three times a day

- **Ginger:** freshly grated to taste in juice daily

- **Goldenseal:** 1 dropperful four times a day

- **Lemon balm:** 1 dropperful four times a day

- **Lomatium root:** 1 dropperful three times a day

- **Mullein leaf:** 1 dropperful four times a day

- **Olive leaf:** 1 dropperful three times a day

- **Propolis:** 1 dropperful four times a day

- **Thyme Tea:** 2 ounces three times a day (use recipe in Chapter 12)

- Vitamin B$_{12}$ (as adenosylcobalamin with methylcobalamin): 6 small drops (not dropperfuls) three times a day

- Vitamin C (as Micro-C or comparable buffered vitamin C): 1 500-milligram capsule three times a day (optional: open capsule and mix into juice or smoothie)

- Zinc (as liquid zinc sulfate): 6 small drops (not dropperfuls) in juice, water, or directly in mouth (with optional water or juice chaser) three times a day

Supplements for Cold, Flu, and COVID in Children Ages 9 to 12

Before applying these, be sure to read Chapter 2, "Golden Rules of Supplements."

- Fresh celery juice: refer to table in Chapter 2 for children's amounts

- Pathogen Exposure: 1 children's portion of Brain Shot daily (see Chapter 8)

- Zinc Shock Therapy: if needed (see children's dosages in Chapter 3)

- Vitamin C Shock Therapy: if needed (see children's dosages in Chapter 3)

- Lemon Balm Shock Therapy: if needed (see children's dosages in Chapter 3)

- Goldenseal Shock Therapy: if needed (see children's dosages in Chapter 3)

- Thyme Tea Shock Therapy: if needed (see children's dosages in Chapter 3)

- Propolis Shock Therapy: if needed (see children's dosages in Chapter 3)

- Aloe Vera Shock Therapy: if needed (see children's dosages in Chapter 3)

- B$_{12}$ Shock Therapy: if needed (see children's dosages in Chapter 3)

- Elderberry syrup: 1 tablespoon four times a day

- Eyebright: 1 dropperful three times a day

- Ginger: freshly grated to taste in juice daily

- Goldenseal: 2 dropperfuls four times a day

- Lemon balm: 2 dropperfuls four times a day

- Lomatium root: 1 dropperful four times a day

- Mullein leaf: 2 dropperfuls four times a day

- Olive leaf: 1 dropperful three times a day

- **Osha:** 2 dropperfuls three times a day

- **Propolis:** 2 dropperfuls four times a day

- **Thyme Tea:** 4 ounces three times a day (use recipe in Chapter 12)

- **Vitamin B$_{12}$ (as adenosylcobalamin with methylcobalamin):** 1 dropperful twice a day

- **Vitamin C (as Micro-C or comparable buffered vitamin C):** 2 500-milligram capsules three times a day (optional: open capsules and mix into juice or smoothie)

- **Zinc (as liquid zinc sulfate):** 10 small drops (not dropperfuls) in juice, water, or directly in mouth (with optional water or juice chaser) three times a day

Supplements for Cold, Flu, and COVID in Children Ages 13 and Up

Before applying these, be sure to read Chapter 2, "Golden Rules of Supplements."

- **Fresh celery juice:** refer to table in Chapter 2 for children's amounts

- **Pathogen Exposure:** 1 children's portion of Brain Shot daily (see Chapter 8)

- **Zinc Shock Therapy:** if needed (see children's dosages in Chapter 3)

- **Vitamin C Shock Therapy:** if needed (see children's dosages in Chapter 3)

- **Lemon Balm Shock Therapy:** if needed (see children's dosages in Chapter 3)

- **Goldenseal Shock Therapy:** if needed (see children's dosages in Chapter 3)

- **Thyme Tea Shock Therapy:** if needed (see children's dosages in Chapter 3)

- **Propolis Shock Therapy:** if needed (see children's dosages in Chapter 3)

- **Aloe Vera Shock Therapy:** if needed (see children's dosages in Chapter 3)

- **B$_{12}$ Shock Therapy:** if needed (see children's dosages in Chapter 3)

- **Elderberry syrup:** 1 to 2 tablespoons four times a day

- **Eyebright:** 3 dropperfuls three times a day

- **Ginger:** freshly grated to taste in juice daily

- **Goldenseal:** 3 dropperfuls four times a day

- **Lemon balm:** 3 dropperfuls four times a day

- **Lomatium root:** 3 dropperfuls four times a day
- **Mullein leaf:** 4 dropperfuls four times a day
- **Olive leaf:** 2 dropperfuls four times a day
- **Osha:** 3 dropperfuls three times a day
- **Propolis:** 3 dropperfuls four times a day
- **Thyme Tea:** 1 cup three times a day (use recipe in Chapter 12)
- **Vitamin B$_{12}$ (as adenosylcobalamin with methylcobalamin):** 1 dropperful twice a day
- **Vitamin C (as Micro-C or comparable buffered vitamin C):** 3 500-milligram capsules three times a day (optional: open capsules and mix into juice or smoothie)
- **Zinc (as liquid zinc sulfate):** 1 dropperful in juice, water, or directly in mouth (with optional water or juice chaser) twice a day

COLD HANDS AND FEET

Refer to Cold Sensitivity protocol.

COLD SENSITIVITY

Before applying these, be sure to read Chapter 2, "Golden Rules of Supplements."

- **Fresh celery juice:** work up to 32 ounces daily
- **Heavy Metal Detox Smoothie:** 1 serving daily (see Chapter 10)
- **Nerve Shifter:** 1 Brain Shot daily (see Chapter 8)
- **5-MTHF:** 1 capsule daily
- **Aloe vera:** 2 or more inches of fresh gel (skin removed) daily
- **Barley grass juice powder:** 1 teaspoon or 3 capsules daily
- **Cat's claw:** 1 dropperful twice a day
- **Celeryforce:** 2 capsules twice a day
- **Chaga mushroom powder:** 1 teaspoon or 3 capsules daily
- **Curcumin:** 3 capsules twice a day
- **Ginger:** 1 cup of tea or freshly grated or juiced to taste daily
- **Glutathione:** 1 capsule daily
- **Lemon balm:** 2 dropperfuls three times a day
- **L-lysine:** 2 500-milligram capsules twice a day
- **Magnesium glycinate:** 2 capsules twice a day

- **MSM:** 1 capsule daily
- **Mullein leaf:** 1 dropperful twice a day
- **Spirulina:** 1 teaspoon or 3 capsules daily
- **Vitamin B$_{12}$ (as adenosylcobalamin with methylcobalamin):** 2 dropperfuls twice a day
- **Vitamin C (as Micro-C or comparable buffered vitamin C):** 4 500-milligram capsules twice a day
- **Vitamin D$_3$:** 1,000 IU daily
- **Wild blueberry:** 2 teaspoons powder or 2 ounces juice daily
- **Zinc (as liquid zinc sulfate):** 1 dropperful twice a day

COLD SORES

Refer to Herpes Simplex 1 and 2 protocol.

CONCUSSION RECOVERY SIDE EFFECTS

Before applying these, be sure to read Chapter 2, "Golden Rules of Supplements."

- **Fresh celery juice:** work up to 32 ounces daily
- **Fresh cucumber juice:** work up to 32 ounces daily

- **Freshly squeezed orange juice:** 16 ounces daily
- **Heavy Metal Detox Smoothie:** 1 serving daily (see Chapter 10)
- **Spinach Soup:** 1 serving daily (see Chapter 12)
- **Vitamin C Shock Therapy:** every two weeks (see Chapter 3)
- **ALA (alpha lipoic acid):** 1 capsule daily
- **Barley grass juice powder:** 1 teaspoon or 3 capsules daily
- **California poppy:** 2 dropperfuls twice a day
- **Curcumin:** 3 capsules twice a day
- **Glutathione:** 1 capsule twice a day
- **Lemon balm:** 4 dropperfuls twice a day
- **Magnesium glycinate:** 3 capsules twice a day
- **Melatonin:** 2 5-milligram capsules at bedtime daily
- **Spirulina:** 1 teaspoon or 3 capsules daily
- **Vitamin B$_{12}$ (as adenosylcobalamin with methylcobalamin):** 4 dropperfuls twice a day
- **Vitamin C (as Micro-C or comparable buffered vitamin

C): 8 500-milligram capsules twice a day

- **Wild blueberry:** 2 tablespoons powder or 4 ounces juice daily
- **Zinc (as liquid zinc sulfate):** 1 dropperful daily

CONNECTIVE TISSUE DISEASE

Refer to Autoimmune Disorders and Diseases protocol.

COVID

Refer to Cold, Flu, and COVID protocol. For long-haul COVID, refer to Mononucleosis protocol and/or Autoimmune Disorders and Diseases protocol.

CRANIAL NERVE ATROPHY

Before applying these, be sure to read Chapter 2, "Golden Rules of Supplements."

- **Fresh celery juice:** work up to 32 ounces daily
- **Heavy Metal Detox Smoothie:** 1 serving daily (see Chapter 10)
- **Nerve Shifter:** 1 Brain Shot daily (see Chapter 8)
- **Pharmaceutical Exposure:** 1 Brain Shot daily (see Chapter 8)
- **Radiation Exposure:** 1 Brain Shot daily (see Chapter 8)

- **5-MTHF:** 1 capsule daily
- **Aloe vera:** 2 or more inches of fresh gel (skin removed) daily
- **Amla berry:** 1 teaspoon daily
- **Barley grass juice powder:** 2 teaspoons or 6 capsules daily
- **Burdock root:** 1 cup of tea or 1 root freshly juiced daily
- **Cat's claw:** 3 dropperfuls twice a day
- **Celeryforce:** 2 capsules twice a day
- **Chaga mushroom powder:** 2 teaspoons or 6 capsules daily
- **Curcumin:** 3 capsules twice a day
- **EPA and DHA (fish-free):** 1 capsule daily (taken with dinner)
- **Glutathione:** 1 capsule daily
- **Lemon balm:** 4 dropperfuls twice a day
- **Licorice root:** 1 dropperful twice a day (two weeks on, two weeks off)
- **L-lysine:** 6 500-milligram capsules twice a day
- **Lomatium root:** 2 dropperfuls twice a day
- **Monolaurin:** 2 capsules daily
- **MSM:** 1 capsule daily
- **Mullein leaf:** 3 dropperfuls twice a day

- **Olive leaf:** 2 dropperfuls twice a day
- **Oregano oil:** 2 capsules daily
- **Rose hips:** 1 cup of tea daily
- **Spirulina:** 2 teaspoons or 6 capsules daily
- **Vitamin B$_{12}$ (as adenosylcobalamin with methylcobalamin):** 2 dropperfuls twice a day
- **Vitamin C (as Micro-C or comparable buffered vitamin C):** 6 500-milligram capsules twice a day
- **Wild blueberry:** 1 tablespoon powder or 2 ounces juice daily
- **Zinc (as liquid zinc sulfate):** 1 dropperful twice a day

CRANIAL NERVE INFLAMMATION

Before applying these, be sure to read Chapter 2, "Golden Rules of Supplements."

- **Fresh celery juice:** work up to 32 ounces daily; then you have the option to work up to 32 ounces twice a day
- **Heavy Metal Detox Smoothie:** 1 serving daily (see Chapter 10)
- **Extractor Smoothie:** 1 serving daily (see Chapter 10)
- **Nerve Shifter:** 1 Brain Shot daily (see Chapter 8)

- **Toxic Fragrances Exposure:** 1 Brain Shot daily (see Chapter 8)
- **Radiation Exposure:** 1 Brain Shot daily (see Chapter 8)
- **Pharmaceutical Exposure:** 1 Brain Shot daily (see Chapter 8)
- **Any Shock Therapies from Chapter 3 can be used if needed**
- **5-MTHF:** 1 capsule twice a day
- **Aloe vera:** 2 or more inches of fresh gel (skin removed) daily
- **Barley grass juice powder:** 2 teaspoons or 6 capsules daily
- **B-complex:** 1 capsule daily
- **Cat's claw:** 2 dropperfuls twice a day
- **Celeryforce:** 3 capsules twice a day
- **Chaga mushroom powder:** 2 teaspoons or 6 capsules daily
- **Curcumin:** 3 capsules twice a day
- **Elderberry syrup:** 1 teaspoon daily
- **EPA and DHA (fish-free):** 1 capsule daily (taken with dinner)
- **GABA:** 1 250-milligram capsule daily
- **Goldenseal:** 1 dropperful twice a day (two weeks on, two weeks off)

- **Lemon balm:** 4 dropperfuls twice a day

- **Licorice root:** 1 dropperful twice a day (two weeks on, two weeks off)

- **L-lysine:** 5 500-milligram capsules twice a day

- **Lomatium root:** 1 dropperful twice a day

- **Magnesium glycinate:** 1 capsule twice a day

- **Melatonin:** 1 5-milligram capsule at bedtime daily

- **Mullein leaf:** 3 dropperfuls twice a day

- **Nettle leaf:** 4 dropperfuls twice a day

- **Olive leaf:** 1 dropperful twice a day

- **Oregano oil:** 1 capsule daily

- **Propolis:** 2 dropperfuls twice a day

- **Spirulina:** 2 teaspoons or 6 capsules daily

- **Vitamin B$_{12}$ (as adenosylcobalamin with methylcobalamin):** 2 dropperfuls twice a day

- **Vitamin C (as Micro-C or comparable buffered vitamin C):** 6 to 8 500-milligram capsules twice a day

- **Vitamin D$_3$:** 1,000 IU twice a week

- **Wild blueberry:** 1 tablespoon powder or 2 ounces juice daily

- **Zinc (as liquid zinc sulfate):** 1 dropperful twice a day

CROHN'S DISEASE

Refer to Stomach Problems protocol.

CROOKED JAW FEELING

Refer to Shingles protocol and/or Herpes Simplex 1 and 2 protocol.

CUSHING'S SYNDROME (HYPERCORTISOLISM)

Before applying these, be sure to read Chapter 2, "Golden Rules of Supplements."

- **Fresh celery juice:** work up to 32 ounces daily

- **Heavy Metal Detox Smoothie:** 1 serving daily (see Chapter 10)

- **Nerve-Gut Acid Stabilizer:** 1 Brain Shot daily (see Chapter 8)

- **Energy Shifter:** 1 Brain Shot daily (see Chapter 8)

- **5-MTHF:** 1 capsule twice a day

- **Aloe vera:** 2 or more inches of fresh gel (skin removed) daily

- **Ashwagandha:** 1 dropperful daily

- **Barley grass juice powder:** 1 teaspoon or 3 capsules daily
- **Chaga mushroom powder:** 2 teaspoons or 6 capsules daily
- **Ginger:** 1 cup of tea or freshly grated or juiced to taste daily
- **Glutathione:** 1 capsule twice a day
- **Magnesium glycinate:** 2 capsules twice a day
- **Milk thistle:** 2 dropperfuls twice a day
- **Raspberry leaf:** 1 cup of tea with 2 tea bags daily
- **Spirulina:** 1 teaspoon or 3 capsules daily
- **Vitamin B$_{12}$ (as adenosylcobalamin with methylcobalamin):** 2 dropperfuls twice a day
- **Vitamin C (as Micro-C or comparable buffered vitamin C):** 6 500-milligram capsules twice a day
- **Wild blueberry:** 1 tablespoon powder or 2 ounces juice daily
- **Zinc (as liquid zinc sulfate):** 1 dropperful twice a day

CYCLOTHYMIC DISORDER

Refer to Bipolar Disorder protocol.

CYSTIC FIBROSIS

Refer to Autoimmune Disorders and Diseases protocol.

DARK SPOTS ON BRAIN

Refer to Brain Lesions protocol.

DARK TONGUE DISCOLORATION

Refer to Brain Fog protocol.

DEMENTIA

Refer to Alzheimer's Disease protocol.

DEPERSONALIZATION

Before applying these, be sure to read Chapter 2, "Golden Rules of Supplements."

- **Fresh celery juice:** work up to 32 ounces daily
- **Heavy Metal Detox Smoothie:** 1 serving daily (see Chapter 10)
- **Mood Shifter:** 1 Brain Shot daily (see Chapter 8)
- **5-HTP:** 1 capsule at bedtime daily
- **Ashwagandha:** 1 dropperful twice a day
- **Barley grass juice powder:** 1 teaspoon or 3 capsules daily

- California poppy: 1 dropperful twice a day
- Celeryforce: 2 capsules twice a day
- GABA: 1 250-milligram capsule daily
- Glutathione: 1 capsule twice a day
- Lemon balm: 2 dropperfuls twice a day
- L-glutamine: 1 500-milligram capsule twice a day
- Magnesium glycinate: 2 capsules twice a day
- Melatonin: 1 5-milligram capsule at bedtime daily
- Raw honey: 1 tablespoon daily
- Skullcap: 1 dropperful twice a day
- Spirulina: 1 teaspoon or 3 capsules daily
- Vitamin B$_{12}$ (as adenosylcobalamin with methylcobalamin): 2 dropperfuls twice a day
- Wild blueberry: 1 tablespoon powder or 2 ounces juice daily

DEPRESSION

Before applying these, be sure to read Chapter 2, "Golden Rules of Supplements."

- Fresh celery juice: work up to 32 ounces daily
- Heavy Metal Detox Smoothie: 1 serving daily (see Chapter 10)
- Extractor Smoothie: 1 serving daily (see Chapter 10)
- Mood Shifter: 1 Brain Shot daily (see Chapter 8)
- Burnout Stabilizer: 1 Brain Shot daily (see Chapter 8)
- Betrayal and Broken Trust Stabilizer: 1 Brain Shot daily (see Chapter 8)
- Lemon Balm Shock Therapy: if needed (see Chapter 3)
- 5-MTHF: 1 capsule daily
- Ashwagandha: 1 dropperful twice a day
- Barley grass juice powder: 2 teaspoons or 6 capsules daily
- B-complex: 1 capsule daily
- Celeryforce: 2 capsules three times a day
- Curcumin: 2 capsules daily
- EPA and DHA (fish-free): 1 capsule daily (taken with dinner)
- GABA: 1 250-milligram capsule daily
- Ginger: 1 cup of tea or freshly grated or juiced to taste daily
- Hibiscus: 1 cup of tea twice a day

- **Lemon balm:** 4 dropperfuls twice a day
- **Licorice root:** 1 dropperful daily (two weeks on, two weeks off)
- **L-lysine:** 2 500-milligram capsules daily
- **Magnesium glycinate:** 2 capsules daily
- **Melatonin:** 1 5-milligram capsule at bedtime daily
- **Nascent iodine:** 3 small drops (not dropperfuls) daily
- **Spirulina:** 2 teaspoons or 6 capsules daily
- **Vitamin B$_{12}$ (as adenosylcobalamin with methylcobalamin):** 2 dropperfuls twice a day
- **Vitamin C (as Micro-C or comparable buffered vitamin C):** 4 500-milligram capsules twice a day
- **Vitamin D$_3$:** 1,000 IU daily
- **Wild blueberry:** 2 teaspoons powder or 2 ounces juice daily
- **Zinc (as liquid zinc sulfate):** 1 dropperful daily

DERMATITIS HERPETIFORMIS (DH)

Refer to Autoimmune Disorders and Diseases protocol and/or Herpes Simplex 1 and 2 protocol.

DEVIC'S DISEASE

Refer to Cranial Nerve Inflammation protocol.

DIFFICULTY COPING

Before applying these, be sure to read Chapter 2, "Golden Rules of Supplements."

- **Fresh celery juice:** work up to 16 ounces daily
- **Heavy Metal Detox Smoothie:** 1 serving daily (see Chapter 10)
- **Energy Shifter:** 1 Brain Shot daily (see Chapter 8)
- **Burnout Stabilizer:** 1 Brain Shot daily (see Chapter 8)
- **Sleep and Recharging Stabilizer:** 1 Brain Shot daily (see Chapter 8)
- **Lemon Balm Shock Therapy:** if needed (see Chapter 3)
- **California Poppy Shock Therapy:** if needed (see Chapter 3)
- **California poppy:** 1 dropperful twice a day
- **Celeryforce:** 3 capsules twice a day
- **GABA:** 1 250-milligram capsule twice a day
- **Lemon balm:** 3 dropperfuls twice a day

- **Magnesium glycinate:** 2 capsules twice a day
- **Vitamin B$_{12}$ (as adenosylcobalamin with methylcobalamin):** 2 dropperfuls twice a day

DIZZINESS

Refer to Vertigo protocol.

DROOPING FACE

Refer to Shingles protocol and/or Herpes Simplex 1 and 2 protocol.

DYSAUTONOMIA

Before applying these, be sure to read Chapter 2, "Golden Rules of Supplements."

- **Fresh celery juice:** work up to 32 ounces daily
- **Heavy Metal Detox Smoothie:** 1 serving daily (see Chapter 10)
- **Extractor Smoothie:** 1 serving daily (see Chapter 10)
- **Nerve Shifter:** 1 Brain Shot daily (see Chapter 8)
- **Lemon Balm Shock Therapy:** if needed (see Chapter 3)
- **5-MTHF:** 1 capsule daily
- **Barley grass juice powder:** 1 teaspoon or 3 capsules daily
- **Cat's claw:** 3 dropperfuls twice a day
- **Celeryforce:** 2 capsules twice a day
- **Curcumin:** 2 capsules twice a day
- **Elderberry syrup:** 1 teaspoon daily
- **GABA:** 1 250-milligram capsule daily
- **Ginger:** 1 cup of tea or freshly grated or juiced to taste daily
- **Goldenseal:** 3 dropperfuls twice a day (two weeks on, two weeks off)
- **Lemon balm:** 3 dropperfuls twice a day
- **Licorice root:** 1 dropperful twice a day (two weeks on, two weeks off)
- **L-lysine:** 2 500-milligram capsules twice a day
- **Magnesium glycinate:** 2 capsules twice a day
- **Monolaurin:** 1 capsule daily
- **Mullein leaf:** 2 dropperfuls twice a day
- **Olive leaf:** 2 dropperfuls twice a day
- **Osha:** 1 dropperful daily
- **Propolis:** 2 dropperfuls twice a day

- **Spirulina:** 1 teaspoon or 3 capsules daily
- **Vitamin B$_{12}$ (as adenosylcobalamin with methylcobalamin):** 3 dropperfuls twice a day
- **Vitamin C (as Micro-C or comparable buffered vitamin C):** 6 500-milligram capsules twice a day
- **Wild blueberry:** 2 teaspoons powder or 2 ounces juice daily
- **Zinc (as liquid zinc sulfate):** 2 dropperfuls twice a day

DYSLEXIA

Before applying these, be sure to read Chapter 2, "Golden Rules of Supplements."

Remember that you can take these adult dosages to your pediatrician to see what dosages are right for your child. Also see Chapter 8, "Brain Shot Therapy," Chapter 10, "Heavy Metal Detox," and Chapter 2, "Golden Rules of Supplements," for adjusted amounts of celery juice, smoothie, and Brain Shot Therapies for children.

- **Fresh celery juice:** work up to 32 ounces daily
- **Heavy Metal Detox Smoothie:** 1 serving daily (see Chapter 10)
- **Extractor Smoothie:** 1 serving daily (see Chapter 10)

- **Pharmaceutical Exposure:** 1 Brain Shot daily (see Chapter 8)
- **5-MTHF:** 1 capsule daily
- **Barley grass juice powder:** 1 teaspoon or 3 capsules daily
- **Burdock root:** 1 cup of tea or 1 root freshly juiced daily
- **Celeryforce:** 2 capsules twice a day
- **L-glutamine:** 1 500-milligram capsule twice a day
- **Magnesium glycinate:** 1 capsule twice a day
- **Spirulina:** 1 teaspoon or 3 capsules daily
- **Vitamin B$_{12}$ (as adenosylcobalamin with methylcobalamin):** 1 dropperful twice a day
- **Wild blueberry:** 2 teaspoons powder or 2 ounces juice daily

DYSPHAGIA

Refer to Vagus Nerve Problems protocol and/or Cranial Nerve Inflammation protocol.

DYSPHORIA

Refer to Depression protocol.

EATING DISORDERS

Before applying these, be sure to read Chapter 2, "Golden Rules of Supplements."

- **Fresh celery juice:** work up to at least 16 ounces daily
- **Fresh cucumber juice:** work up to 16 ounces daily
- **Heavy Metal Detox Smoothie:** 1 serving daily (see Chapter 10)
- **Food Fear Shifter:** 1 Brain Shot daily (see Chapter 8)
- **Cravings Shifter:** 1 Brain Shot daily (see Chapter 8)
- **Trauma, Shock, and Loss Stabilizer:** 1 Brain Shot daily (see Chapter 8)
- **Lemon Balm Shock Therapy:** if needed (see Chapter 3)
- **Aloe Vera Shock Therapy:** if needed (see Chapter 3)
- **5-MTHF:** 1 capsule daily
- **Aloe vera:** 2 or more inches of fresh gel (skin removed) daily
- **Ashwagandha:** 1 dropperful daily (note: if purging is involved, 1 dropperful twice a day)
- **Barley grass juice powder:** 2 teaspoons or 6 capsules daily
- **Cat's claw:** 1 dropperful daily
- **Celeryforce:** 3 capsules twice a day
- **Curcumin:** 1 capsule twice a day
- **D-mannose:** 1 tablespoon in water daily
- **EPA and DHA (fish-free):** 2 capsules daily (taken with dinner)
- **GABA:** 1 250-milligram capsule daily
- **Lemon balm:** 4 dropperfuls twice a day
- **Licorice root:** 1 dropperful daily, or 2 dropperfuls daily if purging is involved (either way, two weeks on, two weeks off)
- **Magnesium glycinate:** 1 capsule twice a day
- **Nascent iodine:** 6 small drops (not dropperfuls) daily
- **Nettle leaf:** 2 dropperfuls daily
- **Raspberry leaf:** 1 cup of tea with 2 tea bags daily
- **Spirulina:** 1 teaspoon or 3 capsules daily
- **Vitamin B$_{12}$ (as adenosylcobalamin with methylcobalamin):** 1 dropperful twice a day
- **Zinc (as liquid zinc sulfate):** 1 dropperful daily

ECTOPIC HEARTBEAT

Refer to Cranial Nerve Inflammation protocol and/or Heart Palpitations (Non-neurological) protocol.

EHLERS-DANLOS SYNDROME

Refer to Autoimmune Disorders and Diseases protocol.

ELECTRIC SHOCK TO THE HEAD FEELING

Refer to Cranial Nerve Inflammation protocol.

ENCEPHALITIS

Refer to Brain Inflammation protocol.

ENCEPHALOPATHY

Before applying these, be sure to read Chapter 2, "Golden Rules of Supplements."

- **Fresh celery juice:** work up to 32 ounces daily; then you have the option to work up to 32 ounces twice a day

- **Heavy Metal Detox Smoothie:** 1 serving daily (see Chapter 10)

- **Pharmaceutical Exposure:** 1 Brain Shot daily (see Chapter 8)

- **Radiation Exposure:** 1 Brain Shot daily (see Chapter 8)

- **Nerve Shifter:** 1 Brain Shot daily (see Chapter 8)

- **5-MTHF:** 1 capsule twice a day

- **Barley grass juice powder:** 1 teaspoon or 3 capsules daily

- **B-complex:** 1 capsule daily

- **Cat's claw:** 3 dropperfuls twice a day

- **Celeryforce:** 3 capsules twice a day

- **CoQ10:** 1 capsule twice a day

- **Curcumin:** 3 capsules twice a day

- **EPA and DHA (fish-free):** 2 capsules daily (taken with dinner)

- **Glutathione:** 2 capsules twice a day

- **Hibiscus tea:** 1 cup daily

- **L-glutamine:** 2 500-milligram capsules twice a day

- **Magnesium glycinate:** 2 capsules twice a day

- **Melatonin:** work up to 80 milligrams at bedtime daily

- **Nettle leaf:** 3 dropperfuls twice a day

- **Raw honey:** 1 tablespoon daily

- **Spirulina:** 1 teaspoon or 3 capsules daily

- **Vitamin B$_{12}$ (as adenosylcobalamin with

methylcobalamin): 3 dropperfuls twice a day

- **Vitamin C (as Micro-C or comparable buffered vitamin C):** 8 500-milligram capsules twice a day
- **Vitamin D$_3$:** 1,000 IU daily
- **Wild blueberry:** 1 tablespoon powder or 2 ounces juice daily
- **Zinc (as liquid zinc sulfate):** 1 dropperful twice a day

ENERGY ISSUES

Refer to Fatigue protocol.

EPILEPSY

Refer to Seizures protocol.

EPSTEIN-BARR VIRUS (EBV) (EARLY STAGE)

Refer to Mononucleosis protocol.

EPSTEIN-BARR VIRUS (EBV) (LATE STAGE)

Refer to Autoimmune Disorders and Diseases protocol.

EPSTEIN-BARR VIRUS (EBV) (REACTIVATED)

Refer to Mononucleosis protocol.

EXCESSIVE SWEATING

Before applying these, be sure to read Chapter 2, "Golden Rules of Supplements."

- **Fresh celery juice:** work up to 32 ounces daily
- **Heavy Metal Detox Smoothie:** 1 serving daily (see Chapter 10)
- **Nerve Shifter:** 1 Brain Shot daily (see Chapter 8)
- **Adrenal Fight or Flight Stabilizer:** 1 Brain Shot daily (see Chapter 8)
- **Lemon Balm Shock Therapy:** if needed (see Chapter 3)
- **5-HTP:** 1 capsule at bedtime daily
- **Ashwagandha:** 2 dropperfuls twice a day
- **Barley grass juice powder:** 1 teaspoon or 3 capsules daily
- **California poppy:** 1 dropperful daily
- **Celeryforce:** 2 capsules twice a day
- **Elderflower:** 1 cup of tea daily
- **GABA:** 1 250-milligram capsule twice a day

- **Glutathione:** 1 capsule daily
- **L-glutamine:** 1 500-milligram capsule twice a day
- **Licorice root:** 1 dropperful twice a day (two weeks on, two weeks off)
- **Magnesium glycinate:** 3 capsules twice a day
- **Melatonin:** 1 5-milligram capsule at bedtime daily
- **Raw honey:** 1 tablespoon daily
- **Skullcap:** 2 dropperfuls twice a day
- **Spirulina:** 1 teaspoon or 3 capsules daily
- **Vitamin B$_{12}$ (as adenosylcobalamin with methylcobalamin):** 2 dropperfuls twice a day

EXTREME FATIGUE

Refer to ME/CFS protocol.

EYEBALL UNUSUAL MOVEMENT (INCLUDING DIFFICULTY WITH MUSCLES AROUND EYES)

Refer to Cranial Nerve Inflammation protocol.

EYE FLOATERS (VISUAL SNOW)

Before applying these, be sure to read Chapter 2, "Golden Rules of Supplements."

- **Fresh celery juice:** work up to 32 ounces daily
- **Heavy Metal Detox Smoothie:** 1 serving daily (see Chapter 10)
- **Nerve Shifter:** 1 Brain Shot daily (see Chapter 8)
- **5-MTHF:** 1 capsule daily
- **Barley grass juice powder:** 1 teaspoon or 3 capsules daily
- **B-complex:** 1 capsule daily
- **Cat's claw:** 2 dropperfuls twice a day
- **Celeryforce:** 2 capsules twice a day
- **Curcumin:** 2 capsules twice a day
- **Dulse liquid:** 1 dropperful daily
- **Glutathione:** 1 capsule daily
- **Lemon balm:** 3 dropperfuls twice a day
- **Licorice root:** 1 dropperful daily (two weeks on, two weeks off)
- **L-lysine:** 4 500-milligram capsules twice a day
- **Lomatium root:** 1 dropperful twice a day
- **Monolaurin:** 2 capsules daily

- **Mullein leaf:** 3 dropperfuls twice a day
- **Nascent iodine:** 3 small drops (not dropperfuls) daily
- **Nettle leaf:** 2 dropperfuls daily
- **Olive leaf:** 2 dropperfuls daily
- **Rose hips:** 1 cup of tea daily
- **Spirulina:** 1 teaspoon or 3 capsules daily
- **Vitamin B$_{12}$ (as adenosylcobalamin with methylcobalamin):** 2 dropperfuls twice a day
- **Vitamin C (as Micro-C or comparable buffered vitamin C):** 4 500-milligram capsules twice a day
- **Wild blueberry:** 2 teaspoons powder or 2 ounces juice daily
- **Zinc (as liquid zinc sulfate):** 2 dropperfuls daily

EYE FOCUS ISSUES

Refer to Cranial Nerve Inflammation protocol.

FACIAL PAIN

Refer to Shingles protocol and/or Herpes Simplex 1 and 2 protocol.

FAINTING

Refer to Cranial Nerve Inflammation protocol.

FATIGUE

Before applying these, be sure to read Chapter 2, "Golden Rules of Supplements."

- **Fresh celery juice:** work up to 32 ounces daily
- **Heavy Metal Detox Smoothie:** 1 serving daily (see Chapter 10)
- **Energy Shifter:** 1 Brain Shot daily (see Chapter 8)
- **Burnout Stabilizer:** 1 Brain Shot daily (see Chapter 8)
- **5-MTHF:** 1 capsule daily
- **Ashwagandha:** 1 dropperful twice a day
- **Barley grass juice powder:** 2 teaspoons or 6 capsules daily
- **Celeryforce:** 3 capsules twice a day
- **Chaga mushroom powder:** 2 teaspoons or 6 capsules daily
- **Ginger:** 1 cup of tea or freshly grated or juiced to taste daily
- **Lemon balm:** 2 dropperfuls daily
- **Licorice root:** 1 dropperful daily (three weeks on, one week off)
- **Mullein leaf:** 2 dropperfuls daily

- **Nascent iodine:** 6 small drops (not dropperfuls) daily
- **Oregon grape root:** 1 dropperful daily (two weeks on, two weeks off)
- **Raw honey:** 1 tablespoon daily
- **Reishi mushroom powder:** 1 teaspoon or 3 capsules daily
- **Spirulina:** 2 teaspoons or 6 capsules daily
- **Turmeric:** 2 capsules daily
- **Vitamin B$_{12}$ (as adenosylcobalamin with methylcobalamin):** 2 dropperfuls twice a day
- **Vitamin C (as Micro-C or comparable buffered vitamin C):** 4 500-milligram capsules daily
- **Zinc (as liquid zinc sulfate):** up to 1 dropperful daily

FEVER BLISTERS

Refer to Herpes Simplex 1 and 2 protocol.

FIBROMYALGIA

Before applying these, be sure to read Chapter 2, "Golden Rules of Supplements."

- **Fresh celery juice:** work up to 32 ounces daily

- **Heavy Metal Detox Smoothie:** 1 serving daily (see Chapter 10)
- **Nerve Shifter:** 1 Brain Shot daily (see Chapter 8)
- **California Poppy Shock Therapy:** if needed (see Chapter 3)
- **Goldenseal Shock Therapy:** if needed (see Chapter 3)
- **Lemon Balm Shock Therapy:** if needed (see Chapter 3)
- **5-MTHF:** 1 capsule daily
- **Ashwagandha:** 1 dropperful daily
- **Barley grass juice powder:** 2 teaspoons or 6 capsules daily
- **Cat's claw:** 1 dropperful twice a day
- **Celeryforce:** 2 capsules twice a day
- **Curcumin:** 2 capsules twice a day
- **EPA and DHA (fish-free):** 1 capsule daily (taken with dinner)
- **Lemon balm:** 4 dropperfuls twice a day
- **Licorice root:** 1 dropperful daily (three weeks on, one week off)
- **L-lysine:** 3 500-milligram capsules twice a day
- **Magnesium glycinate:** 1 capsule twice a day

- Monolaurin: 1 capsule daily
- MSM: 1 capsule daily
- Nettle leaf: 3 dropperfuls twice a day
- Spirulina: 2 teaspoons or 6 capsules daily
- Vitamin B$_{12}$ (as adenosylcobalamin with methylcobalamin): 2 dropperfuls twice a day
- Vitamin C (as Micro-C or comparable buffered vitamin C): 3 500-milligram capsules twice a day
- Vitamin D$_3$: 1,000 IU daily
- Wild blueberry: 1 tablespoon powder or 2 ounces juice daily
- Zinc (as liquid zinc sulfate): 1 dropperful twice a day

FLU

Refer to Cold, Flu, and COVID protocol.

FLUTTERING IN EARS

Refer to Tinnitus protocol.

FOCUS AND CONCENTRATION ISSUES

Refer to Brain Fog protocol.

FOOD POISONING

Refer to Stomach Problems protocol.

FOOD SENSITIVITIES

Refer to Chemical and Food Sensitivities protocol.

FORGETFULNESS

Refer to Brain Fog protocol.

FROZEN SHOULDER

Refer to Shingles protocol.

GAS PAIN

Refer to Stomach Problems protocol.

GASTRIC SPASMS

Refer to Stomach Problems protocol.

GASTRITIS

Refer to Stomach Problems protocol.

GASTRITIS (AUTOIMMUNE)

Refer to Stomach Problems protocol and/or Autoimmune Disorders and Diseases protocol.

GASTROPARESIS (MILD)

Before applying these, be sure to read Chapter 2, "Golden Rules of Supplements."

If you are able to swallow supplements, here are some options:

- **Fresh celery juice:** work up to 32 ounces daily

- **Fresh cucumber juice:** work up to 32 ounces daily

- **Heavy Metal Detox Smoothie:** 1 serving daily (see Chapter 10)

- **Nerve-Gut Acid Stabilizer:** 1 Brain Shot daily (see Chapter 8)

- **Lemon Balm Shock Therapy:** if needed (see Chapter 3)

- **Aloe Vera Shock Therapy:** if needed (see Chapter 3)

- **Aloe vera:** 2 or more inches of fresh gel (skin removed) daily

- **Lemon balm:** 2 dropperfuls twice a day

- **Licorice root:** 1 dropperful twice a day (roughly 21 days total on, 7 days total off per month*)

- **Magnesium glycinate:** 1 capsule twice a day

- **Vitamin B$_{12}$ (as adenosylcobalamin with methylcobalamin):** 2 dropperfuls twice a day

- **Zinc (as liquid zinc sulfate):** 1 dropperful daily

In this particular protocol, your periods on and off licorice root tincture do not need to be continuous. That is, you don't need to take one full week off at a time. You could have several days on licorice, followed by one or two days off, followed by several days on again. You're aiming for roughly 21 days out of every month on licorice and roughly 7 days out of every month off licorice, however you'd like to sequence the on/off days.

Note: If you are able to consume food (blended or solid), consider one of the Mono Eating Cleanse options from *Cleanse to Heal.*

GASTROPARESIS (SEVERE)

Before applying these, be sure to read Chapter 2, "Golden Rules of Supplements."

If you are unable to swallow supplements, you have the option to place these liquid supplements in your mouth for 30 seconds or more, and then spit them out:

- **Lemon balm:** 1 dropperful twice a day

- **Licorice root:** 1 dropperful twice a day (if swallowing, roughly 21 days total on, 7 days total off per month*; if not swallowing, continue past 21 days per month if needed)

- **Vitamin B$_{12}$ (as adenosylcobalamin with methylcobalamin):** 1 dropperful twice a day

- Zinc (as liquid zinc sulfate): 1 dropperful twice a day

In this particular protocol, your periods on and off licorice root tincture do not need to be continuous. That is, you don't need to take one full week off at a time. You could have several days on licorice, followed by one or two days off, followed by several days on again. You're aiming for roughly 21 days out of every month on licorice and roughly 7 days out of every month off licorice, however you'd like to sequence the on/off days.

If you can swallow food-based liquids such as juices, here are some options to work up to:

- **Fresh celery juice:** work up to 32 ounces daily

- **Fresh cucumber juice:** work up to 32 ounces daily

- Aloe Water: 16 ounces daily

Note: If you are able to consume food (blended or solid), consider one of the Mono Eating Cleanse options from *Cleanse to Heal.*

GREEN TEA, MATCHA TEA, AND BLACK TEA WITHDRAWAL

Refer to Addiction protocol.

GUILLAIN-BARRÉ SYNDROME

Refer to Autoimmune Disorders and Diseases protocol.

GUM PAIN (MYSTERY)

Refer to Shingles protocol and/or Herpes Simplex 1 and 2 protocol.

GUT PAINS AND SPASMS

Refer to Vagus Nerve Problems protocol and/or Stomach Problems protocol.

HEADACHES

Refer to Migraines protocol.

HEARING LOSS (UNEXPLAINED)

Refer to Tinnitus protocol.

HEART PALPITATIONS (NEUROLOGICAL)

Refer to Cranial Nerve Inflammation protocol.

HEART PALPITATIONS (NON-NEUROLOGICAL)

Before applying these, be sure to read Chapter 2, "Golden Rules of Supplements."

- **Fresh celery juice:** work up to 32 ounces daily

- **Heavy Metal Detox Smoothie:** 1 serving daily (see Chapter 10)

- **Adrenal Fight or Flight Stabilizer:** 1 Brain Shot daily (see Chapter 8)
- **5-MTHF:** 1 capsule daily
- **Barley grass juice powder:** 1 teaspoon or 3 capsules daily
- **Cat's claw:** 2 dropperfuls daily
- **Celeryforce:** 2 capsules twice a day
- **Chaga mushroom powder:** 2 teaspoons or 6 capsules daily
- **CoQ10:** 2 capsules daily
- **Curcumin:** 2 capsules daily
- **Lemon balm:** 3 dropperfuls daily
- **Magnesium glycinate:** 3 capsules twice a day
- **Nascent iodine:** 4 small drops (not dropperfuls) daily
- **Nettle leaf:** 2 dropperfuls daily
- **Raspberry leaf:** 1 cup of tea with 2 tea bags daily
- **Spirulina:** 2 teaspoons or 6 capsules daily
- **Vitamin B$_{12}$ (as adenosylcobalamin with methylcobalamin):** 2 dropperfuls daily
- **Vitamin C (as Micro-C or comparable buffered vitamin C):** 4 500-milligram capsules daily

- **Wild blueberry:** 1 tablespoon powder or 2 ounces juice daily
- **Zinc (as liquid zinc sulfate):** up to 1 dropperful daily

HEAT SENSITIVITY

Refer to Cold Sensitivity protocol.

HEMISPATIAL NEGLECT

Before applying these, be sure to read Chapter 2, "Golden Rules of Supplements."

- **Fresh celery juice:** work up to 32 ounces daily
- **Heavy Metal Detox Smoothie:** 1 serving daily (see Chapter 10)
- **Extractor Smoothie:** 1 serving daily (see Chapter 10)
- **Radiation Exposure:** 1 Brain Shot daily (see Chapter 8)
- **Pharmaceutical Exposure:** 1 Brain Shot daily (see Chapter 8)
- **Barley grass juice powder:** 1 teaspoon or 3 capsules daily
- **B-complex:** 1 capsule daily
- **Celeryforce:** 2 capsules twice a day
- **CoQ10:** 1 capsule twice a day
- **Elderflower:** 1 cup of tea daily
- **GABA:** 1 250-milligram capsule daily

- **Glutathione:** 1 capsule twice a day
- **Magnesium glycinate:** 2 capsules twice a day
- **Melatonin:** 1 5-milligram capsule at bedtime daily
- **Skullcap:** 1 dropperful twice a day
- **Spirulina:** 1 teaspoon or 3 capsules daily
- **Vitamin C (as Micro-C or comparable buffered vitamin C):** 6 500-milligram capsules twice a day
- **Wild blueberry:** 2 teaspoons powder or 2 ounces juice daily

HEPATITIS (AUTOIMMUNE)

Refer to Autoimmune Disorders and Diseases protocol.

HERPES SIMPLEX (HSV) 1 AND 2

Before applying these, be sure to read Chapter 2, "Golden Rules of Supplements."

- **Fresh celery juice:** work up to 32 ounces daily
- **Heavy Metal Detox Smoothie:** 1 serving daily (see Chapter 10)
- **Nerve Shifter:** 1 Brain Shot daily (see Chapter 8)

- **Any Shock Therapies from Chapter 3 can be used if needed**
- **Aloe vera:** 2 or more inches of fresh gel (skin removed) daily; also apply fresh gel to herpes sores
- **Barley grass juice powder:** 1 teaspoon or 3 capsules daily
- **Cat's claw:** 2 dropperfuls twice a day
- **Curcumin:** 2 capsules twice a day
- **Lemon balm:** 5 dropperfuls twice a day
- **Licorice root:** 2 dropperfuls twice a day (two weeks on, two weeks off)
- **L-lysine:** 8 500-milligram capsules twice a day
- **Lomatium root:** 2 dropperfuls twice a day
- **Mullein leaf:** 4 dropperfuls twice a day
- **Nascent iodine:** 3 small drops (not dropperfuls) twice a day
- **Nettle leaf:** 4 dropperfuls twice a day
- **Oregon grape root:** 2 dropperfuls twice a day (two weeks on, two weeks off)
- **Propolis:** 5 dropperfuls twice a day; also can be dabbed

on herpes sores (body, face, or mouth)

- **Raw honey:** 1 tablespoon daily
- **Spirulina:** 1 teaspoon or 3 capsules daily
- **Thyme:** 2 sprigs of fresh thyme in hot water as tea or 4 sprigs in room temperature water twice a day
- **Vitamin B$_{12}$ (as adenosylcobalamin with methylcobalamin):** 2 dropperfuls twice a day
- **Vitamin C (as Micro-C or comparable buffered vitamin C):** 8 500-milligram capsules twice a day
- **Zinc (as liquid zinc sulfate):** 2 dropperfuls twice a day; also can be dabbed on herpes sores (body, face, or mouth)

HIV (HUMAN IMMUNODEFICIENCY VIRUS)

Refer to Cranial Nerve Inflammation protocol and/or Autoimmune Disorders and Diseases protocol.

HUMIDITY SENSITIVITY

Refer to Cold Sensitivity protocol.

HUNTINGTON'S DISEASE

Refer to Encephalopathy protocol.

HYPERHIDROSIS

Refer to Excessive Sweating protocol.

HYPERPIGMENTATION

Before applying these, be sure to read Chapter 2, "Golden Rules of Supplements."

- **Fresh celery juice:** work up to 32 ounces daily; then you have the option to work up to 32 ounces twice a day
- **Advanced Heavy Metal Detox Smoothie:** 1 serving daily (see Chapter 10)
- **Advanced Extractor Smoothie:** 1 serving daily (see Chapter 10)
- **Pharmaceutical Exposure:** 1 Brain Shot daily (see Chapter 8)
- **Radiation Exposure:** 1 Brain Shot daily (see Chapter 8)
- **Vitamin C Shock Therapy:** if needed (see Chapter 3)
- **Aloe Vera Shock Therapy:** if needed (see Chapter 3)
- **Vitamin B$_{12}$ (as adenosylcobalamin with methylcobalamin):** 2 dropperfuls twice a day

IMPULSE CONTROL ISSUES

Refer to Cranial Nerve Inflammation protocol.

INFLAMMATORY MYOPATHY

Refer to Cranial Nerve Inflammation protocol.

INFLUENZA

Refer to Cold, Flu, and COVID protocol.

INNER EAR DISEASE

Refer to Tinnitus protocol.

INSOMNIA

Before applying these, be sure to read Chapter 2, "Golden Rules of Supplements."

- **Fresh celery juice:** work up to 32 ounces daily
- **Fresh cucumber juice:** 8 ounces daily (within a couple of hours before bed)
- **Heavy Metal Detox Smoothie:** 1 serving daily (see Chapter 10)
- **Sleep and Recharging Stabilizer:** 1 Brain Shot daily (see Chapter 8)
- **Dreams Shifter:** 1 Brain Shot daily (see Chapter 8)

- **Lemon Balm Shock Therapy:** if needed (see Chapter 3)
- **California Poppy Shock Therapy:** if needed (see Chapter 3)
- **5-MTHF:** 1 capsule daily
- **Aloe vera:** 2 or more inches of fresh gel (skin removed) daily
- **Ashwagandha:** 2 dropperfuls twice a day
- **Barley grass juice powder:** 2 teaspoons or 6 capsules daily
- **Cat's claw:** 1 dropperful twice a day
- **Celeryforce:** 3 capsules three times a day
- **Curcumin:** 2 capsules twice a day
- **D-mannose:** 1 tablespoon in water daily
- **GABA:** 1 250-milligram capsule three times a day
- **Ginger:** 2 cups of tea or freshly grated or juiced to taste daily
- **Hibiscus:** 1 cup of tea with 2 tea bags (combined with the lemon balm tea) at bedtime daily
- **Lemon balm:** 4 dropperfuls three times a day plus 1 cup of lemon balm tea (combined with the hibiscus tea) at bedtime daily

- **Licorice root:** 1 dropperful daily (two weeks on, two weeks off)
- **Magnesium glycinate:** 2 capsules twice a day
- **Melatonin:** 5 to 20 milligrams at bedtime daily
- **Raw honey:** 1 tablespoon or more daily, preferably at night (for example, in tea)
- **Spirulina:** 2 teaspoons or 6 capsules daily
- **Vitamin B$_{12}$ (as adenosylcobalamin with methylcobalamin):** 2 dropperfuls twice a day
- **Vitamin C (as Micro-C or comparable buffered vitamin C):** 4 500-milligram capsules twice a day
- **Wild blueberry:** 2 teaspoons powder or 2 ounces juice daily
- **Zinc (as liquid zinc sulfate):** 1 dropperful daily

INTRACRANIAL HYPERTENSION

Refer to Cranial Nerve Inflammation protocol.

IRRITABILITY

Refer to Mood Changes and Mood Swings protocol.

ITCHING AND BURNING (WHEN NO RASH IS PRESENT)

Refer to Cranial Nerve Inflammation protocol.

JAW PAIN (MYSTERY)

Refer to Shingles protocol and/or Herpes Simplex 1 and 2 protocol.

JOINT PAIN

Before applying these, be sure to read Chapter 2, "Golden Rules of Supplements."

- **Fresh celery juice:** work up to 32 ounces daily
- **Heavy Metal Detox Smoothie:** 1 serving daily (see Chapter 10)
- **Nerve Shifter:** 1 Brain Shot daily (see Chapter 8)
- **California Poppy Shock Therapy:** if needed (see Chapter 3)
- **Lemon Balm Shock Therapy:** if needed (see Chapter 3)
- **5-MTHF:** 1 capsule daily
- **Aloe vera:** 2 or more inches of fresh gel (skin removed) daily
- **Barley grass juice powder:** 1 teaspoon or 3 capsules daily
- **B-complex:** 1 capsule daily
- **Cat's claw:** 1 dropperful daily

- **CoQ10:** 1 capsule daily
- **Curcumin:** 3 capsules twice a day
- **Glutathione:** 1 capsule daily
- **Lemon balm:** 3 dropperfuls twice a day
- **Licorice root:** 1 dropperful twice a day (two weeks on, two weeks off)
- **L-lysine:** 4 500-milligram capsules twice a day
- **Magnesium glycinate:** 2 capsules twice a day
- **Milk thistle:** 1 dropperful daily
- **Monolaurin:** 1 capsule daily
- **MSM:** 2 capsules daily
- **Nettle leaf:** 4 dropperfuls twice a day
- **Spirulina:** 1 teaspoon or 3 capsules daily
- **Turmeric:** 4 capsules daily
- **Vitamin B$_{12}$ (as adenosylcobalamin with methylcobalamin):** 2 dropperfuls twice a day
- **Vitamin C (as Micro-C or comparable buffered vitamin C):** 4 500-milligram capsules twice a day
- **Vitamin D$_3$:** 1,000 IU daily
- **Wild blueberry:** 1 tablespoon powder or 2 ounces juice daily

- **Zinc (as liquid zinc sulfate):** 1 dropperful twice a day

LEARNING DISABILITIES AND DISORDERS

Before applying these, be sure to read Chapter 2, "Golden Rules of Supplements." Remember that you can take these adult dosages to your pediatrician to see what dosages are right for your child. Also see Chapter 8, "Brain Shot Therapy," Chapter 10, "Heavy Metal Detox," and Chapter 2, "Golden Rules of Supplements," for adjusted amounts of celery juice, smoothie, and Brain Shot Therapies for children.

- **Fresh celery juice:** work up to 32 ounces daily
- **Heavy Metal Detox Smoothie:** 1 serving daily (see Chapter 10)
- **Extractor Smoothie:** 1 serving daily (see Chapter 10)
- **Burnout Stabilizer:** 1 Brain Shot daily (see Chapter 8)
- **Barley grass juice powder:** 1 teaspoon or 3 capsules daily
- **Celeryforce:** 3 capsules twice a day
- **D-mannose:** 1 teaspoon in water daily
- **Elderberry syrup:** 1 teaspoon daily
- **GABA:** 1 250-milligram capsule daily

- **Glutathione:** 1 capsule twice a day
- **Magnesium glycinate:** 1 capsule twice a day
- **Raw honey:** 1 tablespoon daily
- **Spirulina:** 1 teaspoon or 3 capsules daily
- **Vitamin B$_{12}$ (as adenosylcobalamin with methylcobalamin):** 1 dropperful twice a day
- **Vitamin C (as Micro-C or comparable buffered vitamin C):** 4 500-milligram capsules twice a day
- **Wild blueberry:** 2 teaspoons powder or 2 ounces juice daily

LEFT NEGLECT

Refer to Hemispatial Neglect protocol.

LIVER SPOTS

Refer to Hyperpigmentation protocol.

LONG-HAUL COVID (ALSO CALLED LONG COVID)

Refer to Mononucleosis protocol and/or Autoimmune Disorders and Diseases protocol.

LONG-HAUL FLU

Refer to Mononucleosis protocol and/or Autoimmune Disorders and Diseases protocol.

LOSS OF FACE MOVEMENT

Refer to Shingles protocol and/or Cranial Nerve Inflammation protocol.

LOSS OF SMELL

Refer to Cranial Nerve Inflammation protocol.

LOSS OF TASTE

Refer to Cranial Nerve Inflammation protocol.

LOW VISION

Before applying these, be sure to read Chapter 2, "Golden Rules of Supplements."

- **Fresh celery juice:** work up to at least 16 ounces daily
- **Heavy Metal Detox Smoothie:** 1 serving daily (see Chapter 10)
- **5-MTHF:** 1 capsule daily
- **ALA (alpha lipoic acid):** 1 capsule every other day
- **Amla berry:** 1 teaspoon daily

- **Barley grass juice powder:** 1 teaspoon or 3 capsules daily
- **Cat's claw:** 2 dropperfuls twice a day
- **Celeryforce:** 3 capsules twice a day
- **Curcumin:** 3 capsules twice a day
- **EPA and DHA (fish-free):** 1 capsule daily (taken with dinner)
- **Glutathione:** 1 capsule daily
- **Lemon balm:** 3 dropperfuls twice a day
- **Licorice root:** 1 dropperful daily (two weeks on, two weeks off)
- **L-lysine:** 4 500-milligram capsules twice a day
- **Magnesium glycinate:** 2 capsules twice a day
- **Monolaurin:** 1 capsule daily
- **Mullein leaf:** 2 dropperfuls twice a day
- **Olive leaf:** 2 dropperfuls twice a day
- **Rose hips:** 1 cup of tea daily
- **Spirulina:** 1 teaspoon or 3 capsules daily
- **Vitamin B$_{12}$ (as adenosylcobalamin with methylcobalamin):** 2 dropperfuls twice a day
- **Vitamin C (as Micro-C or comparable buffered vitamin C):** 6 500-milligram capsules twice a day
- **Vitamin D$_3$:** 1,000 IU daily
- **Wild blueberry:** 1 tablespoon powder or 2 ounces juice daily
- **Zinc (as liquid zinc sulfate):** 1 dropperful daily

LOWER BACK PAIN (MYSTERY)

Refer to Shingles protocol and/or Herpes Simplex 1 and 2 protocol.

LUPUS

Refer to Autoimmune Disorders and Diseases protocol.

LYME DISEASE

Before applying these, be sure to read Chapter 2, "Golden Rules of Supplements."

- **Fresh celery juice:** work up to 32 ounces daily; then you have the option to work up to 32 ounces twice a day
- **Fresh cucumber juice:** work up to 16 ounces daily
- **Heavy Metal Detox Smoothie:** 1 serving daily (see Chapter 10)
- **Pathogen Exposure:** 1 Brain Shot daily (see Chapter 8)

- **Pharmaceutical Exposure:** 1 Brain Shot daily (see Chapter 8)
- **Any Shock Therapies from Chapter 3 can be used if needed**
- **5-MTHF:** 1 capsule twice a day
- **Barley grass juice powder:** 2 teaspoons or 6 capsules twice a day
- **Cat's claw:** 3 dropperfuls twice a day
- **Celeryforce:** 4 capsules twice a day
- **Curcumin:** 3 capsules twice a day
- **Eyebright:** 2 dropperfuls twice a day
- **Ginger:** 1 cup of tea or freshly grated or juiced to taste daily
- **Glutathione:** 1 capsule daily
- **Hyssop:** 1 cup of tea daily
- **Lemon balm:** 4 dropperfuls twice a day
- **Licorice root:** 1 dropperful twice a day (two weeks on, two weeks off)
- **L-lysine:** 5 500-milligram capsules twice a day
- **Mullein leaf:** 4 dropperfuls twice a day
- **Nascent iodine:** 3 small drops (not dropperfuls) twice a day
- **Nettle leaf:** 3 dropperfuls twice a day
- **Propolis:** 2 dropperfuls twice a day
- **Raw honey:** 1 to 3 teaspoons daily
- **Spirulina:** 2 teaspoons or 6 capsules daily
- **Vitamin B$_{12}$ (as adenosylcobalamin with methylcobalamin):** 3 dropperfuls twice a day
- **Vitamin C (as Micro-C or comparable buffered vitamin C):** 8 500-milligram capsules twice a day
- **Zinc (as liquid zinc sulfate):** up to 2 dropperfuls twice a day

MANIA

Refer to Bipolar Disorder protocol.

MARIJUANA WITHDRAWAL

Refer to Addiction protocol.

ME/CFS (MYALGIC ENCEPHALOMYELITIS/CHRONIC FATIGUE SYNDROME)

Before applying these, be sure to read Chapter 2, "Golden Rules of Supplements."

- **Fresh celery juice:** work up to 32 ounces daily; then you have the option to work up to 32 ounces twice a day

- **Heavy Metal Detox Smoothie:** 1 serving daily (see Chapter 10)

- **Energy Shifter:** 1 Brain Shot daily (see Chapter 8)

- **Burnout Stabilizer:** 1 Brain Shot daily (see Chapter 8)

- **Any Shock Therapies from Chapter 3 can be used if needed**

- **5-MTHF:** 1 capsule twice a day

- **Ashwagandha:** 1 dropperful daily

- **Barley grass juice powder:** 2 teaspoons or 6 capsules daily

- **Cat's claw:** 2 dropperfuls twice a day

- **Celeryforce:** 2 capsules three times a day

- **Chaga mushroom powder:** 2 teaspoons or 6 capsules daily

- **Curcumin:** 2 capsules twice a day

- **EPA and DHA (fish-free):** 1 capsule daily (taken with dinner)

- **Eyebright:** 1 dropperful daily

- **Glutathione:** 1 capsule daily

- **Goldenseal:** 2 dropperfuls twice a day (two weeks on, two weeks off)

- **Hyssop:** 1 cup of tea daily

- **Lemon balm:** 3 dropperfuls twice a day

- **Licorice root:** 1 dropperful twice a day (two weeks on, two weeks off)

- **L-lysine:** 4 500-milligram capsules twice a day

- **Magnesium glycinate:** 1 capsule twice a day

- **Monolaurin:** 2 capsules twice a day

- **Mullein leaf:** 2 dropperfuls twice a day

- **Oregon grape root:** 1 dropperful daily (two weeks on, two weeks off)

- **Propolis:** 2 dropperfuls twice a day

- **Spirulina:** 2 teaspoons or 6 capsules daily

- **Vitamin B$_{12}$ (as adenosylcobalamin with methylcobalamin):** 2 dropperfuls twice a day

- **Vitamin C (as Micro-C or comparable buffered vitamin C):** 3 500-milligram capsules twice a day

- **Zinc (as liquid zinc sulfate):** 2 dropperfuls twice a day

MELASMA (CHLOASMA)

Refer to Hyperpigmentation protocol.

MEMORY ISSUES

Refer to Brain Fog protocol.

MEMORY LOSS

Refer to Alzheimer's Disease protocol.

MÉNIÈRE'S DISEASE

Refer to Vertigo protocol.

MENINGITIS

Before applying these, be sure to read Chapter 2, "Golden Rules of Supplements."

- **Fresh celery juice:** work up to 32 ounces daily
- **Fresh cucumber juice:** work up to 32 ounces daily
- **Pathogen Exposure:** 1 Brain Shot daily (see Chapter 8)
- **Any Shock Therapies from Chapter 3 can be used if needed**
- **Cat's claw:** 4 dropperfuls twice a day
- **Elderberry syrup:** 1 tablespoon twice a day
- **Eyebright:** 3 dropperfuls twice a day
- **Goldenseal:** 6 dropperfuls twice a day
- **Lemon balm:** 6 dropperfuls twice a day
- **Licorice root:** 4 dropperfuls twice a day (three weeks on, one week off) until meningitis subsides
- **L-lysine:** 4 500-milligram capsules twice a day
- **Lomatium root:** 3 dropperfuls twice a day
- **Mullein leaf:** 6 dropperfuls twice a day
- **Olive leaf:** 4 dropperfuls twice a day
- **Oregon grape root:** 3 dropperfuls twice a day
- **Osha:** 3 dropperfuls twice a day
- **Propolis:** 5 dropperfuls twice a day
- **Thyme:** 2 sprigs fresh thyme in hot water as tea or 4 sprigs in room temperature water daily
- **Vitamin B$_{12}$ (as adenosylcobalamin with methylcobalamin):** 4 dropperfuls twice a day
- **Vitamin C (as Micro-C or comparable buffered vitamin C):** 8 500-milligram capsules three times a day

- Zinc (as liquid zinc sulfate): 3 dropperfuls twice a day

MIGRAINES

Before applying these, be sure to read Chapter 2, "Golden Rules of Supplements."

- Fresh celery juice: work up to 32 ounces daily
- Heavy Metal Detox Smoothie: 1 serving daily (see Chapter 10)
- Nerve Shifter: 1 Brain Shot daily (see Chapter 8)
- Burnout Stabilizer: 1 Brain Shot daily (see Chapter 8)
- Lemon Balm Shock Therapy: if needed (see Chapter 3)
- California Poppy Shock Therapy: if needed (see Chapter 3)
- Ashwagandha: 1 dropperful twice a day
- Barley grass juice powder: 2 teaspoons or 6 capsules daily
- Cat's claw: 2 dropperfuls twice a day
- Celeryforce: 3 capsules three times a day
- CoQ10: 1 capsule daily
- Curcumin: 3 capsules twice a day
- Elderflower: 1 cup of tea daily

- Feverfew: 2 dropperfuls or 2 capsules daily
- GABA: 1 250-milligram capsule twice a day
- Goldenseal: 1 dropperful twice a day (two weeks on, two weeks off)
- Kava kava: 2 dropperfuls or 2 capsules daily
- Lemon balm: 4 dropperfuls twice a day
- L-lysine: 4 500-milligram capsules twice a day
- Magnesium glycinate: 2 capsules twice a day
- Nettle leaf: 4 dropperfuls twice a day
- Oregano oil: 2 capsules daily
- Skullcap: 2 dropperfuls or 2 capsules twice a day
- Spirulina: 2 teaspoons or 6 capsules daily
- Turmeric: 2 capsules twice a day
- Vitamin B_{12} (as adenosylcobalamin with methylcobalamin): 2 dropperfuls twice a day
- Vitamin C (as Micro-C or comparable buffered vitamin C): 4 500-milligram capsules twice a day

- **White willow bark:** 2 dropperfuls or 2 capsules daily
- **Wild blueberry:** 1 tablespoon powder or 2 ounces juice daily

MIND-BODY SYNDROME

Refer to Cranial Nerve Inflammation protocol.

MITOCHONDRIAL MYOPATHY

Refer to Autoimmune Disorders and Diseases protocol.

MONONUCLEOSIS (MONO)

Before applying these, be sure to read Chapter 2, "Golden Rules of Supplements."

- **Fresh celery juice:** work up to 32 ounces daily
- **Pathogen Exposure:** 1 Brain Shot daily (see Chapter 8)
- **Propolis Shock Therapy:** if needed (see Chapter 3)
- **Goldenseal Shock Therapy:** if needed (see Chapter 3)
- **Thyme Tea Shock Therapy:** if needed (see Chapter 3)
- **Vitamin C Shock Therapy:** if needed (see Chapter 3)
- **Zinc Shock Therapy:** if needed (see Chapter 3)

- **Cat's claw:** 3 dropperfuls twice a day
- **Eyebright:** 3 dropperfuls twice a day
- **Ginger:** 1 cup of tea or freshly grated or juiced to taste four times a day
- **Goldenseal:** 4 dropperfuls twice a day (two weeks on, two weeks off)
- **Lemon balm:** 4 dropperfuls twice a day
- **Licorice root:** 1 dropperful twice a day (two weeks on, two weeks off)
- **L-lysine:** 6 500-milligram capsules twice a day
- **Lomatium root:** 3 dropperfuls twice a day
- **Monolaurin:** 2 capsules twice a day
- **Mullein leaf:** 4 dropperfuls twice a day
- **Oregon grape root:** 2 dropperfuls twice a day (two weeks on, two weeks off)
- **Osha:** 3 dropperfuls twice a day
- **Thyme:** 2 sprigs fresh thyme in hot water as tea or 4 sprigs in room temperature water daily
- **Vitamin C (as Micro-C or comparable buffered vitamin C):** 10 500-milligram capsules twice a day

- Zinc (as liquid zinc sulfate): 3 dropperfuls twice a day

MOOD CHANGES AND MOOD SWINGS

Before applying these, be sure to read Chapter 2, "Golden Rules of Supplements."

- **Fresh celery juice:** work up to 32 ounces daily
- **Heavy Metal Detox Smoothie:** 1 serving daily (see Chapter 10)
- **Mood Shifter:** 1 Brain Shot daily (see Chapter 8)
- **Lemon Balm Shock Therapy:** if needed (see Chapter 3)
- **Aloe vera:** 2 or more inches of fresh gel (skin removed) daily
- **Barley grass juice powder:** 2 teaspoons or 6 capsules daily
- **Celeryforce:** 2 capsules twice a day
- **GABA:** 1 250-milligram capsule daily
- **Hibiscus:** 1 cup of tea twice a day
- **Lemon balm:** 4 dropperfuls twice a day
- **Magnesium glycinate:** 2 capsules twice a day
- **Nascent iodine:** 3 small drops (not dropperfuls) daily

- **Nettle leaf:** 1 dropperful or 1 cup of tea twice a day
- **Spirulina:** 2 teaspoons or 6 capsules daily
- **Vitamin B$_{12}$ (as adenosylcobalamin with methylcobalamin):** 1 dropperful twice a day
- **Vitamin C (as Micro-C or comparable buffered vitamin C):** 2 500-milligram capsules twice a day
- **Vitamin D$_3$:** 1,000 IU daily
- **Wild blueberry:** 1 tablespoon powder or 2 ounces juice daily
- **Zinc (as liquid zinc sulfate):** up to 1 dropperful daily

MOTOR SKILLS DISORDER (ALSO KNOWN AS DEVELOPMENTAL DYSPRAXIA)

Before applying these, be sure to read Chapter 2, "Golden Rules of Supplements."

Remember that you can take these adult dosages to your pediatrician to see what dosages are right for your child. Also see Chapter 8, "Brain Shot Therapy," Chapter 10, "Heavy Metal Detox," and Chapter 2, "Golden Rules of Supplements," for adjusted amounts of celery juice, smoothie, and Brain Shot Therapies for children.

- **Fresh celery juice:** work up to 32 ounces daily

- **Heavy Metal Detox Smoothie:** 1 serving daily (see Chapter 10)

- **Extractor Smoothie:** 1 serving daily (see Chapter 10)

- **Nerve Shifter:** 1 Brain Shot daily (see Chapter 8)

- **5-HTP:** 1 capsule at bedtime daily

- **5-MTHF:** 1 capsule daily

- **Barley grass juice powder:** 1 teaspoon or 3 capsules daily

- **Cat's claw:** 1 dropperful daily

- **Celeryforce:** 2 capsules twice a day

- **GABA:** 1 250-milligram capsule daily

- **Glutathione:** 1 capsule twice a day

- **L-glutamine:** 1 500-milligram capsule daily

- **Magnesium glycinate:** 2 capsules twice a day

- **Melatonin:** 1 5-milligram capsule at bedtime daily

- **MSM:** 1 capsule daily

- **Silica:** 1 teaspoon daily

- **Spirulina:** 1 teaspoon or 3 capsules daily

- **Vitamin B$_{12}$ (as adenosylcobalamin with methylcobalamin):** 1 dropperful twice a day

- **Vitamin C (as Micro-C or comparable buffered vitamin C):** 4 500-milligram capsules twice a day

- **Wild blueberry:** 2 teaspoons powder or 2 ounces juice daily

- **Zinc (as liquid zinc sulfate):** 1 dropperful daily

MULTIPLE SCLEROSIS (MS)

Before applying these, be sure to read Chapter 2, "Golden Rules of Supplements."

- **Fresh celery juice:** work up to 32 ounces daily; then you have the option to work up to 32 ounces twice a day

- **Heavy Metal Detox Smoothie:** 1 serving daily (see Chapter 10)

- **Extractor Smoothie:** 1 serving daily (see Chapter 10)

- **Pharmaceutical Exposure:** 1 Brain Shot daily (see Chapter 8)

- **Radiation Exposure:** 1 Brain Shot daily (see Chapter 8)

- **Nerve Shifter:** 1 Brain Shot daily (see Chapter 8)

- **Any Shock Therapies** from Chapter 3 can be used if needed

- **5-MTHF:** 2 capsules twice a day

- **ALA (alpha lipoic acid):** 1 capsule daily

- Barley grass juice powder: 1 to 3 teaspoons or 3 to 9 capsules daily

- B-complex: 1 capsule daily

- Cat's claw: 3 dropperfuls twice a day

- Celeryforce: 2 capsules three times a day

- CoQ10: 1 capsule daily

- Curcumin: 3 capsules twice a day

- EPA and DHA (fish-free): 1 capsule daily (taken with dinner)

- GABA: 1 250-milligram capsule daily

- Glutathione: 1 capsule daily

- Goldenseal: 2 dropperfuls twice a day (two weeks on, two weeks off)

- Lemon balm: 4 dropperfuls twice a day

- L-glutamine: 1 capsule twice a day

- Licorice root: 2 dropperfuls twice a day (two weeks on, two weeks off)

- L-lysine: 4 500-milligram capsules twice a day

- Magnesium glycinate: 2 capsules twice a day

- Monolaurin: 1 capsule twice a day

- MSM: 1 capsule twice a day

- Mullein leaf: 3 dropperfuls twice a day

- Nettle leaf: 4 dropperfuls twice a day

- Propolis: 2 dropperfuls twice a day

- Spirulina: 2 teaspoons or 6 capsules daily

- Vitamin B_{12} (as adenosylcobalamin with methylcobalamin): 2 dropperfuls twice a day

- Vitamin C (as Micro-C or comparable buffered vitamin C): 6 500-milligram capsules twice a day

- Wild blueberry: 2 teaspoons powder or 2 ounces juice daily

- Zinc (as liquid zinc sulfate): 2 dropperfuls twice a day

MUSCLE PAIN (MYSTERY)

Refer to Fibromyalgia protocol.

MUSCLE SPASMS

Refer to Cranial Nerve Inflammation protocol.

MUSCLE WEAKNESS

Refer to Cranial Nerve Inflammation protocol.

MUSCULAR DYSTROPHY

Refer to Multiple Sclerosis protocol.

MYASTHENIA GRAVIS

Refer to Autoimmune Disorders and Diseases protocol.

MYELIN NERVE SHEATH DAMAGE

Refer to Cranial Nerve Inflammation protocol.

MYOCARDITIS

Refer to Autoimmune Disorders and Diseases protocol.

MYSTERY FEARS AND WORRIES

Before applying these, be sure to read Chapter 2, "Golden Rules of Supplements."

- Fresh celery juice: work up to 32 ounces daily
- Heavy Metal Detox Smoothie: 1 serving daily (see Chapter 10)
- Obsessive Thoughts Shifter: 1 Brain Shot daily (see Chapter 8)
- Energy Shifter: 1 Brain Shot daily (see Chapter 8)
- Trauma, Shock, and Loss Stabilizer: 1 Brain Shot daily (see Chapter 8)
- Betrayal and Broken Trust Stabilizer: 1 Brain Shot daily (see Chapter 8)
- GABA: 1 250-milligram capsule twice a day
- Magnesium glycinate: 2 capsules twice a day
- Vitamin B_{12} (as adenosylcobalamin with methylcobalamin): 2 dropperfuls twice a day

MYSTERY HUNGER

Before applying these, be sure to read Chapter 2, "Golden Rules of Supplements."

- Fresh celery juice: work up to 32 ounces daily
- Heavy Metal Detox Smoothie: 1 serving daily (see Chapter 10)
- Food Fear Shifter: 1 Brain Shot daily (see Chapter 8)
- Cravings Shifter: 1 Brain Shot daily (see Chapter 8)
- Nerve-Gut Acid Stabilizer: 1 Brain Shot daily (see Chapter 8)
- 5-MTHF: 1 capsule daily

- Barley grass juice powder: 1 teaspoon or 3 capsules daily
- Cardamom: sprinkle on food to taste daily
- Celeryforce: 2 capsules twice a day
- Chaga mushroom powder: 2 teaspoons or 6 capsules daily
- Chicory root: 1 cup of tea daily
- Chestnuts: 2 ounces packaged edible chestnuts (preservative-free) eaten daily
- Curcumin: 2 capsules daily
- Dulse liquid: 2 dropperfuls daily
- Ginger: 1 cup of tea or freshly grated or juiced to taste daily
- Lemon balm: 2 dropperfuls twice a day
- Licorice root: 1 dropperful daily (two weeks on, two weeks off)
- Magnesium glycinate: 2 capsules daily
- Peppermint: 1 cup of tea daily
- Spirulina: 1 teaspoon or 3 capsules daily
- Vitamin B$_{12}$ (as adenosylcobalamin with methylcobalamin): 1 dropperful daily

NARCOLEPSY

Before applying these, be sure to read Chapter 2, "Golden Rules of Supplements."

- Fresh celery juice: work up to 32 ounces daily
- Heavy Metal Detox Smoothie: 1 serving daily (see Chapter 10)
- Extractor Smoothie: 1 serving daily (see Chapter 10)
- Energy Shifter: 1 Brain Shot daily (see Chapter 8)
- 5-MTHF: 1 capsule daily
- ALA (alpha lipoic acid): 1 capsule daily
- Amla berry: 1 teaspoon or 3 capsules daily
- Ashwagandha: 1 dropperful twice a day
- Barley grass juice powder: 1 teaspoon or 3 capsules daily
- Cat's claw: 1 dropperful twice a day
- Celeryforce: 3 capsules twice a day
- CoQ10: 1 capsule daily
- EPA and DHA (fish-free): 1 capsule daily (taken with dinner)
- Glutathione: 1 capsule twice a day
- L-glutamine: 1 500-milligram capsule twice a day

- **Licorice root:** 1 dropperful twice a day (two weeks on, two weeks off)
- **Magnesium glycinate:** 1 capsule twice a day
- **Nettle leaf:** 1 dropperful twice a day
- **Spirulina:** 1 teaspoon or 3 capsules daily
- **Vitamin C (as Micro-C or comparable buffered vitamin C):** 8 500-milligram capsules twice a day
- **Zinc (as liquid zinc sulfate):** 1 dropperful twice a day

NAUSEA (MYSTERY)

Refer to Vagus Nerve Problems protocol and/or Stomach Problems protocol.

NECK PAIN (MYSTERY)

Refer to Shingles protocol and/or Herpes Simplex 1 and 2 protocol.

NEURALGIA

Refer to Herpes Simplex 1 and 2 protocol and/or Shingles protocol.

NEURITIS

Refer to Shingles protocol.

NEUROLOGICAL FATIGUE

Refer to ME/CFS protocol.

NEUROLOGICAL GASTROPARESIS

Refer to Gastroparesis (Mild) protocol and/or Gastroparesis (Severe) protocol.

NEUROLOGICAL LYME

Refer to Lyme Disease protocol.

NEUROLOGICAL SYMPTOMS

Refer to Cranial Nerve Inflammation protocol.

NEUROMUSCULAR DISEASE

Refer to Autoimmune Disorders and Diseases protocol.

NEUROPATHY

Refer to Shingles protocol.

NEUROSIS

Refer to Depression protocol, Anxiety protocol, OCD protocol, and/or Bipolar Disorder protocol.

NUMBNESS

Refer to Cranial Nerve Inflammation protocol.

OBSESSIVE-COMPULSIVE DISORDER (OCD)

Before applying these, be sure to read Chapter 2, "Golden Rules of Supplements."

- **Fresh celery juice:** work up to 32 ounces daily

- **Heavy Metal Detox Smoothie:** 1 serving daily (see Chapter 10)

- **Extractor Smoothie:** 1 serving daily (see Chapter 10)

- **Obsessive Thoughts Shifter:** 1 Brain Shot daily (see Chapter 8)

- **Lemon Balm Shock Therapy:** if needed (see Chapter 3)

- **Barley grass juice powder:** 1 teaspoon or 3 capsules daily

- **B-complex:** 1 capsule daily

- **Cat's claw:** 1 dropperful daily

- **Celeryforce:** 3 capsules twice a day

- **CoQ10:** 1 capsule daily

- **Curcumin:** 1 capsule twice a day

- **Elderflower:** 1 cup of tea daily

- **EPA and DHA (fish-free):** 1 capsule daily (taken with dinner)

- **GABA:** 1 250-milligram capsule daily

- **Lemon balm:** 3 dropperfuls twice a day

- **L-glutamine:** 1 capsule twice a day

- **Magnesium glycinate:** 1 capsule twice a day

- **Melatonin:** 2 5-milligram capsules at bedtime daily

- **Spirulina:** 1 teaspoon or 3 capsules daily

- **Vitamin B$_{12}$ (as adenosylcobalamin with methylcobalamin):** 1 dropperful twice a day

- **Vitamin C (as Micro-C or comparable buffered vitamin C):** 2 500-milligram capsules twice a day

- **Wild blueberry:** 1 tablespoon powder or 2 ounces juice daily

OCCIPITAL NEURALGIA

Refer to Herpes Simplex 1 and 2 protocol and/or Shingles protocol.

OPTIC NERVE ATROPHY

Refer to Cranial Nerve Atrophy protocol.

OPTIC NEURITIS

Refer to Cranial Nerve Inflammation protocol.

ORTHOREXIA

Before applying these, be sure to read Chapter 2, "Golden Rules of Supplements."

- **Food Fear Shifter:** 1 Brain Shot daily (see Chapter 8)
- **Negative Energy Exposure:** 1 Brain Shot daily (see Chapter 8)
- **Guilt and Shame Shifter:** 1 Brain Shot daily (see Chapter 8)

If you are struggling emotionally with food, refer to Obsessive-Compulsive Disorder protocol and/or Chronic Mystery Guilt protocol.

If you are struggling physically with food, refer to Stomach Problems protocol, Gastroparesis (Mild) protocol, and/or Gastroparesis (Severe) protocol.

OTHER SPECIFIED FEEDING AND EATING DISORDER (OSFED)

Refer to Eating Disorders protocol.

OVEREATING

Refer to Eating Disorders protocol and/or Mystery Hunger protocol.

PAIN IN BACK OF HEAD (MYSTERY)

Refer to Shingles protocol and/or Herpes Simplex 1 and 2 protocol.

PAIN INSIDE OR AROUND EAR(S)

Refer to Shingles protocol and/or Herpes Simplex 1 and 2 protocol.

PANCREATITIS (AUTOIMMUNE) (AIP)

Refer to Autoimmune Disorders and Diseases protocol.

PANDAS (PEDIATRIC AUTOIMMUNE NEUROPSYCHIATRIC DISORDERS ASSOCIATED WITH STREPTOCOCCAL INFECTIONS)

This is an instance where dosages are geared to children.

Before applying these, be sure to read Chapter 2, "Golden Rules of Supplements."

- **Fresh celery juice:** refer to table in Chapter 2 for children's amounts
- **Heavy Metal Detox Smoothie:** 1 children's serving daily (see Chapter 10 for guidance)

- **Zinc Shock Therapy:** if needed (see children's dosages in Chapter 3)

- **Vitamin C Shock Therapy:** if needed (see children's dosages in Chapter 3)

- **Lemon Balm Shock Therapy:** if needed (see children's dosages in Chapter 3)

- **Goldenseal Shock Therapy:** if needed (see children's dosages in Chapter 3)

- **Thyme Tea Shock Therapy:** if needed (see children's dosages in Chapter 3)

- **Propolis Shock Therapy:** if needed (see children's dosages in Chapter 3)

- **Aloe Vera Shock Therapy:** if needed (see children's dosages in Chapter 3)

- **B$_{12}$ Shock Therapy:** if needed (see children's dosages in Chapter 3)

- **Cat's claw:** 4 small drops (not dropperfuls) twice a day

- **D-mannose:** 1 teaspoon in water twice a day

- **Eyebright:** 4 small drops (not dropperfuls) twice a day

- **Goldenseal:** 10 small drops (not dropperfuls) twice a day (two weeks on, two weeks off)

- **Lemon balm:** 10 small drops (not dropperfuls) twice a day

- **Licorice root:** 10 small drops (not dropperfuls) twice a day (two weeks on, two weeks off)

- **Mullein leaf:** 10 small drops (not dropperfuls) twice a day

- **Olive leaf:** 10 small drops (not dropperfuls) twice a day

- **Spirulina:** ½ teaspoon daily

- **Vitamin B$_{12}$ (as adenosylcobalamin with methylcobalamin):** 10 small drops (not dropperfuls) daily

- **Vitamin C (as Micro-C or comparable buffered vitamin C):** 2 500-milligram capsules twice a day (if needed, open capsules and mix contents into juice, smoothie, or water)

- **Wild blueberry:** 1 teaspoon powder or 1 ounce juice daily

- **Zinc (as liquid zinc sulfate):** up to 6 small drops (not dropperfuls) in juice, water, or directly in mouth (with optional water or juice chaser) twice a day

PANIC ATTACKS

Refer to Anxiety protocol.

PARALYSIS OF FACIAL NERVES (TEMPORARY)

Refer to Cranial Nerve Inflammation protocol.

PARANEOPLASTIC CEREBELLAR DEGENERATION (PCD)

Refer to Multiple Sclerosis protocol.

PARASITES

Refer to Cranial Nerve Inflammation protocol, Autoimmune Disorders and Diseases protocol, and/or Stomach Problems protocol.

PARKINSON'S DISEASE

Before applying these, be sure to read Chapter 2, "Golden Rules of Supplements."

- **Fresh celery juice:** work up to 32 ounces daily; then you have the option to work up to 32 ounces twice a day
- **Fresh cucumber juice:** work up to 32 ounces daily
- **Heavy Metal Detox Smoothie:** 1 serving daily (see Chapter 10)
- **Nerve Shifter:** 1 Brain Shot daily (see Chapter 8)
- **Pharmaceutical Exposure:** 1 Brain Shot daily (see Chapter 8)

- **Radiation Exposure:** 1 Brain Shot daily (see Chapter 8)
- **Lemon Balm Shock Therapy:** if needed (see Chapter 3)
- **5-MTHF:** 1 capsule daily
- **Amla berry:** 2 teaspoons daily
- **Ashwagandha:** 1 dropperful twice a day
- **Barley grass juice powder:** 2 teaspoons or 6 capsules daily
- **California poppy:** 4 dropperfuls daily
- **Celeryforce:** 3 capsules three times a day
- **CoQ10:** 1 capsule daily
- **Curcumin:** 3 capsules twice a day
- **EPA and DHA (fish-free):** 1 capsule daily (taken with dinner)
- **GABA:** 1 250-milligram capsule twice a day
- **Kava kava:** 1 capsule or 1 dropperful twice a day
- **Lemon balm:** 4 dropperfuls twice a day
- **L-glutamine:** 2 capsules twice a day
- **Magnesium glycinate:** 3 capsules twice a day
- **Melatonin:** work up to 20 milligrams at bedtime daily
- **MSM:** 1 capsule daily

- **Nettle leaf:** 2 dropperfuls twice a day
- **Raw honey:** 1 tablespoon daily
- **Selenium:** 1 capsule daily
- **Spirulina:** 2 teaspoons or 6 capsules daily
- **Turmeric:** 4 capsules daily
- **Vitamin B$_{12}$ (as adenosylcobalamin with methylcobalamin):** 3 dropperfuls twice a day
- **Vitamin C (as Micro-C or comparable buffered vitamin C):** 4 500-milligram capsules twice a day
- **Wild blueberry:** 1 tablespoon powder or 2 ounces juice daily
- **Zinc (as liquid zinc sulfate):** 1 dropperful daily

PARSONAGE-TURNER SYNDROME (PTS)

Refer to Cranial Nerve Inflammation protocol and/or Multiple Sclerosis protocol.

PERISTALTIC ISSUES

Refer to Vagus Nerve Problems protocol and/or Stomach Problems protocol.

PERSONALITY DISORDERS

Refer to Depersonalization protocol.

PICA EATING DISORDER

Refer to Eating Disorders protocol.

POLYMYALGIA RHEUMATICA

Refer to Fibromyalgia protocol.

POPPING IN EARS

Refer to Tinnitus protocol.

POST-POLIO SYNDROME

Refer to Cranial Nerve Inflammation protocol.

POTS (POSTURAL ORTHOSTATIC TACHYCARDIA SYNDROME)

Refer to Autoimmune Disorders and Diseases protocol.

PRESSURE IN CHEST (MYSTERY)

Refer to Vagus Nerve Problems protocol.

PSYCHEDELIC MUSHROOM WITHDRAWAL

Refer to Addiction protocol.

PSYCHOSIS

Before applying these, be sure to read Chapter 2, "Golden Rules of Supplements."

- **Fresh celery juice:** work up to 32 ounces daily
- **Heavy Metal Detox Smoothie:** 1 serving daily (see Chapter 10)
- **Extractor Smoothie:** 1 serving daily (see Chapter 10)
- **Pharmaceutical Exposure:** 1 Brain Shot daily (see Chapter 8)
- **Negative Energy Exposure:** 1 Brain Shot daily (see Chapter 8)
- **Obsessive Thoughts Exposure:** 1 Brain Shot daily (see Chapter 8)
- **California Poppy Shock Therapy:** if needed (see Chapter 3)
- **Lemon Balm Shock Therapy:** if needed (see Chapter 3)
- **Ashwagandha:** 2 dropperfuls twice a day
- **Celeryforce:** 3 capsules twice a day
- **GABA:** 1 250-milligram capsule twice a day

- **Lemon balm:** 4 dropperfuls twice a day
- **Magnesium glycinate:** 3 capsules twice a day
- **Melatonin:** 20 milligrams at bedtime daily
- **Vitamin B$_{12}$ (as adenosylcobalamin with methylcobalamin):** 2 dropperfuls twice a day

PTSD (POSTTRAUMATIC STRESS DISORDER) / PTSS (POSTTRAUMATIC STRESS SYMPTOMS)

Before applying these, be sure to read Chapter 2, "Golden Rules of Supplements."

- **Fresh celery juice:** work up to 32 ounces daily
- **Heavy Metal Detox Smoothie:** 1 serving daily (see Chapter 10)
- **Adrenal Fight or Flight Stabilizer:** 1 Brain Shot daily (see Chapter 8)
- **Dreams Shifter:** 1 Brain Shot daily (see Chapter 8)
- **Trauma, Shock, and Loss Stabilizer:** 1 Brain Shot daily (see Chapter 8)
- **Betrayal and Broken Trust Stabilizer:** 1 Brain Shot daily (see Chapter 8)

- **Lemon Balm Shock Therapy:** if needed (see Chapter 3)
- **California Poppy Shock Therapy:** if needed (see Chapter 3)
- **5-MTHF:** 1 capsule daily
- **Aloe vera:** 2 or more inches of fresh gel (skin removed) daily
- **Ashwagandha:** 2 dropperfuls twice a day
- **Barley grass juice powder:** 2 teaspoons or 6 capsules daily
- **B-complex:** 1 capsule daily
- **California poppy:** 3 dropperfuls at bedtime daily
- **Cat's claw:** 1 dropperful daily
- **Celeryforce:** 3 capsules three times a day
- **Chrysanthemum:** 1 cup of tea daily
- **CoQ10:** 1 capsule daily
- **Curcumin:** 2 capsules twice a day
- **D-mannose:** 1 tablespoon in water daily
- **Elderflower:** 1 cup of tea daily
- **EPA and DHA (fish-free):** 1 capsule daily (taken with dinner)
- **GABA:** 1 250-milligram capsule daily
- **Lemon balm:** 5 dropperfuls three times a day
- **Licorice root:** 1 dropperful daily (two weeks on, two weeks off)
- **Magnesium glycinate:** 2 capsules twice a day
- **Melatonin:** 1 5-milligram capsule at bedtime daily
- **NAC:** 1 capsule daily
- **Nascent iodine:** 4 small drops (not dropperfuls) daily
- **Nettle leaf:** 3 dropperfuls twice a day
- **Peppermint:** 1 cup of tea twice a day
- **Spirulina:** 2 teaspoons or 6 capsules daily
- **Vitamin B$_{12}$ (as adenosylcobalamin with methylcobalamin):** 3 dropperfuls twice a day
- **Vitamin C (as Micro-C or comparable buffered vitamin C):** 2 500-milligram capsules twice a day
- **Wild blueberry:** 1 tablespoon powder or 2 ounces juice daily

PULLING SENSATION IN THE FACE (SUCH AS NOSE, EYES, OR FOREHEAD)

Refer to Cranial Nerve Inflammation protocol.

PULSATING SENSATIONS IN THE HEAD

Refer to Cranial Nerve Inflammation protocol.

RECREATIONAL DRUG WITHDRAWAL

Refer to Addiction protocol.

REPETITIVE STRAIN INJURIES (RSI)

Refer to Fibromyalgia protocol.

RESTLESS LEGS SYNDROME

Refer to Cranial Nerve Inflammation protocol and/or Shingles protocol.

RESTLESSNESS

Refer to Cranial Nerve Inflammation protocol.

RHEUMATOID ARTHRITIS (RA)

Refer to Autoimmune Disorders and Diseases protocol.

RIGHT NEGLECT

Refer to Hemispatial Neglect protocol.

RINGING IN EARS

Refer to Tinnitus protocol.

ROVING PAIN

Refer to Cranial Nerve Inflammation protocol.

SADNESS

Refer to Depression protocol and/or Chronic Mystery Guilt protocol.

SARCOIDOSIS

Refer to Autoimmune Disorders and Diseases protocol.

SCAR TISSUE ON BRAIN

Refer to Brain Lesions protocol.

SCHIZOPHRENIA

Before applying these, be sure to read Chapter 2, "Golden Rules of Supplements."

- **Fresh celery juice:** work up to 32 ounces daily

- **Heavy Metal Detox Smoothie:** 1 serving daily (see Chapter 10)

- **Extractor Smoothie:** 1 serving daily (see Chapter 10)

- **Pharmaceutical Exposure:** 1 Brain Shot daily (see Chapter 8)

- **Negative Energy Exposure:** 1 Brain Shot daily (see Chapter 8)

- **Obsessive Thoughts Exposure:** 1 Brain Shot daily (see Chapter 8)

- **Mood Shifter:** 1 Brain Shot daily (see Chapter 8)

- **Lemon Balm Shock Therapy:** if needed (see Chapter 3)

- **California Poppy Shock Therapy:** if needed (see Chapter 3)

- **Ashwagandha:** 2 dropperfuls twice a day

- **Kava kava:** 2 dropperfuls twice a day

- **Lemon balm:** 6 dropperfuls twice a day

- **Magnesium glycinate:** 3 capsules twice a day

- **Melatonin:** work up to 60 milligrams at bedtime daily

- **Milk thistle:** 2 dropperfuls twice a day

- **Nascent iodine:** 6 small drops (not dropperfuls) daily

- **Skullcap:** 2 dropperfuls twice a day

- **Vitamin B$_{12}$ (as adenosylcobalamin with methylcobalamin):** 2 dropperfuls twice a day

SCIATICA

Refer to Shingles protocol.

SEASONAL AFFECTIVE DISORDER (SAD)

Before applying these, be sure to read Chapter 2, "Golden Rules of Supplements."

- **Fresh celery juice:** work up to 32 ounces daily

- **Heavy Metal Detox Smoothie:** 1 serving daily (see Chapter 10)

- **Mood Shifter:** 1 Brain Shot daily (see Chapter 8)

- **Lemon Balm Shock Therapy:** if needed (see Chapter 3)

- **5-MTHF:** 1 capsule daily

- **Ashwagandha:** 1 dropperful daily

- **Barley grass juice powder:** 1 teaspoon or 3 capsules daily

- **B-complex:** 1 capsule daily

- **Celeryforce:** 3 capsules three times a day

- **Curcumin:** 2 capsules twice a day

- **EPA and DHA (fish-free):** 1 capsule daily (taken with dinner)

- Elderflower: 1 cup of tea daily
- Lemon balm: 4 dropperfuls twice a day
- Melatonin: 1 5-milligram capsule at bedtime daily
- Nascent iodine: 6 small drops (not dropperfuls) daily
- Raw honey: 1 tablespoon daily
- Red clover: 1 cup of tea daily
- Spirulina: 1 teaspoon or 3 capsules daily
- Turmeric: 2 capsules daily
- Vitamin B_{12} (as adenosylcobalamin with methylcobalamin): 2 dropperfuls twice a day
- Vitamin C (as Micro-C or comparable buffered vitamin C): 6 500-milligram capsules daily
- Vitamin D_3: 2,000 IU daily
- Wild blueberry: 1 tablespoon powder or 2 ounces juice daily
- Zinc (as liquid zinc sulfate): up to 2 dropperfuls daily

SEIZURES

Before applying these, be sure to read Chapter 2, "Golden Rules of Supplements."

- Fresh celery juice: work up to 32 ounces daily; then you have

the option to work up to 32 ounces twice a day

- Fresh cucumber juice: work up to 32 ounces daily
- Heavy Metal Detox Smoothie: 1 serving daily (see Chapter 10)
- Extractor Smoothie: 1 serving daily (see Chapter 10)
- Pharmaceutical Exposure: 1 Brain Shot daily (see Chapter 8)
- Radiation Exposure: 1 Brain Shot daily (see Chapter 8)
- Nerve Shifter: 1 Brain Shot daily (see Chapter 8)
- Lemon Balm Shock Therapy: if needed (see Chapter 3)
- B_{12} Shock Therapy: if needed (see Chapter 3)
- Curcumin: 2 capsules twice a day
- EPA and DHA (fish-free): 1 capsule daily (taken with dinner)
- Lemon balm: 1 dropperful twice a day
- Magnesium glycinate: 3 capsules twice a day
- Vitamin B_{12} (as adenosylcobalamin with methylcobalamin): 1 dropperful daily
- Vitamin C (as Micro-C or comparable buffered vitamin

C): 4 500-milligram capsules twice a day

- **Vitamin D$_3$:** 1,000 IU daily
- **Zinc (as liquid zinc sulfate):** 1 dropperful twice a day

SENSE OF NOT DIGESTING WELL

Refer to Vagus Nerve Problems protocol.

SHINGLES

Before applying these, be sure to read Chapter 2, "Golden Rules of Supplements."

- **Fresh celery juice:** work up to 32 ounces daily
- **Heavy Metal Detox Smoothie:** 1 serving daily (see Chapter 10)
- **Nerve Shifter:** 1 Brain Shot daily (see Chapter 8)
- **Any Shock Therapies from Chapter 3 can be used if needed**
- **Aloe vera:** 2 or more inches of fresh gel (skin removed) daily; also apply fresh gel to shingles rash
- **Barley grass juice powder:** 1 teaspoon or 3 capsules daily
- **California poppy:** 3 dropperfuls twice a day
- **Cat's claw:** 2 dropperfuls twice a day

- **Curcumin:** 3 capsules three times a day
- **Hyssop:** 1 cup of tea twice a day
- **Lemon balm:** 4 dropperfuls three times a day
- **Licorice root:** 2 dropperfuls twice a day (two weeks on, two weeks off)
- **L-lysine:** 6 500-milligram capsules twice a day
- **Mullein leaf:** 4 dropperfuls twice a day
- **Nettle leaf:** 4 dropperfuls twice a day
- **Propolis:** 3 dropperfuls three times a day
- **Spirulina:** 1 teaspoon or 3 capsules daily
- **Vitamin B$_{12}$ (as adenosylcobalamin with methylcobalamin):** 3 dropperfuls twice a day
- **Vitamin C (as Micro-C or comparable buffered vitamin C):** 8 500-milligram capsules twice a day
- **Wild blueberry:** 2 teaspoons powder or 2 ounces juice daily
- **Zinc (as liquid zinc sulfate):** 2 dropperfuls twice a day

SJÖGREN'S SYNDROME

Refer to Autoimmune Disorders and Diseases protocol.

SLEEP APNEA

Refer to Cranial Nerve Inflammation protocol.

SLEEP ISSUES

Refer to Insomnia protocol and/or Narcolepsy protocol.

SLURRED SPEECH

Refer to Cranial Nerve Inflammation protocol.

SPASMS

Refer to Cranial Nerve Inflammation protocol.

SPEECH DIFFICULTIES

Refer to Cranial Nerve Inflammation protocol, ADHD protocol, and/or Tourette's Syndrome protocol. There are multiple protocols as an option because there are multiple causes.

STIFFNESS (INCLUDING STIFF PERSON SYNDROME)

Refer to Cranial Nerve Inflammation protocol.

STOMACH BURNING

Refer to Stomach Problems protocol.

STOMACH FLIPPING

Refer to Vagus Nerve Problems protocol.

STOMACH PAIN

Refer to Stomach Problems protocol.

STOMACH PROBLEMS

Before applying these, be sure to read Chapter 2, "Golden Rules of Supplements."

- **Fresh celery juice:** work up to 32 ounces daily

- **Fresh cucumber juice:** work up to 32 ounces daily

- **Aloe Vera Shock Therapy:** if needed (see Chapter 3)

- **Mono Eating Cleanse:** consider one of the options from *Cleanse to Heal*

- **Aloe vera:** 2 or more inches of fresh gel (skin removed) daily, or work up to 16 ounces Aloe Water daily (see Chapter 12)

- **Licorice root:** 2 dropperfuls twice a day (three weeks on, one week off), plus option of 1 cup of tea daily as well (on same on/off schedule)

- **Lemon balm:** 1 cup of tea twice a day

- **Ginger:** 1 cup of tea or freshly grated or juiced to taste twice a day

- **Peppermint:** 1 cup of tea daily

- **Vitamin B$_{12}$ (as adenosylcobalamin with methylcobalamin):** 2 dropperfuls twice a day

- **Zinc (as liquid zinc sulfate):** 1 dropperful daily (can be swallowed or held in the mouth for 30 seconds or more and then spat out)

STROKES

Before applying these, be sure to read Chapter 2, "Golden Rules of Supplements."

- **Fresh celery juice:** work up to 32 ounces daily

- **Fresh cucumber juice:** work up to 32 ounces daily

- **Heavy Metal Detox Smoothie:** 1 serving daily (see Chapter 10)

- **Radiation Exposure:** 1 Brain Shot daily (see Chapter 8)

- **Toxic Heavy Metals Exposure:** 1 Brain Shot twice a day for three days after medical testing (see Chapter 8)

- **Pathogen Exposure:** 1 Brain Shot daily (see Chapter 8)

- **5-HTP:** 1 capsule at bedtime daily

- **5-MTHF:** 1 capsule daily

- **Amla berry:** 1 teaspoon or 3 capsules daily

- **Barley grass juice powder:** 1 teaspoon or 3 capsules daily

- **Celeryforce:** 3 capsules twice a day

- **CoQ10:** 1 capsule twice a day

- **Curcumin:** 3 capsules twice a day

- **Glutathione:** 2 capsules twice a day

- **Hawthorn berry:** 1 dropperful twice a day

- **Hibiscus:** 1 cup of tea with 2 tea bags daily

- **Lemon balm:** 4 dropperfuls twice a day

- **L-glutamine:** 1 500-milligram capsule twice a day

- **Magnesium glycinate:** 3 capsules twice a day

- **Melatonin:** 1 5-milligram capsule at bedtime daily
- **Reishi mushroom powder:** 1 teaspoon or 3 capsules daily
- **Selenium:** 1 capsule twice a week
- **Spirulina:** 1 teaspoon or 3 capsules daily
- **Vitamin B$_{12}$ (as adenosylcobalamin with methylcobalamin):** 2 dropperfuls twice a day
- **Vitamin C (as Micro-C or comparable buffered vitamin C):** 6 500-milligram capsules twice a day
- **Wild blueberry:** 2 teaspoons powder or 2 ounces juice daily
- **Zinc (as liquid zinc sulfate):** 1 dropperful daily

SUN SENSITIVITY

Refer to Cold Sensitivity protocol.

SUNSPOTS

Refer to Hyperpigmentation protocol.

SWALLOWING DIFFICULTY

Refer to Vagus Nerve Problems protocol.

SYSTEMIC EXERTION INTOLERANCE DISEASE (SEID)

Refer to ME/CFS protocol.

TENDONITIS

Refer to Fibromyalgia protocol.

TENNIS ELBOW

Refer to Fibromyalgia protocol.

THROAT PAIN, PRESSURE, OR TIGHTNESS (MYSTERY)

Refer to Vagus Nerve Problems protocol.

TICS

Refer to Cranial Nerve Inflammation protocol.

TINGLES

Refer to Cranial Nerve Inflammation protocol.

TINNITUS

Before applying these, be sure to read Chapter 2, "Golden Rules of Supplements."

- **Fresh celery juice:** work up to 32 ounces daily; then you have the option to work up to 32 ounces twice a day

- **Heavy Metal Detox Smoothie:** 1 serving daily (see Chapter 10)

- **Sleep and Recharging Stabilizer:** 1 Brain Shot daily (see Chapter 8)

- **Nerve Shifter:** 1 Brain Shot daily (see Chapter 8)

- **Any Shock Therapies from Chapter 3 can be used if needed**

- **5-MTHF:** 1 capsule daily

- **ALA (alpha lipoic acid):** 1 capsule twice a week

- **Barley grass juice powder:** 2 teaspoons or 6 capsules daily

- **Cat's claw:** 2 dropperfuls twice a day

- **Celeryforce:** 1 capsule twice a day

- **Chaga mushroom powder:** 2 teaspoons or 6 capsules daily

- **Curcumin:** 3 capsules twice a day

- **Lemon balm:** 4 dropperfuls twice a day

- **Licorice root:** 1 dropperful twice a day (two weeks on, two weeks off)

- **L-lysine:** 6 500-milligram capsules twice a day

- **Lomatium root:** 2 dropperfuls twice a day

- **Magnesium glycinate:** 1 capsule twice a day

- **Monolaurin:** 1 capsule daily

- **Mullein leaf:** 3 dropperfuls twice a day

- **Nettle leaf:** 3 dropperfuls twice a day

- **Olive leaf:** 1 dropperful twice a day

- **Oregano oil:** 1 capsule twice a day

- **Propolis:** 1 dropperful twice a day

- **Spirulina:** 2 teaspoons or 6 capsules daily

- **Vitamin B$_{12}$ (as adenosylcobalamin with methylcobalamin):** 3 dropperfuls twice a day

- **Vitamin C (as Micro-C or comparable buffered vitamin C):** 6 500-milligram capsules twice a day

- **Wild blueberry:** 1 tablespoon powder or 2 ounces juice daily

- **Zinc (as liquid zinc sulfate):** 2 dropperfuls twice a day

TMJ (TEMPOROMANDIBULAR JOINT DYSFUNCTION)

Refer to Shingles protocol.

TONGUE PAIN (MYSTERY)

Refer to Shingles protocol and/or Herpes Simplex 1 and 2 protocol.

TOOTH GRINDING

Refer to Shingles protocol and/or Herpes Simplex 1 and 2 protocol.

TOOTH PAIN (MYSTERY)

Refer to Shingles protocol and/or Herpes Simplex 1 and 2 protocol.

TOURETTE'S SYNDROME

Before applying these, be sure to read Chapter 2, "Golden Rules of Supplements."

- **Fresh celery juice:** work up to 32 ounces daily
- **Fresh cucumber juice:** work up to 32 ounces daily
- **Heavy Metal Detox Smoothie:** 1 serving daily (see Chapter 10)
- **Extractor Smoothie:** 1 serving daily (see Chapter 10)
- **Nerve Shifter:** 1 Brain Shot daily (see Chapter 8)

- **Lemon Balm Shock Therapy:** if needed (see Chapter 3)
- **Aloe vera:** 2 or more inches of fresh gel (skin removed) daily
- **Barley grass juice powder:** 1 teaspoon or 3 capsules daily
- **B-complex:** 1 capsule daily
- **Celeryforce:** 1 capsule twice a day
- **Chaga mushroom powder:** 1 teaspoon or 3 capsules daily
- **Elderflower:** 1 cup of tea daily
- **EPA and DHA (fish-free):** 1 capsule daily (taken with dinner)
- **Glutathione:** 1 capsule daily
- **Lemon balm:** 2 dropperfuls twice a day
- **L-glutamine:** 1 500-milligram capsule twice a day
- **Magnesium glycinate:** 1 capsule twice a day
- **Rose hips:** 1 cup of tea daily
- **Silica:** 1 teaspoon daily
- **Spirulina:** 1 teaspoon or 3 capsules daily
- **Vitamin B$_{12}$ (as adenosylcobalamin with methylcobalamin):** 1 dropperful twice a day
- **Vitamin C (as Micro-C or comparable buffered vitamin C):** 2 500-milligram capsules twice a day

- **Wild blueberry:** 2 teaspoons powder or 2 ounces juice daily

TRANSIENT ISCHEMIC ATTACK (TIA)

Refer to Strokes protocol.

TREMBLING HANDS

Refer to Cranial Nerve Inflammation protocol.

TREMORS

Refer to Cranial Nerve Inflammation protocol.

TRIGEMINAL NEURALGIA

Refer to Shingles protocol and/or Herpes Simplex 1 and 2 protocol.

TRIGGER FINGER

Refer to Fibromyalgia protocol.

TWITCHES, INCLUDING TWITCHING AROUND HEAD AND FACE

Refer to Cranial Nerve Inflammation protocol.

ULCERATIVE COLITIS

Refer to Shingles protocol.

ULCERS

Refer to Stomach Problems protocol.

UNSPECIFIED FEEDING OR EATING DISORDER (UFED)

Refer to Eating Disorders protocol.

VAGUS NERVE PROBLEMS

Before applying these, be sure to read Chapter 2, "Golden Rules of Supplements."

- **Fresh celery juice:** work up to 32 ounces daily
- **Heavy Metal Detox Smoothie:** 1 serving daily (see Chapter 10)
- **Toxic Fragrances Exposure:** 1 Brain Shot daily (see Chapter 8)
- **Nerve Shifter:** 1 Brain Shot daily (see Chapter 8)
- **Lemon Balm Shock Therapy:** if needed (see Chapter 3)
- **Aloe Vera Shock Therapy:** if needed (see Chapter 3)
- **Aloe vera:** 2 or more inches of fresh gel (skin removed) daily
- **GABA:** 1 250-milligram capsule daily

- **Ginger:** 1 cup of tea or freshly grated or juiced to taste daily

- **Hops:** 1 cup of tea daily

- **Lemon balm:** 3 dropperfuls twice a day

- **Licorice root:** 2 dropperfuls twice a day plus 1 cup of tea daily (both on same schedule of three weeks on, one week off)

- **Magnesium glycinate:** 2 capsules twice a day

- **Peppermint:** 1 cup of tea daily

- **Raw honey:** 1 tablespoon daily

- **Skullcap:** 1 dropperful twice a day

- **Vitamin B$_{12}$ (as adenosylcobalamin with methylcobalamin):** 1 dropperful twice a day

- **Mono Eating Cleanses:** if needed, any of the Medical Medium Mono Eating Cleanse options from *Cleanse to Heal*

VASCULITIS

Refer to Autoimmune Disorders and Diseases protocol.

VERTIGO

Before applying these, be sure to read Chapter 2, "Golden Rules of Supplements."

You can integrate the Vagus Nerve Problems protocol with this list or apply the Vagus Nerve Problems protocol instead of this list if you desire.

- **Fresh celery juice:** work up to 32 ounces daily

- **Heavy Metal Detox Smoothie:** 1 serving daily (see Chapter 10)

- **Nerve Shifter:** 1 Brain Shot daily (see Chapter 8)

- **Lemon Balm Shock Therapy:** if needed (see Chapter 3)

- **Barley grass juice powder:** 2 teaspoons or 6 capsules daily

- **B-complex:** 1 capsule daily

- **Cat's claw:** 2 dropperfuls twice a day

- **Celeryforce:** 2 capsules twice a day

- **Chaga mushroom powder:** 2 teaspoons or 6 capsules daily

- **Curcumin:** 2 capsules twice a day

- **EPA and DHA (fish-free):** 1 capsule daily (taken with dinner)

- **Eyebright:** 1 dropperful daily

- **Ginger:** 1 cup of tea or freshly grated or juiced to taste daily

- **Lemon balm:** 3 dropperfuls three times a day

- **L-glutamine:** 1 capsule daily

- **Licorice root:** 1 dropperful daily (two weeks on, two weeks off)

- **L-lysine:** 5 500-milligram capsules twice a day
- **Lomatium root:** 2 dropperfuls twice a day
- **Magnesium glycinate:** 1 capsule daily
- **Monolaurin:** 1 capsule daily
- **Mullein leaf:** 3 dropperfuls twice a day
- **Olive leaf:** 1 dropperful twice a day
- **Spirulina:** 2 teaspoons or 6 capsules daily
- **Vitamin B$_{12}$ (as adenosylcobalamin with methylcobalamin):** 2 dropperfuls twice a day
- **Vitamin C (as Micro-C or comparable buffered vitamin C):** 4 500-milligram capsules twice a day
- **Wild blueberry:** 2 teaspoons powder or 2 ounces juice daily
- **Zinc (as liquid zinc sulfate):** 2 dropperfuls twice a day

VIBRATING FACE AND/OR HEAD

Refer to Cranial Nerve Inflammation protocol.

VIBRATING IN EARS

Refer to Tinnitus protocol.

VIRAL INFECTION FATIGUE

Refer to ME/CFS protocol.

VISUAL DISTURBANCES

Refer to Cranial Nerve Inflammation protocol.

VOMITING (MYSTERY)

Refer to Vagus Nerve Problems protocol and/or Stomach Problems protocol.

WEAKNESS OF LIMBS

Refer to Cranial Nerve Inflammation protocol.

WHITE SPOTS ON BRAIN

Refer to Brain Lesions protocol.

WHOOSHING SOUNDS IN EARS

Refer to Tinnitus protocol.

WILLIS-EKBOM DISEASE

Refer to Cranial Nerve Inflammation protocol and/or Shingles protocol.

WILSON'S DISEASE

Refer to Cranial Nerve Inflammation protocol.

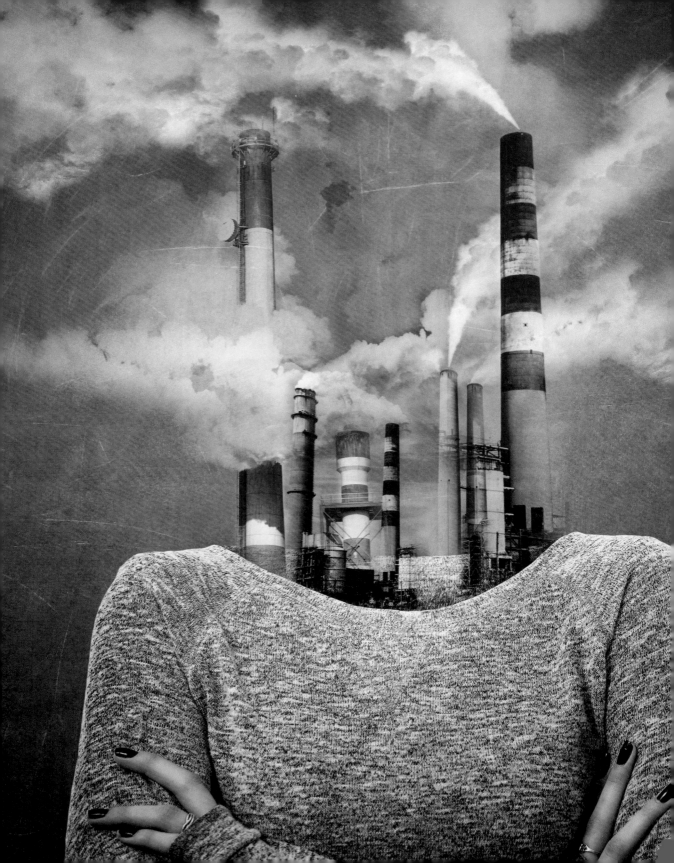

PART II

BRAIN BETRAYERS

"People are afraid of lemons, bananas, grapes, fruit sugars eroding their teeth . . . yet have they consumed 10,000 or even 1,000 lemons or bananas or grapes in their lifetime? No. They *have* had chocolate or coffee 10,000 times or more. Say you regularly consume vinegar. You could have consumed well over 20 gallons of vinegar in 10 years. And still, it's the bananas and lemons and grapes— the healing options we could all benefit from bringing into our lives in greater quantities—that we're warned away from, not the coffee, chocolate, or vinegar."

— Anthony William, Medical Medium

CHAPTER 5

Brain Betrayer Foods

You may look at this list of brain betrayer foods and think, *This is a list of what I should be eating.* That's how misleading food trends and food advice can be. Some of the foods in this chapter slow down, interfere with, or even stop the healing process. Some of the foods accelerate neurological symptoms and chronic illness. And some of these foods start additional health problems.

While it may seem overwhelming to try to avoid one or more of the brain betrayer foods, know that the restored health you get out of it will be more than worth it. It's not about deprivation or judgment. You're not a good or bad person based on what you eat.

Go slowly if you want:

Experiment with replacing a few of the top items on this list with some of the healing options in Chapter 12, "Medical Medium Brain Saver Recipes."

Check out the Cravings Shifter Brain Shot in Chapter 8, "Medical Medium Brain Shot Therapy," for support.

Consider a 10-day Brain Shot Therapy Cleanse option from Chapter 9, or a 15-day Heavy Metal Detox Cleanse option from Chapter 11, knowing that you could someday work up to any of the longer cleanse options in those chapters if you wish.

You can also find a handy list of health-promoting foods in the chapter "Brain Cell Food and Filler Food" in this book's companion title, *Brain Saver.* Keeping that list nearby, along with the Brain Saver Recipes in this book, will remind you that you have delicious alternatives to the brain betrayer foods in this chapter.

These foods are listed with the worst at the top. If you're sick or suffering and looking for relief, start by avoiding the foods at the top of this list. As you seek more healing, you can continue to work your way down the list.

1. Eggs

2. Dairy (including milk, cheese, butter, ghee, yogurt, cream, and kefir)

3. Gluten

4. Caffeine (including coffee, green tea, matcha, chocolate, and cacao)

5. Alcohol (consumed more than occasionally)

6. Vinegar (including apple cider vinegar, or ACV)

7. Pork products (including ham, bacon, sausage, pancetta, canned pork product, lard, pulled pork, pork chops, pork belly, and pork rinds)

8. Tuna

9. Corn (including corn products such as corn syrup and corn starch)

10. Industrial food oils (including vegetable oil, palm oil, palm kernel oil, canola [rapeseed] oil, corn oil, safflower oil, soybean oil, cottonseed oil, peanut oil, hydrogenated oils, and margarine)

11. Kombucha

12. Nutritional yeast

13. Soy (including tofu, edamame, soy milk, soy sauce, miso, soybeans, soy nuts, texturized vegetable protein [TVP], soy protein powder, and artificial meat products made with soy)

14. GMO (bioengineered) foods

15. Bone broth

16. Problematic fish and seafood (including catfish, red snapper, striped bass, bluefish, swordfish, grouper, clams, oysters, mussels, shrimp, crab, lobster, squid, octopus, scallops, flounder, tilapia, and shark)

17. Lamb

18. Salt

19. Fermented foods (including sauerkraut, pickled preserves, sourdough, cheese, and yogurt [animal- or plant-based])

20. Grains eaten in an unproductive way

It's no mystery how brain betrayer foods enter our lives: we eat and drink them. What does sometimes sneak up on us is how much of them we eat. For example, it's easy to eat a high-fat diet because we've been dazzled by the high-protein trend, not stopping to think or even realizing that protein sources are almost always fat sources too. On top of which, now we're being told that lots of fat is good for us, so we pile more fats onto our plates, or into our blenders as we make our trendy smoothies, with no idea that we're doing our brains a disservice.

Some of these items, such as canola oil, nutritional yeast, and corn, frequently make it into our meals without our knowledge. Any time you see that an oil *blend* is being used, beware—there's a good chance it contains one of these brain betrayers. Even oils labeled as pure are sometimes diluted with canola or corn oil, so seek out high-quality oil whenever possible and even better, limit your use of oil in general to keep your fat consumption lower to protect your body and brain.

The main issue with most of these brain betrayer foods is that they feed viruses in the body such as EBV and bacteria such as *Streptococcus*—viruses and bacteria that many, many people unknowingly harbor in dormant form. These viruses and bacteria can come out of dormancy if they receive the right fuel. Some of these foods don't directly feed viruses and bacteria. Instead, usually because of their high fat content, these other foods foster an environment in our body that allows pathogens to thrive. Either way, whether a food directly feeds pathogens or fosters a hospitable environment for pathogens, the food doesn't help *us* thrive. Viruses and bacteria especially proliferate when we're eating eggs, milk, cheese, butter, all other dairy products, gluten, soy, pork, corn, or an overall high-fat diet.

As you can read more about in the *Brain Saver* chapter "Your Viral Brain," publicly known medical research and science aren't aware that viruses "eat." Viruses do eat,

and that's how they stay alive. They don't exist on mystical energy; viruses stay active by absorbing unproductive chemical compounds through their outer membranes. Viruses then process whatever they take in and release it as waste matter such as neurotoxins and dermatoxins. When they reach the central nervous system, these neurotoxins cause hundreds of symptoms and conditions.

Some of these brain betrayer foods themselves are also not good for the brain. We're often told eggs are good for the brain because of their omegas. We're not told that because eggs are filled with hormones that intercept healthy hormones involved with the brain, any benefit is outweighed. Same goes for dairy. Even eggs and dairy sourced farm fresh from organic, grass-fed, pasture-raised, and/or free-range cows and chickens contain hormones that intercept and confuse the hormones involved in our systems.

1. Eggs

Circa 1910, classified medical research and science discovered that the undeveloped protein inside eggs fed viruses and bacteria. This led to a method for the past 100 years of raising pathogens on eggs and then releasing the pathogens into our environment. Autoimmune and chronic neurological symptoms, many of which are involved with brain inflammation, are caused by viruses. When we eat eggs, we can feed the very viruses keeping us sick with chronic neurological symptoms and conditions.

2. Dairy (including milk, cheese, butter, ghee, yogurt, cream, and kefir)

Dairy's combination of both fat and sugar weakens the liver and pancreas, causing insulin resistance. At the same time, dairy allows pathogens to thrive in two ways: (1) the lactose and dairy proteins in dairy products feed viruses such as EBV, HIV, HPV, and many more, as well as bad bacteria such as *Streptococcus* and *H. pylori* inside the intestinal tract and liver. Meanwhile, (2) the fat from dairy causes high blood fat, limiting oxygen and allowing pathogens to proliferate and colonize inside the bloodstream and organs, in turn leading to worsened neurological symptoms and conditions.

(While plant-based cheese is a tempting alternative to cheese made from dairy milk, keep this in mind: even though it's not made out of animal products, plant-based cheese can be so similar to dairy cheese that it does cause problems. Plant-based cheese can mimic dairy cheese so closely that it can be just as inflammatory, trip up signals to the brain's emotional centers, and open the floodgates to degrading our health as if it were a dairy product. Plus, plant-based cheese is a fermented product with many fillers and additives. As you'll read in a few pages, fermentation can have its own disrupting effect on our health.)

3. Gluten

Gluten itself is not inflammatory to the body. This is why many people can consume gluten and not have any difficulties with their health. It's pathogens such as viruses and bacteria that cause inflammation inside the body and autoimmune disorders and diseases, and those viruses and bacteria use gluten as a food. This allows pathogens to grow in number, eventually causing the symptoms and conditions that people struggle with, including conditions they believe are gluten-caused. Intestinal conditions that worsen because of consuming gluten do so because bad, unproductive bacteria and viruses inside the intestinal tract are feeding on the gluten, creating the symptoms.

4. Caffeine (including coffee, green tea, matcha, chocolate, and cacao)

What makes caffeine a psychoactive drug? Caffeine is not a psychoactive drug simply because it's a substance that changes behavior and mood. In order for a substance to be a psychoactive drug, it has to be poisonous to the brain. It has to be toxic, causing chemical imbalances and chemical disturbances. It's this intoxication of our brain cells that creates emotional and mental changes as the drug stimulates our brain cells to react to the poisonous substance.

So caffeine creates a brain reaction. This reaction is to try to expel the caffeine because it's a poison. When brain cells try to expel caffeine as caffeine enters them, brain cells also expel critically needed chemical compounds and nutrients. The expelling process destroys amino acids too. (The brain contains a small amount of naturally occurring amino acids, some created in the liver, some that we ingest from our foods. Caffeine destroys naturally occurring amino acids in the brain.)

This reaction creates excitement within the brain: excitement and stimulation that take us out of mundane states. Caffeine causes brain cells to vibrate—a subtle shaking occurs in brain cells on a microscopic level. This is a reaction when a brain cell is poisoned. It's the same reaction that occurs with a venomous snake bite, spider bite, or neurotoxic substance. Caffeine puts the brain cells in a state of crisis, requiring a signal from the brain to the adrenal glands. This is how caffeine prompts adrenaline: by poisoning the brain, which in turn sends an alarm bell to the adrenals to release adrenaline (epinephrine). It's the crisis alarm of a psychoactive, neurotoxic drug.

Adrenaline enters the brain, allowing somebody to wake up or stay awake, become alert, and think more clearly. Adrenaline calms the shaking and rattling of the brain cells because it's steroidal and suppresses the toxic reaction of the caffeine, and gives somebody a euphoric caffeine and adrenaline high. (If the adrenaline high were missing, the caffeine would feel uncomfortable. This is why so many people who have adrenal fatigue are more sensitive to caffeine. Their adrenals don't produce enough adrenaline to override the

poisonous effects.) What goes up must come down. Over time, as the adrenaline leaves the brain, it leaves with much of the caffeine, getting you ready to do it all over again the same day or the next day.

It often takes someone taking a break from caffeine to realize the disruptive effect it was having on them. Read more about caffeine's brain and nervous system effects in *Brain Saver*'s "Caffeine" chapter.

5. Alcohol (consumed more than occasionally)

Refer to "Alcohol" in Chapter 7, "Brain Betrayer Food and Supplement Chemicals" for a glimpse into alcohol as a brain betrayer. Find in-depth information on recreational alcohol use in the "Alcohol" chapter in *Brain Saver*.

6. Vinegar (including apple cider vinegar, or ACV)

The acetic acid in vinegar diminishes neurotransmitter activity and slows down the renewal process of glial cells in the brain by dehydrating them. The acidity of vinegar also accelerates the oxidation process of toxic heavy metals by corroding them more quickly, causing the toxic heavy metals in the brain to erupt and flake, accelerating the spread of toxic heavy metal byproduct to adjacent brain tissue.

People are already chronically acidic, with all body systems on the acidic side of the scale, so the body is already in a fight for homeostasis to try to at least become neutral. Vinegar derails that fight for homeostasis. Even when including vinegar in a trendy plant-derived or animal protein diet that's said to be alkalizing, vinegar makes it nearly impossible for all body systems to become alkaline. You can have a completely plant-based diet and still be acidic. Do not get fooled by acidity/alkalinity testing with pH strips. Vinegar leaches calcium out of our bones and teeth in order to buffer the acidic shock that vinegar creates inside the body. Calcium is alkaline. As we urinate calcium out of our body onto a pH strip, we sometimes see an alkaline reading, when in reality, we're losing our alkalinity and the body is more acidic than ever. You can't get an accurate reading on a pH strip with vinegar and other brain betrayers in the diet.

We need a certain amount of living, beneficial sodium from plant sources inside our bloodstream and a certain amount of living, beneficial sodium inside our spinal fluid as part of the critical electrolyte complex that sustains our brain and body. For example, living, beneficial sodium is meant to help replenish neurotransmitter chemicals, strengthen neurons, and fortify every brain cell. Vinegar disturbs this balance by hijacking sodium, forcing sodium to do vinegar's bidding. Vinegar turns living, beneficial sodium against the body by causing that sodium to dehydrate cells, versus living sodium's purpose of helping with hydration of cells.

Naturally occurring sodium from plant foods doesn't have a message or information within it to turn against cells and force dehydration within the cell. Only added salt in the diet (including healthier salts such as sea salt or rock salt) is inherently dehydrating. Vinegar turns even naturally occurring trace mineral salts in fruits, leafy greens, herbs, wild foods, and vegetables into small bioweapons. The acetic acid in vinegar attaches itself to sodium, not allowing sodium to do what it's meant to do. With acetic acid attached to sodium entering cells, cells are forced to excrete fluid, dehydrating cells in the brain—and essentially pickling the brain.

By the way, vinegar coupled with added salt is even more dehydrating—and rarely does anyone enjoy vinegar without added salt. Salt is traditionally in every recipe where vinegar is.

7. Pork Products (including ham, bacon, sausage, pancetta, canned pork product, lard, pulled pork, pork chops, pork belly, and pork rinds)

Pork's high fat content suffocates the brain by diminishing oxygen levels to brain cells. When fat from pork enters the brain through the bloodstream, it accelerates oxidation of toxic heavy metals in the brain. Pork fat also accelerates brain atrophy, shrinking the brain in one's older years, because fat from pork doesn't allow glucose—the brain's number one fuel source—to easily enter brain cells. That is, pork is a glucose inhibitor: fat from pork contributes to starving brain cells of what they need.

Pork fat also weakens the pancreas, diminishing digestive strength and lowering insulin production and insulin reserves.

8. Tuna

We often think of tuna as only a mercury-ridden fish, when in reality, tuna is an all-toxic-heavy-metals fish. Tuna is high in mercury, toxic copper, aluminum, cadmium, and even lead. Metals from tuna find their way to the liver easily, eventually oxidizing there. That oxidation and toxic heavy metal byproduct is then released back into the bloodstream and into the bile fluid traveling to other areas of the body. Next, the oxidized material can travel through the bloodstream to the brain.

The viruses and other pathogens that live inside our livers love mercury and other toxic heavy metals. Tuna provides pathogens with an abundance of food so they can thrive and proliferate. For example, feeding on mercury allows a virus to produce mercury-based neurotoxins that accelerate neurological brain diseases.

There are fish that have lower amounts of oil and fish that have higher amounts of oil. When you're eating a fish such as tuna, which has higher oil, it allows mercury and other toxic heavy metals to escape directly into the bloodstream through the intestinal tract lining too. That's because when you're eating tuna, you're getting accelerated bile production to break down its oil. That bile is dispersing the tuna's oil, and mercury is in that oil. As the oil gets dispersed, it spreads

mercury. So tuna's high fat content works against you, allowing mercury to easily enter the bloodstream through the intestinal lining and, via the bloodstream, reach the brain. This happens in addition to tuna's mercury and other toxic heavy metals entering the liver through the hepatic portal vein.

9. Corn (including corn products such as corn syrup and corn starch)

It's unfortunate that corn is in this list. Corn would not be a brain betrayer if it weren't contaminated by the GMO and pharmaceutical industries. Industries have weaponized corn going back a hundred years. Corn is currently used in all pharmaceuticals—GMO (bioengineered) medical-grade industrial corn is produced for manufactured GMO drugs.

Whether we're consuming our corn in food products or pharmaceuticals, GMO glucose confuses the brain. It's like somebody spiking your gasoline with diesel. Your engine would quickly become confused in that scenario, if it could think. GMO glucose confuses the brain because it's missing components that non-GMO glucose contains. Glucose is not just glucose. It's a chemical compound with more complexities than medical research and science understand. Glucose has never been studied properly or efficiently. GMO glucose is lacking components that fuel brain cells at the same time it provides components that are foreign to brain cells. It's Frankensteined glucose, missing things the brain needs while delivering things the brain doesn't need.

Corn eaten by itself, without butter or any fats or oils, would be a beneficial food if not for GMO contamination. The glucose from corn would actually be a good glucose for the brain in a perfect world without cross-contamination or GMOs. Even organic corn can be cross-contaminated. If you're not struggling with symptoms or conditions and you choose to eat organic heirloom corn and you feel it's safer than other varieties, eat it without the oil and butter and fat. Eat it in a mono fashion, or eat it in a salad without oil or fats, and then you can utilize the benefits of the corn.

10. Industrial Food Oils (including vegetable oil, palm oil, palm kernel oil, canola [rapeseed] oil, corn oil, safflower oil, soybean oil, cottonseed oil, peanut oil, hydrogenated oils, and margarine)

Industrial oils are not natural to our body systems. If someone receives a healthy oil, like when they're chewing a walnut and naturally extract the healthy oil out of that walnut, their body systems don't see this as a foreign invader. Just because industrial oils are originally derived from natural sources before they were industrialized—just because they're not synthesized oils—does not mean our bodies invite them with open arms as a natural food source that the body can utilize and see as healthy.

Industrial oils stop electrolytes from getting to the brain and even swallow up electrolytes. Industrial oils are sticky and attach to brain tissue, so when industrial oils enter the brain, they do not always leave the brain. When oil from an olive or walnut or coconut travels to the brain, most of the oil will travel back out of the brain. Why? These oils have less ability to bind on to tissue because the fruit and nut they come from carry anti-binding compounds undiscovered by research and science. Industrial oils, on the other hand, tend to block passageways, plump, congeal, cling to brain tissue, and interfere with neurons and neurotransmitters while blocking nutrients from absorbing into the brain because they interfere with glucose absorption.

A lifelong diet of industrial oils can lead to a fatty brain while simultaneously causing atrophy and deterioration of brain tissue. It's a shrinking of the brain while replacing what's lost with fat deposits in and around the brain. These fat deposits are often found in a cadaver's brain without the understanding of why they are there. This is similar to a heart that's collecting fat deposits in the valves and arteries and ventricles.

As problematic as industrial food oils are in their "normal" form, frying and cooking them takes it to another level of denaturing the oil. These low-grade oils are already denatured and rancid from industrial processing. Cooking and frying makes them radically foreign to the body.

11. Kombucha

There's confusion about kombucha. People hear it prevents disease, when in reality it does the opposite. All symptoms and conditions resulting in disease accelerate when all body systems become acidic, and kombucha contributes to acidity. The funny thing is, you see people who know the body should be alkaline drinking their acidifying kombucha.

Kombucha tea contains acetic acid, which is harmful to the brain. The environment in and around the brain has to be alkaline in order to protect the brain and allow the brain to thrive, produce new brain cells, and keep away disease. Every time kombucha tea is consumed, the brain environment becomes acidic—which halts the brain's process of rejuvenating or healing and instead flips a switch to the opposite direction of allowing any kind of disease state to press forward.

Acetic acid in kombucha tea is different from acetic acid in vinegar, though they are similar. They're both bad. Yet the acetic acid in kombucha tea is attached to glutamic acid (which is a foundation of MSG) and traces of alcohol. All three of these (acetic acid, glutamic acid, and alcohol) are biohazards to your brain. The kombucha tea industry will fight hard to convince you there's no glutamic acid in it. The simple truth is that glutamic acid can't be avoided whenever yeast is involved.

Acetic acid in kombucha tea accelerates the oxidation of toxic heavy metals in the brain, which can lead to more depression and anxiety. Someone likely doesn't know kombucha tea is harming them. If they're drinking kombucha tea, they're usually into health, which means that most likely they're consuming other items that are countering the immediate ill effects from kombucha tea. For example, they're most likely consuming green smoothies, occasional green juices, occasional celery juice, avocado toast, healthier fats such as nuts and seeds, more vegetables, more water, and occasionally a little bit of fruit. They're not eating lots of fast foods and they're not eating as much processed food. If someone didn't unknowingly counterbalance kombucha with these measures, they would truly feel how detrimental kombucha tea's acetic acid–glutamic acid–alcohol composition is to the brain. If someone were to live on kombucha tea for a month versus living on bananas for a month, you would see how much harm is caused by the kombucha.

There's also caffeine present in kombucha tea, which results in an adrenaline surge. Once again, the caffeine industry has addicted people to a product. Kombucha tea survives not just because of the marketing and money behind it. Kombucha tea survives because its caffeine gives people added energy, which is a false added energy.

Just because kombucha tea was used in ancient times doesn't mean it was ever good for us. Any and all fermented foods were survival foods that kept people alive when no other food was available. Kombucha wasn't a key to living a longer, healthier life. It was a choice made in survival mode, when there was a lack of fresh fruits, leafy greens, herbs, wild foods, or vegetables available to promote well-being.

12. Nutritional Yeast

People think nutritional yeast has beneficial vitamin B_{12}. It doesn't. Any B_{12} in nutritional yeast has been added, and it's the wrong B_{12} that's added, one that's not beneficial to the brain or nervous system. When they manufacture processed white bread, they strip the nutrients from the grain and then "fortify" the bread by putting nutrients back in. Nutritional yeast is similar. It needs to be fortified because it's lacking so many nutrients.

Nutritional yeast also has a naturally occurring MSG, a variety of glutamic acid that is different from glutamic acid in other foods. When any yeast grows, glutamic acid forms. This glutamic acid is specifically designed for the yeast itself, not designed for the human body. It's yeast-personalized. So this glutamic acid becomes a foreign invader to the brain, a byproduct that's hard to cleanse or detox or remove because the glutamic acid crystallizes on and around neurons.

Imagine tiny crystals that harden. These tiny crystals don't perform as badly as toxic heavy metal deposits in the brain do because they are not conductors like metals. The glutamic acid crystals cause excessive heating of neurons when someone gets excited, in a happy way or an unhappy way, because the crystals are insulating the neurons. The additional heat created from electricity running through neurons coated with these hardened, crystallized MSG deposits can cause headaches, weaknesses in the central nervous system, mild fatigue,

inconsistencies when blood sugar drops (making someone more temperamental, likely to blow a fuse faster). Also, MSG deposits can help accelerate all manner of brain diseases by heating the neurons. Glutamic acid is an electrical dampener for the brain.

If someone is already dealing with brain and neurological problems for any reason, glutamic acid crystals can amplify the problems if enough crystals are present. Excessive nutritional yeast consumption can bring someone to that larger amount of glutamic acid crystal buildup, bringing about larger deposits and more of them. Too many years of nutritional yeast consumption can be detrimental for somebody's health, especially if they're already susceptible from living with a symptom or condition.

13. Soy (including tofu, edamame, soy milk, soy sauce, miso, soybeans, soy nuts, texturized vegetable protein [TVP], soy protein powder, and artificial meat products made with soy)

The brain is an organ that gathers and disseminates information. It's the organ that sends signals throughout the body. All food has information in it as well. Since the beginning of humankind, our brains have communicated with the food we've ingested.

Natural foods on the planet need to stay natural, not be tampered with to the point that they become unnatural, because there's communication between these natural foods and the brain that allows information in those foods to communicate with the brain and body. GMO (bioengineered) foods such as soy break those communication lines. Our brain does not adapt to GMO foods. Our brain is not man-made. The first human being wasn't created as a science project in a GMO lab, and neither were the foods that fed our brains up until this time in history. All GMO foods are brain disruptors. They are the ultimate brain betrayers because the messaging inside that GMO food is destructive. It's designed to dismantle balance and continuity of brain health. Our brain understands this destructive message.

All soy is cross-contaminated at this point. When we grow natural food, the plants are designing their edible components for human and animal consumption, so the nutrients and phytochemical compounds within are designed to give the human body an opportunity to heal, perform, and grow. GMO foods are not designed for human consumption. GMO foods are designed to protect themselves, not the person consuming them. GMO plants are not designed to nurture and feed. The natural mission of the plant changes when it's genetically modified.

We consume foods to feed our brain and protect our brain from oxidative stress and free radicals. GMO foods such as soy do the opposite. Instead of protecting the brain, they leave our brain vulnerable. GMO soy can feed viruses and bacteria. And because organic soy is cross-contaminated now, soy is not something you want to play with.

Soy is misleading. We see it as a protein source. Really, it's high in fat, and not healthy fat. Soy oil is not a healthy fat. Soy should be considered an overt, radical fat rather than a protein source. As a result of this fat content, soy is a glucose inhibitor.

Plus, soy is usually not eaten on its own. There's usually added fat with soy, such as canola oil or olive oil added to soy products. Many soy products also contain MSG, and this MSG factor is reason enough to stay away from all soy products.

In small dosages, non-GMO soy may not cause a problem for someone who's not struggling yet with any kind of condition. For anyone struggling with a symptom or condition related to the brain or nervous system, soy can be disruptive as it inhibits or suppresses neurotransmitter hormones, important amino acids, enzymes, and chemical compounds that keep the brain healthy.

14. GMO (Bioengineered) Foods

The term *bioengineered* is starting to replace the term *GMO* (genetically modified organism), especially on food labels. The information here applies just the same whether a food is called GMO, bioengineered, or any new term(s) in the future.

GMO foods are designed to deplete and rob nutrients from the body. Our brain sees GMO foods the same way it sees industrialized chemicals. Just because a food is edible and we can chew it, consume it, and utilize some of it doesn't mean the brain accepts it as a natural source of fuel.

As industrialized food formulated by the chemical industry, GMO food is different from non-GMO fast food or processed food. Every structure of every single chemical compound in a GMO food is foreign to the body. The brain views these as foreign, synthesized chemicals. Our brain sees GMO foods as synthesized, factory-made substances even though they came from a plant or a tree growing in the earth. Every GMO food consumed triggers a response by our brain to our adrenal glands to release a specific blend of adrenaline that warns of a genetic chemical invasion occurring inside the body.

GMO foods are not antiviral and antibacterial. They lose the ability to fight viruses, bacteria, and pathogens. For example, the vitamin C produced in a GMO fruit or vegetable is foreign to the human body. Even if a lab might show that a GMO food is abundant in vitamin C, if people relied upon it as their only source of vitamin C, every vitamin C deficiency disease would accelerate.

GMO foods are hormone disruptors. Hormone disruption is the engineered plant's survival method to destroy the consumer's hormones as a means of protecting the plant's hormones—so the consumer has a shorter lifespan to consume the engineered plant. It's kill-or-be-killed genetic plant survival. Because GMO foods contain hormone inhibitors, which enter endocrine glands such as the adrenals, thyroid, and pancreas, GMO foods create a struggle for these glands to produce hormones properly. This can be detrimental to the brain. If the chemical compounds from GMO foods enter the hypothalamus or pituitary gland, a dampening of hormone production occurs there too, reducing the percentage of proper hormone production.

The hypothalamus and pituitary gland are also involved with information that extends past our own consciousness. These glands are involved with our intuition, our ability to receive information from outside our body. For instance, these glands involve tapping into our abilities that understand weather patterns, our abilities to be insightful with what's going on with us on the planet. So the effect of GMO foods is not just a dampening, a hampering, a lowering in the amount of hormone production. If someone is eating a lot of GMO, it can really interfere with intuition.

15. Bone Broth

When a cow is slaughtered, the cow's large adrenal glands expel an entire lifetime's worth of adrenaline into the bloodstream to try to save the cow's life as it's dying. This is intended to give the cow supernatural strength to survive the attack. In order for a creature to possess supernatural strength, the adrenaline must go into the bones, not just the muscles, brain, and nervous system. So as the cow's brain starts to die, adrenaline cycles rapidly into deeper parts of the cow, and eventually most of the adrenaline settles in the bones as a natural defense mechanism, in a last-ditch effort to try to resurrect the cow (or other creature). This means that as we consume bone broth, we're consuming the cow's last-ditch effort to survive. We're consuming the messaging inside that adrenaline that's stored in the bone marrow.

That adrenaline is a steroid. Bone broth is basically a steroid treatment, one that is not helpful for our recovery or healing. This steroid effect is why some people may seem to feel better when consuming bone broth.

Yet our brain understands adrenaline, even when it's not our own. Our brain knows how to interpret fight-or-flight when it receives an adrenaline burst from our own adrenals, so when we're consuming an adrenaline steroid–based product from a creature such as a cow, our brain receives the information of fear and chaos from that adrenaline. Our brain does not want to be treated with steroids that contain information for another creature's fight-or-flight that ended in death. This steroid is not a human steroid, so it signals neurotransmitter hormones to be released under false pretenses. These steroids are highly toxic to the brain. Steroids mean a withdrawal process, and our brain has to go through that withdrawal process after every time we consume them because the steroids numb out our neurons' ability to respond to a toxin. As that numbness wears off, it stimulates a craving for more. This steroid cycle helps accelerate degenerative brain diseases.

Bone broth is also high in fat, which slows down glucose absorption in brain cells, essentially starving the brain. This is why bone broth consumers have more cravings for sweet treats at the end of the day. Bone broth often contains vinegar too. Bone broth with vinegar is a double whammy.

16. Problematic Fish and Seafood (including catfish, red snapper, striped bass, bluefish, swordfish, grouper, clams, oysters, mussels, shrimp, crab, lobster, squid, octopus, scallops, flounder, tilapia, and shark)

These varieties of fish and seafood are a source of mercury, copper, lead, barium, fluoride, dioxins, and radioactive isotopes of strontium and uranium.

Fish and seafood can also contain microorganisms such as parasites and worms. Violent allergic reactions to seafood occur when someone reacts to cooked microorganisms within the seafood. This is different from food poisoning from uncooked or undercooked seafood or seafood juices, where the microorganisms such as parasites or worms are still alive. Both forms of exposure—to either live or cooked microorganisms inhabiting seafood—can be injurious to the brain. (Read more about how and why in Brain Saver's "Bacteria and Other Microbes" chapter.)

17. Lamb

The trend is to say lamb is healthy. This is deceiving. Lamb is high in fat. This means that lamb causes the liver to be stagnant and sluggish and allows the brain to become more toxic from brain betrayers. Lamb fat also starves the brain of glucose by interfering with glucose, making it another glucose inhibitor.

18. Salt

In the health world, we're under the impression that every time we consume salt, it all leaves our body. So if someone is indulging one night for dinner by eating a lot of salty foods, eventually—whether that night or the next day—they'll just urinate all that salt out. In reality, you only urinate out most of the salt, not all of it. There's still a substantial percentage of salt that accumulates inside the body. The first place where salt accumulates is the liver. That's our first line of defense, so the liver is where salt deposits start to build. Eventually salt deposits can accumulate in the brain.

When we eat even the highest-quality salt, our body has a different reaction than it does to sodium that naturally occurs in fruits, leafy greens, herbs, wild foods, and vegetables. Salt that we add to food has a concentration level that sends us into salt shock. So you don't get the benefits of salt that you're told within health communities you're getting. The benefits don't really become bioavailable because your body sees over-salting as a threat.

Salt draws moisture out of cell tissue. When salt squeezes water out of a healthy cell, the salt disperses along with the fluid in the cell. That cell can rehydrate and restore itself shortly afterward, even hours afterward. Yet when cells inside organs are damaged by other toxins and pathogens and there's excessive salt consumption in a person's diet, the salt can crystallize and accumulate in areas that have damaged tissue. That's because when salt enters damaged tissue—broken cells, scar tissue, injured blood vessels—the water that the salt squeezes out of these damaged areas isn't enough to disperse and wash away the salt. So the salt clings and starts to crystallize.

This means injuries in the body, including injuries in the brain, start to accumulate salt deposits. Salt deposits can lead to mysterious white spots on brain MRIs; the salt deposits reflect the magnetic resonance imaging. Tiny microstrokes and tiny micro-blood clots in the brain, which people often live with, are vulnerable areas where salt deposits accumulate quickly when people are consuming excess salt. Or if someone has dehydrated, weakened neurotransmitter chemicals, sodium can accumulate around the weakened neurotransmitters. If someone has damaged, weakened neurons, salt deposits can accumulate around the weakened neurons. After 20 to 30 years of consuming larger quantities of salt than we're supposed to, we can gather salt deposits all through the body, including our brain. We can become one big salt lick. Salt accelerates the aging process.

19. Fermented Foods (including sauerkraut, pickled preserves, sourdough, cheese, and yogurt [animal- or plant-based])

More and more people, including medical doctors, are getting sold on the mistaken theory that if you're sick, it's all about the gut and that "fixing" gut flora with fermented foods fixes your brain.

Fermented foods are a false solution for brain health for two reasons: (1) the real threats against our brain and inside our gut are pathogens and the poisons and toxins those pathogens release from feeding on brain betrayers, and (2) fermented foods and products do not contain beneficial bacteria anyway. The microorganisms in fermented foods are not the good bacteria and other beneficial microorganisms, such as beneficial fungus, that we have inside our guts naturally.

Fermented foods actually contain unproductive microorganisms, so when we consume them, our hydrochloric acid is meant to destroy and disperse the microorganisms quickly. Most people have very low hydrochloric acid, so the majority of these unproductive microorganisms escape death in the stomach, pass through, and temporarily land in the intestinal tract until they die. Either way, these unproductive microorganisms' lifespan is short in the gastrointestinal environment, and as these unproductive microorganisms die off, they become food for bad bacteria.

Even if fermented foods did contain beneficial bacteria, that wouldn't be the winning answer for our health because good bacteria do not battle bad bacteria. Trying to crowd out bad bacteria with good bacteria is not how our microbiome works. Good bacteria do not kill bad bacteria. No matter the quantity of good bacteria present in the gut, bad bacteria thrive unless you remove what feeds bad bacteria—and have learned the tools needed to kill bad bacteria. Bad bacteria will always remain there, regardless

of how many probiotics or fermented foods with theoretically beneficial microorganisms you take. Given that pathogens and the toxins they consume are the real threat against our brain—and the real threat living in our gut—removing foods that feed these unproductive bacteria and viruses does more to benefit our microflora than adding trillions of recommended beneficial bacteria.

Why do people think they're getting benefits from fermented foods? Very few people simply add fermented foods to a standard American or standard European diet without making other changes. They usually change many other habits at the same time as they pursue their fermented food journey. They go from not eating well into all kinds of healthy practices at once, such as removing gluten, removing dairy, consuming green juice, and lowering their calories. This gives them the false impression that the sauerkraut they eat offers extreme benefits.

Here's another reason fermented foods don't help us: our brain needs electrolytes in order to function, and fermented foods lose their electrolytes through the fermentation process. Trace mineral salts' composition is such that they deactivate and change when plant matter is decaying. Any other nutrients that were in the plant, such as phytochemical compounds, are also deactivated and destroyed during the fermentation process. A fermented food becomes an empty food for the brain.

Many brain conditions are caused by toxic heavy metals. Fermented foods are not remedying that. Many brain conditions are caused by viruses. Fermented foods are not remedying that. Fermented foods are neither stopping toxic heavy metals in the brain from oxidizing nor fixing neurotoxins trapped in the brain from viruses. Nor are fermented foods getting viruses or toxic heavy metals out of the gut.

While plant-based fermented foods themselves won't feed viruses and bad bacteria and unproductive fungus, they won't starve or stop or kill them either. And some microorganisms that die in your gut from these fermented foods will feed viruses and bad bacteria and unproductive fungus—not enough to substantially increase a viral load or bacterial colony or fungus explosion but enough to feed them, keeping them alive. A living plant food that once contained antiviral and antibacterial compounds loses the antiviral and antibacterial compounds during the fermentation process because fermentation is a form of plant death that changes the structure of all phytochemical compounds originally in the living plant.

Meanwhile, the fat in fermented dairy or fermented meats and fish makes these foods the perfect environment for bacteria to increase in numbers. The fats in fermented meats are even denser than the fats rendered from cooking non-fermented meats because the fats harden as they go rancid. The fat in fermented meats makes it much more difficult for bile to disperse and break down the hardened fat, allowing bad bugs in the gut to proliferate.

20. Grains Eaten in an Unproductive Way

Grains are not an antiviral, antibacterial food. The carbohydrates in grains don't easily reach the brain. Instead the carbohydrates in grains reach the liver and tend to spend more time in the liver than what's needed.

For example, when someone is eating oats—even though oats are better than most other grains—they don't create a quick, reliable glucose for the brain. The same is true of rice and other grains. The carbohydrates from grains, even gluten-free grains, are not dispersed into the bloodstream quickly and aren't 100 percent bioavailable until they're converted into a bioavailable sugar that can be used for the brain. To become usable, their glucose has to be converted by the liver, and almost everyone's liver is partially sick in some way, stagnant and sluggish and filled with pathogens and toxins.

A weakened liver can't convert grain without a struggle, which leads to the grains becoming gummy and sticky and lingering in the liver longer, acting almost like a protective coating for pathogens, because these grains are not antiviral or antibacterial. By the time the liver does convert grains' carbohydrates into valuable glucose, the carbohydrates have spent far too long inside the body before reaching the brain. When the carbohydrates are released from the liver, they've already had too many hours inside the body of not being useful, so the chemical structure of the carbohydrates has changed.

The brain is seeking viable fuel that's been absorbed into the bloodstream or released by the liver quickly. If the brain is receiving two fuel sources—that is, the brain is getting the highly bioavailable glucose it wants from one source plus it's getting the not-so-bioavailable glucose from grains—the fuel sources clash. The grains get in the way of the brain receiving the bioavailable glucose from the other fuel source, which leads to overeating the grain, because the brain is hungry and not receiving what it needs. This is what makes grains addictive. When fats like oil, avocado, pork, dairy, cheese, or eggs are added to the grain, it's even more addictive.

If someone is eating grains, millet is the best option. Millet causes the least amount of trouble because it's converted more easily by the liver. Oats are the second-best choice for grains. Quinoa, which can be scratchy on the intestinal linings, is third. Rice is okay sparingly because it is less nutrient-dense. Even brown rice is less nutrient-dense than millet, oats, and quinoa. (People are sometimes worried about arsenic with rice. That's only one variety of rice that's conventionally sprayed.)

Do not have your grains with fats if you're someone who is trying to heal. Combining a less bioavailable form of glucose that hasn't been converted properly by the liver with a fat of any kind, whether plant fat or animal fat, will stop the brain from receiving the majority of glucose from the grain. Because of this, some people are hungry shortly after they eat. Weight gain can also occur from the combination of fat and glucose because the liver becomes overburdened, processing even more than normal with both the fat and the grains' carbohydrates.

"People are told that 70 to 90 percent cacao is better for you—'the more potency, the better'—when in reality, a higher cacao percentage means more caffeine, which is more damaging to the adrenals."

— Anthony William, Medical Medium

CHAPTER 6

Brain Betrayer Supplements

These supplements fall into four main categories:

A. Problematic and damaging supplements

B. Mildly problematic supplements

C. Overrated or overused supplements

D. Quality concerns (supplements where it's especially important to seek out high-quality forms because they're frequently produced with low-quality ingredients or problematic additives such as preservatives)

The following supplements are listed alphabetically within each category:

A. Problematic and Damaging

1. Alkaline ionizer water machines
2. Apple cider vinegar (ACV) and ACV supplements taken internally
3. Bentonite and other clays taken internally
4. Caffeine-based energy supplements
5. Charcoal taken internally
6. Chlorella
7. Chlorine dioxide (sodium chlorite)
8. Cod liver oil and shark liver oil
9. Colostrum
10. Deer antler (also called deer velvet and antler velvet)
11. Diatomaceous earth (DE)
12. Digestive bitters
13. Essential oils taken internally
14. Fat burners
15. Fish oil and krill oil
16. Gut powder blends
17. Herbal tinctures in alcohol

18. Hydrochloric acid (HCl or HCL) supplements
19. L-carnitine and L-arginine
20. Mineral oil
21. Mushroom coffee (with caffeine)
22. Oyster supplements
23. Pearl powder
24. Sodium bicarbonate (baking soda) when taken internally in large amounts
25. Turpentine oil
26. Whey protein powder
27. Zeolites

B. Mildly Problematic

28. Amino acid supplement combinations
29. Chicken cartilage
30. Desiccated animal organs and glandular supplements (including liver, adrenal gland, spleen, kidney, stomach, pancreas, brain, tongue, and heart; also including bovine serum)
31. Electrolyte powders and beverages
32. Herbal combination powders
33. Iron supplements (that are not plant-based)
34. Neem oil (taken internally)
35. Oil pulling
36. Pine needle tea
37. Pre-workout supplements
38. Senna leaf

C. Overrated or Overused

39. CBD (cannabidiol)
40. Chlorophyll
41. Collagen
42. Fruit and vegetable powders
43. Fulvic minerals, fulvic acid, humic acid, humic minerals, and shilajit
44. Maca root
45. Plant protein powder
46. Prebiotics (including inulin powder)
47. Probiotics
48. Vitamin D overuse or megadoses

D. Quality Concerns

49. Cyanocobalamin (low-quality vitamin B_{12})
50. Low-quality colloidal silver
51. Low-quality zinc
52. MCT oil

53. Multivitamins and hair-skin-nail supplements
54. Oregano oil
55. Prenatals

A. PROBLEMATIC AND DAMAGING SUPPLEMENTS

1. Alkaline Ionizer Water Machines

Metal plates inside these machines corrode and oxidize over time, slowly leaching oxidized metal byproduct and metal nanoparticles into the water, regardless of the brand of machine. Oxidized metal byproduct and metal nanoparticles eventually lead to neurological symptoms. Alkaline ionizer water machines are not water purifiers. Their filtration is limited. Water becomes dead water as it's being destructured by the electricity of these machines. The water becomes foreign to the human body.

2. Apple Cider Vinegar (ACV) and ACV Supplements (taken internally)

Causes teeth deterioration. Refer to "Vinegar" in the previous chapter, "Brain Betrayer Foods," for more.

3. Bentonite and Other Clays (taken internally)

These clays do not remove toxic heavy metals; they are too harsh and aggressive on the intestinal lining. They act as sandpaper in your intestinal tract. Clays irritate sensitive nerves that connect in and around the intestinal tract. People with sensitive or inflamed vagus nerves should not ingest clays. Clays can also disrupt the microbiome: bentonite and other clays suffocate good bacteria and microorganisms and allow bad bacteria and microorganisms to thrive because clays remove oxygen inside the intestinal tract. Good bacteria and microorganisms need higher levels of oxygen to survive. Bad bacteria and microorganisms need lower levels of oxygen to survive. Clays can create a chronic dehydration within the intestinal tract.

4. Caffeine-Based Energy Supplements

Caffeine lowers the immune system, weakens the adrenals, is neurotoxic to the brain, depletes bones and teeth of precious minerals, and is highly addictive as a psychoactive drug. For more, refer to *Brain Saver*'s "Caffeine" chapter.

5. Charcoal (taken internally)

Charcoal, including activated charcoal, suffocates intestinal linings, not allowing nutrients to absorb, assimilate, or easily pass through the intestinal linings to the hepatic portal vein. This causes nutritional deficiencies, suffocating good bacteria and microorganisms while allowing bad bacteria and microorganisms to thrive. Charcoal does not remove toxic heavy metals. Charcoal is not a binder for toxic heavy metals. Charcoal does the opposite; charcoal can keep toxic heavy metals from leaving the intestinal tract, because the metals get buried under the charcoal as it coats the intestinal tract lining. Charcoal, even activated charcoal, stains the walls of the intestinal tract and takes weeks to completely eliminate. Charcoal is toxic to the body because it keeps toxins inside the body. It is helpful to brush your teeth with an activated charcoal supplement periodically. Make sure you do not swallow and instead spit out the charcoal, then rinse your mouth as much as you can.

6. Chlorella

Does not bind onto toxic heavy metals properly. Spreads toxic heavy metals into adjacent tissue, accelerating brain conditions. Chlorella does not have the ability to remove toxic heavy metals from the body. Chlorella is not antibacterial or antiviral. Rather, it often contains bad bacteria, resulting in foodborne illness.

7. Chlorine Dioxide (Sodium Chlorite)

An irritant on the intestinal tract that can kill more good bacteria and microorganisms than bad bacteria and microorganisms. When entering the bloodstream in larger dosages, it's toxic to the brain because chlorine dioxide in high dosages is damaging to neurons. When nausea occurs after ingestion of chlorine dioxide, this is the vagus nerves reacting to the toxicity.

8. Cod Liver Oil and Shark Liver Oil

Contain high concentrations of toxins, including mercury and other toxic heavy metals.

9. Colostrum

Colostrum is a dairy product that feeds pathogens such as viruses and bacteria, accelerating chronic illness. Classified medical research and science used dairy products, colostrum included, as a fuel source to feed and raise pathogens in labs. (Human colostrum does not feed pathogens because human colostrum was not used as a fuel source in labs.)

10. Deer Antler (also called deer velvet and antler velvet)

Not helpful for someone living with chronic illness. The hormones in deer antler disrupt naturally produced and occurring hormones in the body—deer antler's steroid compounds interfere with human hormone production. The larger the dosage of deer antler supplements, the more interference with the endocrine system occurs. The higher the dosage and the longer the dosage is taken, the more withdrawal can occur, eventually causing adrenal fatigue and hair loss.

11. Diatomaceous Earth (DE)

Agitates and clings to the intestinal linings and does not leave the intestinal tract quickly. Abrasive to sensitive nerves throughout the stomach, duodenum, and intestinal tract, triggering symptoms of sensitive vagus nerves.

Also be cautious not to inhale diatomaceous earth, due to its ability to lower the immune system when caught in the lungs. White blood cells see diatomaceous earth particles as foreign invaders and have to consume them, which can lead to an overburdened lymphatic immune system, allowing pathogens such as viruses to take advantage and create a flare-up of a chronic condition.

12. Digestive Bitters

Normally contain alcohol. Read about the problem with alcohol in supplements in the next chapter, "Brain Betrayer Food and Supplement Chemicals." Also refer to *Brain Saver*'s "Alcohol" chapter.

13. Essential Oils (taken internally)

When ingested, especially in higher quantities, essential oils can trigger vagus nerves into spasm, resulting in heightened symptoms such as anxiety, panic, burning sensations, and overexcited senses. Essential oil therapies should not be ingested or used internally for people with symptoms and conditions involving a sensitive nervous system.

Be cautious of excessive external use of essential oils in carriers and body lotions. The oils rub onto mattresses, sheets, blankets, couches, chairs, and even walls, leading these objects and surfaces to harbor oil dampness, which can collect dust, dirt, sand, and food particles. This makes a perfect environment for mold to proliferate throughout areas of the home. It's best to use essential oils sparingly and wipe off the excess oil. This is true for any oils, even without essential oils added to them.

14. Fat Burners

Often contain fillers, preservatives, MSG, caffeine. Fat burners do not help someone rid or burn fat. Instead, they burden an already stagnant and sluggish liver, accelerating fat storage. Most fat burners are stimulants to allow the person who is taking the supplements to run on adrenaline and get through longer durations of not eating.

15. Fish Oil and Krill Oil

Contains a homeopathic version of mercury—the essence of mercury—left over after mercury removal from many fish oils, allowing methylmercury to enter the brain, easily accelerating brain diseases. Most fish oils are manufactured with unwanted fish byproduct and waste from various varieties of fish brought to the processing centers and mixed-matched together during the oil extraction process. One fish oil capsule can be filled with fish oil that was derived from dozens of fishes.

When a fish dies, the mercury and other toxic heavy metals oxidize and expand more quickly in the dying fish oil, due to gases being produced because the fish is decomposing. This is why it is much safer to eat a fish than to take a fish oil supplement. You would never eat as much oil eating a piece of fish as you would concentrated into a fish oil capsule. As is noted in *Brain Saver*'s "Toxic Heavy Metals" chapter, mercury is less concentrated in the muscle of the fish than in the fat and oil.

16. Gut Powder Blends

Abrasive, scratchy combinations of irritants that do not balance the microbiome and do quite the opposite: scramble up the microbiome. This worsens intestinal tract conditions for sensitive people, especially when dealing with nervous system issues such as vagus and phrenic nerve inflammation, resulting in increased anxiety and digestive distress. Gut powder blends can throw an intestinal tract into spasm, creating cramping, gastrointestinal pain, gastritis, and bloating. Health practitioners will often mistake these reactions for a healing or detox of some sort, when in reality, it's the opposite.

17. Herbal Tinctures in Alcohol

See "Alcohol" in the next chapter, "Brain Betrayer Food and Supplement Chemicals." Seek out alcohol-free herbal tinctures.

18. Hydrochloric Acid (HCl or HCL) Supplements

Not the same as the hydrochloric acid produced by your stomach glands. Hydrochloric acid supplements are aggressive on the stomach, duodenum, and intestinal tract linings, causing irritation. They do not solve a low hydrochloric acid problem, only confuse and weaken stomach glands and worsen a hydrochloric acid problem. Hydrochloric acid supplements are made from just one variety of acid. Our natural hydrochloric acid inside our stomach is composed of multiple acids and is far more complex than research and science are aware of. Hydrochloric acid supplements do not break down protein in the food that enters the stomach because the supplements are missing the other critical gastric acids that make up the authentic hydrochloric acid blend produced by our own stomach glands. Our natural hydrochloric acid cannot be replicated with a supplement.

19. L-carnitine and L-arginine

Amino acids can be antiviral—L-lysine is a prime example of this type of beneficial amino acid. In contrast, L-carnitine and L-arginine are not antiviral. They can, especially in high dosages of supplemental form, feed and promote viral proliferation because viruses were raised in labs on eggs, which are high in L-arginine and L-carnitine.

20. Mineral Oil

Made from petroleum and often contains a variety of industrial toxins. Avoid ingesting and using as a moisturizer.

21. Mushroom Coffee (with caffeine)

Mushrooms such as reishi, chaga, cordyceps, shiitake, and lion's mane are beneficial. When coffee with caffeine is added to them, the brew becomes problematic. Now you're getting a false sense of energy from the psychoactive drug caffeine in the coffee, so that makers of mushroom coffee products get additional sales from the person being addicted to their coffee product. That consumer is being tricked into thinking the mushrooms are giving them that clarity and energy, when really the buzz is coming from caffeine addiction. It's best to enjoy the mushrooms without the coffee.

22. Oyster Supplements

Bottom dwellers such as oysters contain mercury, dioxins, strontium, uranium, petrochemicals, and other toxic heavy metals. Not a good source of zinc. While oysters do contain some zinc, zinc gets diminished and depleted from toxins. The toxins in oysters cancel out the zinc that oysters provide. Consuming oysters, oyster supplements, or oyster extracts does not restore zinc levels and clear up zinc deficiencies.

23. Pearl Powder

An irritant that's abrasive to the intestinal linings, triggering vagus nerves, which can elevate anxiety. Pearl powder does not leave the intestinal tract quickly; it accumulates and cakes inside pockets of the intestinal tract lining. Avoid if you have any type of intestinal tract disorder. Pearl powder carries traces of mercury. The accumulation of pearl powder on the intestinal linings can eventually cause bloating due to the powder not allowing gas to flow through the intestinal tract properly.

24. Sodium Bicarbonate (Baking Soda) (taken internally in large amounts)

Too abrasive on the intestinal tract linings when used as a therapy or supplement. (Occasionally used in baked goods or food recipes, baking soda is vastly different and safe. Sodium bicarbonate therapies use much larger amounts.) People with intestinal tract disorders worsen when using sodium bicarbonate supplement products and therapies, as it causes intestinal spasms, aggravating vagus nerves and all other nerves inside and around the intestinal tract, also overexciting the vagus nerves, which can increase anxiety.

25. Turpentine Oil

Scorches the intestinal tract linings, killing off more good bacteria and microorganisms than bad bacteria and microorganisms. When entering the bloodstream, raises blood toxicity, which stresses and intoxicates the liver and brain. Turpentine oil has a very high astringency factor that almost brings it to a solvent level.

26. Whey Protein Powder

Feeds viruses, bad bacteria, unproductive fungus, yeast, and mold inside the body, accelerating symptoms and condi-tions. Whey protein powder is inflamma-tory because it fuels pathogens that create inflammation. Whey protein is not a useful source of protein because it doesn't break down inside our stomachs and small intes-tinal tracts. Naturally human-produced hydrochloric acid does not dismantle whey protein so our bodies can utilize it.

27. Zeolites

In recent years inedible varieties of zeolites have been unearthed and manufactured in the same places as edible zeolites, causing cross-contamination. Neither edible nor inedible zeolites cross the blood-brain barrier, nor do they enter the brain. Cross-contaminated zeolite varieties stay in the intestinal tract and irritate the lining, causing dehydration and vagus nerve sensitivities.

Edible zeolites, even if you have every assurance that they're not cross-contaminated, should not be taken in high dosages or long term because even edible zeolite varieties build up inside the gut, cre-ating imbalances and dehydration. Large dosages of zeolites can create a trace min-eral imbalance because zeolites don't have a discernment between what's a toxic heavy metal and what's a precious trace mineral. Zeolites do not travel into the bloodstream, binding onto toxic heavy metals there. Zeo-lites are not a reliable binder. Zeolites only stay in the intestinal tract, just like clay. As zeolites sit inside the intestinal tract, they can interrupt trace minerals from leaving the intestinal tract and entering the liver.

B. MILDLY PROBLEMATIC SUPPLEMENTS

28. Amino Acid Supplement Combinations

A variety of amino acids put together without the understanding of what causes chronic illness. Many amino acids can insti-gate and trigger pathogens out of dor-mancy, some amino acids can work against the immune system, some amino acids can alter an immune cell's response, while some amino acids help defend against pathogens. The makers of amino acid supplements don't know the difference; therefore, amino acid supplements can trigger someone into a bout of illness.

29. Chicken Cartilage

Offers nothing for the body. Chicken car-tilage raises blood acids, supporting chronic acidosis in all body systems. These acids force the body to release calcium storage to neutralize the acid, which depletes bones and can cause kidney stones and gallstones.

30. Desiccated Animal Organs and Glandular Supplements (including liver, adrenal gland, spleen, kidney, stomach, pancreas, brain, tongue, and heart; also including bovine serum)

Contain toxic heavy metals, dehydrated adrenaline, pathogen material, and hor-mones foreign to the human body. These products increase brain toxicity because organs and glands used to make these supplements have concentrated amounts of toxins stored in them. The organs and glands shouldn't be consumed whether desiccated or eaten in their whole form.

31. Electrolyte Powders and Beverages

Accelerate dehydration within the brain and body because of low-quality sodium (that is not found naturally occurring in whole foods) being added to the powder or beverage. Low-quality macro minerals do not equate or even compare to electrolytes found in fruits, leafy greens, herbs, wild foods, and vegetables. Manufactured electrolyte compositions are greatly different from naturally occurring electrolytes and do not restore neurotransmitters or neurons because they are man-made concoctions that can never equal coconut water or celery juice, for example.

32. Herbal Combination Powders

Herbal combinations that are low quality, often containing toxic heavy metals. Often these herbal combination powders contain non-herbal additives such as clays and probiotics that can be either irritating to the gastrointestinal linings or just not beneficial to the brain and body. The herbs that are chosen are not for specific conditions and symptoms. Rather, the herbs chosen are hit-and-miss. Even if there is an herb that can be helpful for a condition, it's not in enough quantity because it's merely a smidgen of that herb mixed with a dozen or more other herbs and/or additives.

33. Iron Supplements (that are not plant-based)

Iron supplements are a false "fix" to a deeper problem caused by viruses such as EBV. If you're seeking iron, search for plant-based iron supplements and/or supplement your diet with iron-rich foods such as spinach, barley grass, parsley, wild blueberries, grapes (black, purple, or red), blackberries, cilantro, burdock root (juiced), potatoes (with skins), kale, sprouts, squash, pumpkin seeds (in small amounts), asparagus, and sulfur-free dried apricots and raisins. Also consider seeking out antiviral Medical Medium protocols such as the Autoimmune Disorders and Diseases protocol from Chapter 4, "Medical Medium Protocols."

34. Neem Oil (taken internally)

Avoid taking neem internally. It's too astringent; its chemical compounds are aggressive on the stomach and intestinal linings. Because of this, neem is also irritating to the vagus nerves.

35. Oil Pulling

Whether swishing or brushing your teeth with oil such as coconut oil, this practice coats and protects bad bacteria in and around the gums, keeping oxygen away from the bacteria, which allows the bacteria to thrive. Swishing or brushing any variety of oil around inside the mouth does not pull or remove toxins. Meanwhile, the oil slick on your teeth makes you feel like they're smooth and glistening. If you're still devoted to this practice, make sure you brush again afterward without using any oil to get the oil off your teeth and gums.

36. Pine Needle Tea

Does not help with anything related to COVID. The resin from pine needle tea is an irritant to the intestinal tract lining. If someone has sensitive vagus nerves or a sensitive nervous system, pine needle tea can be triggering and may heighten symptoms such as anxiety. The irritation in someone's intestinal tract can be confusing, making someone believe they're cleansing contaminants.

37. Pre-workout Supplements

Don't provide what the body truly needs before working out—instead contribute to dehydration—and often contain MSG and sometimes caffeine.

38. Senna Leaf

Senna is an irritant to the intestinal tract, causing an intestinal tract spasm that sometimes stimulates peristaltic action for people who have difficulties with constipation or other gastrointestinal symptoms. There are more productive ways to stimulate peristalsis. Refer to the Vagus Nerve Problems protocol and/or Stomach

Problems protocol in Chapter 4, "Medical Medium Protocols."

C. OVERRATED OR OVERUSED SUPPLEMENTS

39. CBD (Cannabidiol)

Most chronic illnesses are caused by pathogens and toxins. CBD is neither anti-viral nor detoxifying. In the past, CBD was commonly sold as a treatment on its own. The lack of results with CBD then spurred on a change with its usage. The strategy for CBD has evolved, and CBD is now being sold mixed in with other medicinals such as herbs, vitamins, and nutrients that offer better results for individuals living with various symptoms. This can be misleading for CBD users because CBD gets the spotlight, while it's the other constituents in the combinations that are providing more benefits.

40. Chlorophyll

The body does not utilize chlorophyll that's been processed and singled out from its original source because the chlorophyll is missing key components that are intertwined when chlorophyll is part of a complete, whole food. Separating chlorophyll is a processing method, stripping other phytochemical compounds that make chlorophyll usable and potent when it enters into the body as part of a whole food. Chlorophyll cannot be isolated and still serve a purpose. Chlorophyll can only be utilized if still in its natural source with other phytochemical compounds and nutrients.

It's becoming a trend to add a few drops of chlorophyll to your water to turn it green, as if you were adding food coloring. As a healing and beneficial alternative, add some drops of parsley juice or barley grass juice powder to your water.

41. Collagen

Collagen products help clog an already stagnant and sluggish liver, resulting in lowered conversion abilities when the liver is converting vitamins and nutrients for the brain to assimilate. Other vitamins and nutrients are the true building blocks to collagen. Taking collagen does the reverse of restoring collagen. It causes you to lose collagen because it burdens an already stagnant, sluggish liver. Collagen products never worked; you can't create new collagen in the body by consuming collagen itself. You have to consume plant foods such as leafy greens, herbs, and fruits to give you the building blocks to create collagen. Collagen products are starting to change because of Medical Medium–published material: they are now including silica, vitamin C, nettle leaf, and other herbs and plant food–based compounds and vitamins. If collagen is still an ingredient in the supplement, it's not ideal. Eventually collagen products won't have any collagen in them at all.

42. Fruit and Vegetable Powders

Fruit and vegetable powder supplements are the result of taking a few specks of dehydrated or freeze-dried fruits and vegetables, compiling dozens of different types into a capsule, and thinking that offers a better benefit than consuming fresh fruits and vegetables. One whole radish, orange, or tomato on its own will offer more nutrition than a mixed fruit and vegetable capsule or powder—because that whole radish, orange, or tomato will contain more phytochemical compounds, nutrients, living water, and antioxidants than a gram or two of dehydrated or freeze-dried mixed fruit and vegetable powder. In order for a capsule or powder of a fruit or vegetable to offer a benefit, one item needs to be the focus, not a mix, and preferably that capsule or powder should be made from a wild, close-to-wild, or highly nutritious food.

43. Fulvic Minerals, Fulvic Acid, Humic Acid, Humic Minerals, and Shilajit

Anyone who has been sick long enough with chronic illness has stumbled across these products in desperation, only to find that they are not the health panacea that they were told. When these products are in combination with other therapies or supplements that are helpful, they can be confused as being the reason for health improvements. On their own, they are mostly disappointing.

These irritants provide a false sense of getting your minerals and "This is going to get me better." Not all plant matter is non-toxic or safe to use. Not every part of every plant can be used for human consumption. This isn't taken into account when fulvic products, humic products, and shilajit are manufactured into a supplement form. The reliability of where these ingredients are being sourced and what is even being used for ingredients is in question. Full disclosure is usually not occurring.

Anyone with a gastrointestinal disorder should be cautious since these are irritants to the intestinal tract lining. Fulvic products, humic products, and shilajit are not antiviral or antibacterial in nature and do not remove toxic heavy metals or assist the body in detoxing. They are not binders. They are not natural for human consumption; they need to be manipulated through manufacturing to make them theoretically assimilable or absorbable. These products can be very dehydrating when taken in higher dosages.

44. Maca Root

Contains endocrine gland disruptors, which enter glands and suppress hormone-producing cells inside the glands, altering the endocrine glands' natural patterns of hormone production. Maca root taken every day long term confuses endocrine glands, causing an overproduction of hormones when not needed, or an underproduction of hormones. Maca can provide a temporary feel-good sensation due to its mild steroidal effect, which eventually wears off, leading you to increase your maca consumption to get the same feel-good effect. Eventually you get no feel-good effect at all, no matter how high you increase your maca root dosages.

45. Plant Protein Powder

If you're sensitive, the abrasiveness of protein powders can irritate vagus nerves extending into the intestinal tract. Look out for MSG, which is disguised as "natural flavors" in protein powders. Look out for hidden sugars and hidden fats, which are there to give someone a false satiation. Look out for protein powders that have a mix of many different ingredients. Protein is not an important nutrient for preventing or reversing brain diseases and chronic illness.

46. Prebiotics (including inulin powder)

Not the panacea everybody believes this type of supplement to be. All fresh fruits, leafy greens, herbs, wild foods, and vegetables are prebiotics in their raw form. Anything bottled, packaged, industrialized, or manufactured and not in its whole, living, fresh source is acting as a ghost of a prebiotic, not the whole thing.

47. Probiotics

Probiotics do not have a record of fixing chronic illness. Probiotics do not rid bad bacteria and microorganisms from the gut. Probiotics often contain negative ingredients that are toxic to the body.

Recently, probiotics makers have started to change their formulas by adding in Medical Medium recommendations such as zinc, B_{12}, vitamin C, and herbs such as nettle leaf, lemon balm, and goldenseal to the probiotic formulas. This is because probiotic companies realize they need more in order to provide any kind of benefit, and the new healing ingredients are starting to bring some mild relief to consumers. The probiotics themselves are still not the answer to fixing autoimmune disorders and diseases, chronic illness, neurological symptoms, and digestive symptoms such as bloating. The microorganisms in probiotic supplements are not the beneficial microorganisms that we rely upon in our guts for assimilation and absorption.

Even if probiotics did provide the real beneficial microorganisms, that's not the answer. Good bacteria don't battle bad bacteria. (See Brain Saver's chapter "Bacteria and Other Microbes.")

48. Vitamin D Overuse or Megadoses

High doses of vitamin D burden the liver, especially when someone is experiencing symptoms caused by a stagnant and sluggish liver. Health authorities take pride in their vitamin D recommendations without knowing the true cause of symptoms and conditions and that vitamin D is not the most important tool for fighting those conditions. Vitamin D is not an antiviral or antibacterial nutrient. Large dosages of vitamin D are often prescribed to improve someone's immune system and actually do the opposite because they place a stress upon some of the body systems.

Vitamin D does not assimilate or absorb any better when it's combined with vitamin K. Vitamin K is one of the most accessible nutrients and is in virtually every food we eat. Some foods are exceptionally high in vitamin K. It's one of the most abundant vitamins in the human diet, and there isn't a need to supplement it.

Vitamin D is beneficial to our overall health when kept in the 1,000 IU to 5,000 IU range. If someone is very deficient, 10,000 IU can be used periodically. Look out for poor sources of vitamin D.

D. QUALITY CONCERNS

In this list, you'll see references to some supplements, such as zinc, that are problematic in low-quality form and beneficial in high-quality form. For the best, most bioavailable forms of supplements such as zinc, visit the supplement directory at www.medicalmedium.com. Supplements often have lots of fillers, preservatives, chemicals, binders, and undisclosed additives.

49. Cyanocobalamin (low-quality vitamin B_{12})

B_{12} that the human body does not recognize as a viable, usable, natural form. The liver has to convert your nutrients and vitamins and can't convert cyanocobalamin.

50. Low-Quality Colloidal Silver

Be cautious of low-quality colloidal silvers, which may contain higher amounts of copper and nickel and are not made from pure silver. Low-quality colloidal silver is not activated or nano-sized enough.

51. Low-Quality Zinc

There are aggressive zinc supplements out there that make people vomit if they are sensitive. These zincs are not stabilized. Your best option is liquid zinc sulfate. Watch out for citric acid and other preservatives.

52. MCT Oil

Like other oils, MCT oil by the teaspoon or tablespoon interferes with glucose absorption in the brain. Just like any other processed oil, MCT oil still causes insulin resistance when consumed in these large amounts. (In tiny droplets, MCT oil is harmless.) Be especially cautious of MCT oil made from palm kernel oil. It's not a quality source.

53. Multivitamins and Hair-Skin-Nail Supplements

Made from low-quality and sometimes old, outdated, expired warehouse ingredients in small amounts mixed together to fill space and make supplement companies maximum money while offering minimum benefits to the consumer. One capsule or tablet contains specks of each vitamin, mineral, and other nutrient, which is not enough to make a substantial difference when battling brain and chronic illnesses. These products are usually vitamins, minerals, and nutrients theoretically placed together without the understanding of what causes chronic illness.

54. Oregano Oil

Oregano oil needs to be in the right form and used at the right time and place. Oregano oil's best use is for foodborne pathogens: for example, before someone eats in a restaurant, if they're concerned about acquiring food poisoning. Or if someone has a chronic condition shortly after food poisoning that's persistent for more than a week. Oregano is helpful for bad bacteria in the intestinal tract. It does not fix symptoms and conditions of chronic illness that's brain-related. People often make the mistake of taking essential oil of oregano internally, which is different from the supplemental form of oregano oil designed to be taken internally.

55. Prenatals

Made from small amounts of low-quality ingredients that are not in the most bioavailable forms, prenatals provide a false sense of security, coming across as authentic, prescriptive, hard-core science when they're not. Try not to be under the illusion that with prenatals, you're covering your bases. There's no medical research or science going into these prenatal supplement formulas that addresses what a baby needs from the pregnant mother. When taking a prenatal, it's best to supplement alongside it with spirulina, barley grass juice powder, wild blueberry in any form, methylfolate, vitamin B_{12}, and non–ascorbic acid vitamin C in consultation with your doctor.

CHAPTER 7

Brain Betrayer Food and Supplement Chemicals

Keep a close eye on food, drink, and supplement ingredient labels to avoid these brain betrayers.

Some of these additives, such as ammonia, won't appear on labeling, so it helps to gain the inside knowledge in this chapter about where these chemicals sneak into food and supplements.

1. **Aspartame and other artificial sweeteners**

2. **Monosodium glutamate (MSG)** (including seasoning with MSG, fake meats, bottled or packaged sauces, cold cuts, and hot dogs)

3. **Flavors** (natural and artificial)

4. **Alcohol**

5. **Citric acid**

6. **Soft drinks** (conventional and natural)

7. **Preservatives, ammonia, formaldehyde, and nitrates** (including sodium nitrate)

These additives creep into our lives. Often disguised as "*flavors*" or "*flavorings*" on labels, whether natural or artificial, they're much less innocent than they appear. The fact that these ingredients often appear at the end of a food or supplement's ingredient list doesn't make them unthreatening. They're that potent, even in a small amount.

Accountability still has a long way to go when it comes to food labeling. Even if you take care to buy foods and supplements that don't list preservatives as ingredients, it doesn't mean these chemicals don't make their way into your food, or haven't been present in food you ate in the past and then stuck around in your brain, liver, and body. If we're not actively cleansing these brain betrayers, they can stay in our brains, livers, and bodies for decades. For example, the additives in a hot dog and soda you ate at a sports game when you were a kid could still be affecting you today.

Food additives were never supposed to be in the brain. These problematic food and supplement chemicals heighten sensitivities and also create diseased tissue because they're so highly toxic: These chemicals can kill brain cells by eating away at brain tissue, creating pits in the brain, little crevices and craters, similar to how toxic heavy metals work. These chemicals can create lesions, white spots, gray spots, and black spots in brain tissue. These chemicals can spur along brain atrophy.

Problematic food chemicals are toxic invaders that tend to affect the emotional centers of the brain. The emotional centers of the brain are sacred spaces. Humans are constantly struggling to keep emotional stamina strong and balanced. The more aspartame, MSG, or other items from the list above that are in the brain, the more unstable someone can become. What's more, these brain betrayers are highly addictive, making us dependent without even realizing it. That's even more damaging because it means we walk around with the false perception that our brain needs these chemicals, so we consume more and more of them.

1. Aspartame and Other Artificial Sweeteners

When aspartame and other artificial sweeteners enter blood vessels, they weaken the vessels. In the case of tiny blood vessels, this can cause the vessels to burst, prompting the body to create fluid to surround the bursting blood vessels. Often this heals rather quickly because the body compensates and mends this reaction.

A larger consumption of aspartame can create, over time, multiple blood vessel injuries. If a person is compromised in other ways, whether with a weakened immune system or high toxic heavy metal loads or undergoing tremendous stress, the body can't compensate and repair these tiny blood vessels, so mild scar tissue can occur. Larger consumption of aspartame can eventually cause a mild stroke.

Aspartame is also neurotoxic. This means it's toxic to neurons and toxic to nerves such as the vagus nerves and other nerves stemming from the brain. People who have neurological conditions of any kind should steer clear of aspartame.

2. Monosodium Glutamate (MSG) (including seasoning with MSG, fake meats, bottled or packaged sauces, cold cuts, and hot dogs)

MSG is added to products to make people addicted. It's even sprayed on our food chain, which can get us addicted. When MSG enters the brain, it does not leave the brain unless we work to cleanse it out.

MSG is a brain conductor. This means it reacts to electrical currents traveling through brain tissue, even though it is not a toxic heavy metal. MSG tends to pocket itself in specific areas, causing a type of crystallization that's different from the crystallizations from salt or toxic calcium because it doesn't harden like salt or calcium. Because MSG is very sticky, when it settles in a pathway, it tends to attach itself. Any other MSG traveling through tends to stick to it, causing MSG globules in the brain. It takes years' worth of MSG consumption to get to this point, sometimes a lifetime.

MSG globules in the brain are highly toxic and even have a weight behind them that eventually puts pressure on adjacent brain tissue. This is one reason why MSG causes headaches: MSG creates pressure inside the brain because MSG creates tiny little cyst-like formations. MSG becomes reflective and glossy, unlike calcium and salt deposits. These cystic globule formations also heighten electrical sparks, so electricity hitting these globules tends to bounce off the globules, flare out, and burn hotter for a quick moment. This can allow someone to become drained more easily by the end of the day or have difficulty processing thoughts at moments, or it could even give somebody a sense of pressure in their head when they're thinking too hard. MSG interferes with neurotransmitters and neurons receiving information.

3. Flavors
(Natural and Artificial)

Artificial flavors have always contained MSG. Then natural flavors came on the scene, seeming like a friendly alternative.

MSG is still a hidden demon among natural flavors.

Natural flavors are another great deception in alternative medicine, both in supplementation and in natural foods. The reason natural flavors are in supplement products and packaged foods and drinks is that anyone who wants to start a product company has to go to a manufacturer and rely on what the food and supplement chemists at the manufacturing facility tell them. The person starting the supplement or food product company ends up unaware of what's really going into their product. They go to taste the product, or they don't even get a chance to taste it, and they remain unaware of what's really in their product. Even if they're told natural flavors were added to alter the taste of the food or supplement, the person running the company remains unaware of what's in the "natural" flavor. They entrust the manufacturing facility or food chemist's lab that's affiliated with the facility to make a product they can be proud to sell.

Unfortunately, so many foods, beverages, and supplements are contaminated with MSG. "Natural flavors" is the new label to hide MSG and other chemicals that are not good for us. (It's similar to the hidden labels "fragrance" or "perfume," which industries use to hide other chemicals that are not disclosed so no one knows they're there.) Anything with "flavor" or "flavoring" in the ingredient list is a red flag: "berry flavor," "lemon flavor," "vanilla flavor," "chocolate flavor," "strawberry flavor"—even if the label says the flavorings are "natural" or "organic"—still contain MSG. Be cautious.

When supplements have these flavors added, they have a larger amount of MSG than food products that say "natural flavors." Flavorings in supplements are more concentrated to hide the bad tastes of their other ingredients.

4. Alcohol

Alcohol in tinctures is not necessary in many ways. Alcohol was an old way to create a liquid extraction of herbal nutrients. It's not necessary anymore, and to begin with, it wasn't ever truly necessary. Water extraction, such as an herbal tea, is still more beneficial than alcohol extraction of herbs where the tinctures still contain alcohol. The alcohol damages and diminishes the phytochemical compounds extracted. Alcohol (also called ethanol) has been relied upon as a preservative, yet it's a damaging one, both to the constituents of the plant and to the human body.

Most everyone who's sick with a weakened immune system doesn't fare well with alcohol in tinctures. Alcohol lowers the immune system for people who already have lowered immune systems to begin with. Alcohol causes hydrochloric acid deficiencies because alcohol from tinctures enters the stomach glands that produce your hydrochloric acid and injures the glands over time, causing lower hydrochloric acid production. This is why people who have gastric distress and take alcohol in tinctures have difficulties. Alcohol also causes stress upon the liver.

The argument for alcohol in tinctures is that it's the only way to extract phytochemical compounds from the herbs. There are very rare situations where a trace amount of a certain type of alcohol in a medicinal doesn't outweigh the benefits of that medicinal—for example, with propolis. Keep in mind, these situations are few and far between. The vast majority of the time, it isn't true that alcohol is needed for an extraction, especially since the alcohol damages the phytochemical compounds. Burning off the alcohol in your tincture before you consume the tincture still doesn't remove the leftover residue from the alcohol within the tincture or fix the problem of denatured phytochemical compounds. This is why tinctures haven't had a good history of fixing people who are sick with chronic illness. Herbalists and natural doctors who have been recommending herbal tinctures with alcohol in them for years for Lyme, myalgic encephalomyelitis/chronic fatigue syndrome (ME/CFS), and other conditions have not seen enough results, or have even seen no results. Tinctures without alcohol have taken healing to a new level in the chronic illness community—when the tinctures are of high quality, with the appropriate herbs for the appropriate condition: for example, in Medical Medium protocols.

5. Citric Acid

Be wary of any product that lists "citric acid" in its ingredients. The citric acid in most every product that contains it is derived from GMO corn or other GMO sources. It's a very small percentage of products that use concentrated citric acid from actual citrus, and even that form of citric acid is still far from eating an orange, grapefruit, or lemon. It's a factory-made composition that denatures the citric acid, turns the citric acid into something far different from what's in citrus itself.

Because of its concentrated nature, citric acid is an irritant to the stomach lining and intestinal tract. Citric acid contains additives that are not listed alongside *"citric acid"* in an ingredients list—additives that are highly irritating to the gastrointestinal lining. The intestinal tract has a nerve highway attached to it: the vagus nerves. When we irritate the linings of our intestinal tract, we irritate our vagus and other nerves.

Corn-derived citric acid for industrial use is by far the most aggressive. That's the one specifically used in supplementation. Supplement companies have made a ghastly mistake of putting citric acid in zinc and other products, causing the person consuming it to sicken with multiple varieties of stomach issues, including nausea, vomiting, and pain.

Citric acid should be avoided whenever possible, unless it's in a product that's helping someone so much that it's superseding citric acid's problematic and irritating effects.

6. Soft Drinks
(conventional and natural)

Soft drinks on a whole are never any good for the brain. There's always something in the soft drink that is harmful for brain cells, that can increase brain toxicity levels, whether it's corn syrup, aspartame, MSG within natural or artificial flavoring, coloring, carbonation, caffeine, preservatives, or low-quality ingredients that contain toxic heavy metals. And a guaranteed percentage of mystery ingredients are not labeled on the can or bottle. Soft drinks should be avoided.

(When soft drinks are in a can, the acidity of the soft drinks eats away at the epoxy or plastic liner inside the can, if they even have a liner. Most cans do not have that plastic liner. Read more about cans in *Brain Saver's* "Toxic Heavy Metals" chapter.)

7. Preservatives, Ammonia, Formaldehyde, and Nitrates (including sodium nitrate)

Often found in processed and fast foods, these brain betrayers enter the brain in two ways: through the blood and the spinal fluid. These chemicals, which can cross the blood-brain barrier, are neurotransmitter interceptors. Phytochemical compounds from plants, electrolytes, and enzymes are meant to communicate with and enter neurotransmitters. Ammonia, nitrates, formaldehyde, and many varieties of preservatives interrupt this communication. These chemicals coat neurotransmitters, creating a shield that blocks neurotransmitters from receiving information, phytochemical compounds, electrolytes, and enzymes that would sustain the neurotransmitters and help them last longer.

"Finding ways to limit or remove these items from your life can have a profound healing effect all its own. This isn't about condemning comfort food or associating what we eat with shame. It's about bringing you the ultimate comfort: freedom to make choices based on an understanding of what does and doesn't serve your health."

— Anthony William, Medical Medium

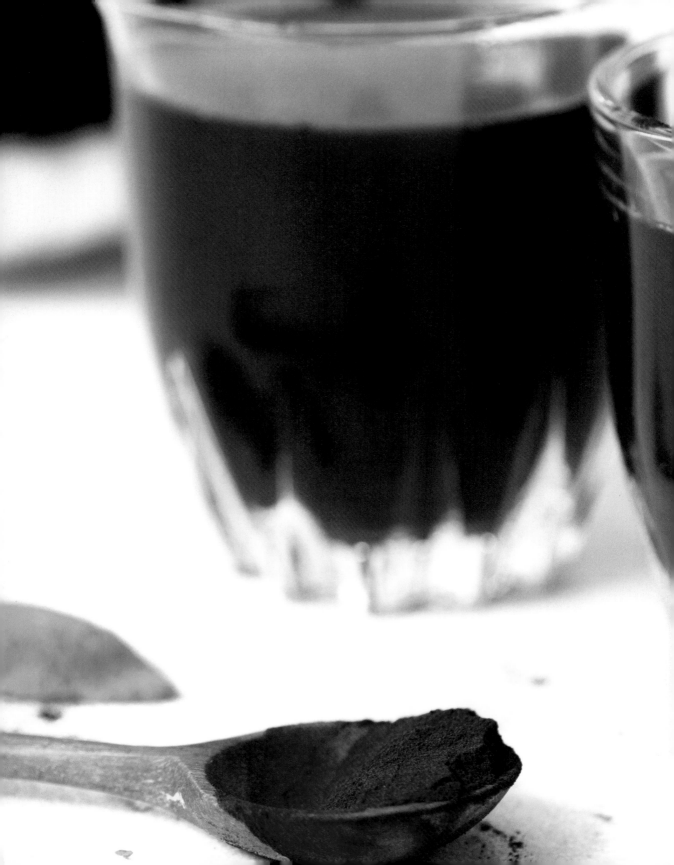

PART III

BRAIN SHOT THERAPY

"Your healing process partly depends on what was done in the past. The world of guessing games can set you back in your healing process. And that's okay. You're going in the other direction now. You're putting what you have tried in the past behind you."

— Anthony William, Medical Medium

CHAPTER 8

Medical Medium Brain Shot Therapy

Medical Medium Brain Shot Therapy offers instant relief while you're working to fix problems at a deeper level in your brain, nervous system, and body. Your brain and body have a quick response to medicinals delivered in liquid form, what I call a "shot." Designed to be highly absorbable in the mouth, these Brain Shots' valuable healing components can reach the brain fast. These specially formulated shots have the ability to reset and rewire the brain, to shock it out of patterns while at the same time reducing triggers.

Medical Medium Brain Shot Therapy is uncharted territory. These are special configurations synergistically combined just right to crack the code of how fruits, herbs, leafy greens, wild foods, and vegetables can work as medicine. While creative juice concoctions have their place, and human creativity in the kitchen should be honored, that's not what you'll find here. These Brain Shots aren't tasty delights thrown together for fun and experimentation.

The healing shots of Medical Medium Brain Shot Therapy are tools that come from above. These Brain Shots are composed of specific combinations of ingredients working together systematically for specific reasons that only a source above could know. The relationships among these ingredients are intricate and unknown to anyone. Until now, this knowledge from above has remained untapped.

THE BRAIN SHOT THERAPY LIST

Exposures

1. Pathogens
2. Toxic Fragrances
3. Negative Energy
4. Mold
5. EMF and 5G
6. Radiation

7. Toxic Heavy Metals

8. Pesticides, Herbicides, and Fungicides

9. Pharmaceuticals

10. Chem Trails

Shifters

1. Obsessive Thoughts

2. Mood

3. Nerve

4. Energy

5. Food Fear

6. Cravings

7. Anger

8. Guilt and Shame

9. Ego

10. Dreams

Stabilizers

1. Nerve-Gut Acid

2. Trauma, Shock, and Loss

3. Adrenal Fight or Flight

4. Burnout

5. Betrayal and Broken Trust

6. Relationship Breakups

7. Sleep and Recharging

8. Speaking Your Truth

9. Finding Your Purpose

10. Wisdom and Intuition

HOW TO USE MEDICAL MEDIUM BRAIN SHOT THERAPY

Medical Medium Brain Shot Therapy is highly adaptable to your needs. You have two main options:

- **Use these shots as stand-alone Medical Medium Brain Shot Therapy.** Apply the Brain Shots as needed or desired, based on whichever specific form of relief you're seeking. Just like with any other Medical Medium therapy, you may also want to incorporate various other Medical Medium tools as part of your customized healing protocol.

- **Use these shots in a Medical Medium Brain Shot Therapy Cleanse.** Systematically work your way through the Brain Shots as part of a 10-, 20-, or 30-day cleanse. Find details for how to do this in the next chapter, "Medical Medium Brain Shot Therapy Cleanses."

Choosing Your Therapeutic Tools

If you're using stand-alone Medical Medium Brain Shot Therapy, you may know simply from looking at the names which Brain Shots you'd like to try. Or you may discover what resonates once you read the suggested uses. Or you may want to explore, trying them all.

Keep in mind, the descriptions of the Brain Shots are only examples. You may be up against an issue that's not listed. Don't let that deter you—the shot still applies to you. For instance, you may decide from the names "Mood Shifter" or "Burnout Stabilizer" or "Toxic Fragrances Exposure" that these shots are supportive for your situation, then perhaps not see your exact situation in the explanations. The Brain Shots still hold just as much merit for you.

When it comes to Medical Medium Brain Shot Therapy, it's good to explore. Any Brain Shot can apply to anyone. Feel free to experiment with which shots you choose. Use them as therapeutic tools whether you're targeting a specific need or not—because whether you're aware or not, you probably do have a cause and a reason for needing these Brain Shots. For example, you may not know you have a trust issue, yet when you try the "Betrayal and Broken Trust Stabilizer," enlightenment follows.

Many people don't know what issues they have within. They don't know what's broken. With Medical Medium Brain Shot Therapy, you don't need to know what's wrong for these shots to help you. Even if you don't believe you have a need, these shots will find a way to help you. That's one reason why the Medical Medium Brain Shot Therapy Cleanses, some of which methodically take you through the different Brain Shots, can be such a revelation.

With Medical Medium Brain Shot Therapy, however you decide to use it, you venture into uncharted territory with your healing.

When to Take Your Shots

If you're doing stand-alone Medical Medium Brain Shot Therapy, you can take your shots at any time of day as long as you follow this one golden rule: **drink your Brain Shots at least 15 to 30 minutes before or after celery juice**. In other words, drink your shots separately from celery juice, waiting at least 15 to 30 minutes in between drinking the shot and the celery juice. You don't want to disrupt pure celery juice's efficacy as it does its work inside your brain and body.

Ideally, drink your Brain Shots 15 to 30 minutes apart from any other food and drink too. That is, wait a minimum of 15 to 30 minutes after consuming anything else before you have a shot, then wait a minimum of 15 to 30 minutes after consuming a shot before you consume anything else. You want to give yourself time to resonate with each Brain Shot, letting the therapy enter the bloodstream and allowing yourself to pick up the frequency of the shot metaphysically and physically.

If you're doing a Medical Medium Brain Shot Therapy Cleanse, you'll find specific guidance about when to take your shots in the next chapter.

Frequency

For stand-alone Medical Medium Brain Shot Therapy, it's up to you how often you take these shots. You may decide to take the Brain Shots daily. If your need for exposure protection, shifting, or stabilization is great or you're dealing with an aggressive situation, you can take the shots multiple times a day.

You're also welcome to try different shots within a day or different shots from day to day.

For the Medical Medium Brain Shot Therapy Cleanses, there's specific guidance about frequency in the next chapter.

Preparation and Storage

You are welcome to make your Brain Shots fresh or ahead of time. If prepping ahead, you may decide to make them the night before or to juice multiple shots in the morning for the day ahead. If you won't be drinking your shots right away, store them in an airtight container in the fridge or in a cooler or insulated lunch bag if you're on the go. Consume within 24 hours of juicing.

Notes on Juicing

- While you can use any juicer for these recipes, a cold press, masticating juicer will be more effective at extracting all the juice nutrients, especially from herbs and leafy greens. If you're using a centrifugal juicer, you may need to increase ingredient quantities a little to get full shots.

- When juicing herbs and greens in a centrifugal juicer, you may have the most success if you wrap your leafy greens and herbs around some of the firmer ingredients, such as apples, rather than sending the greens and herbs down the juicer chute separately.

- If your juicer is not producing a full shot, you can try running a tiny bit of water or coconut water through your juicer, after the other ingredients, to top off your shot. This isn't ideal. If you can, it's better to try increasing the ingredient quantities a little if your juicer isn't producing enough when following these recipes.

- It's best to follow the listed recipes if at all possible. If you can't use or access any of the ingredients, use the listed ingredients that you can or focus on Brain Shots for which all the ingredients are available to you. If you're missing a particular ingredient because you can't source it at the moment, you may come across it another time or decide to grow it yourself. When you can finally make the complete shot recipe, that Brain Shot will be all the more precious.

Adjustments for Children

Depending on the age and size of your child, serve a small portion of a given Brain Shot, whether that means reducing to a 1 ounce serving or even as little as a teaspoon.

Exposure Shots

These Brain Shots can be administered before an exposure, during an exposure, shortly after an exposure, or even days, weeks, or months after an exposure.

PATHOGEN EXPOSURE

(Viruses, Bacteria, and Viral/Bacterial Byproduct)

Makes 1 to 2 shots

This shot can be useful if:

- You feel you've been around others who could be contagious due to COVID, the flu, or mono
- You're concerned about having shared bodily fluids with another person through shared glasses, bottles, food, utensils, or plates
- You're concerned about having shared bodily fluids through public restrooms or sexual activity
- You believe you might have been exposed to foodborne pathogens and you're concerned about getting food poisoning

Also consider trying this shot before attending an event where there will be a crowd of people and/or before eating out in restaurants.

6 sprigs fresh thyme
2 sprigs fresh rosemary
1 small garlic clove (optional)
2 raw medium asparagus spears
   (¼ cup chopped)
2 raw brussels sprouts
1 to 2 stalks celery

Run each ingredient through a juicer in the order listed from top to bottom.

Pour into a glass and serve.

TIPS

- For the fresh thyme and rosemary, if the stems are woody, you can use just the leaves. If the stems are soft, you can juice them too.

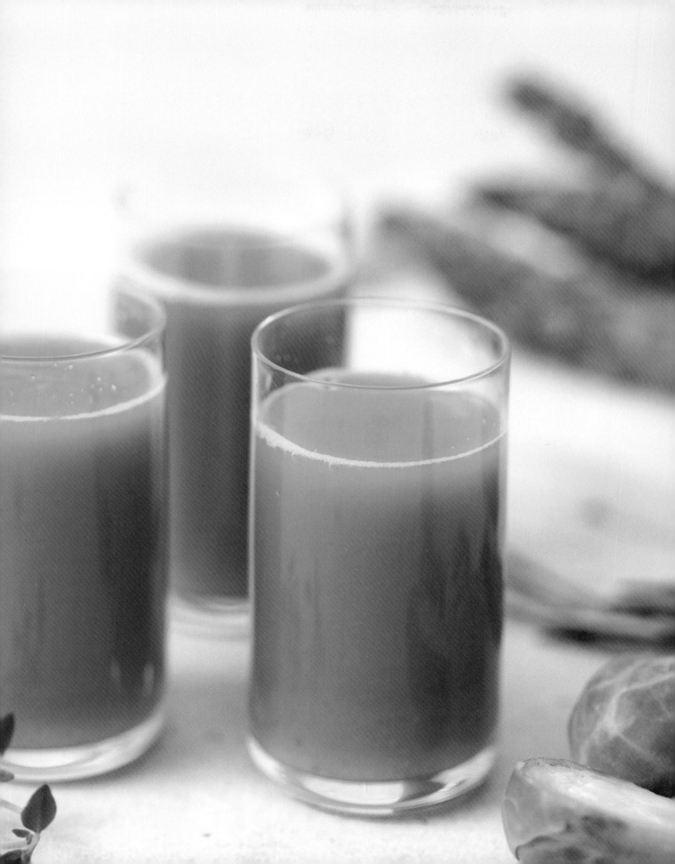

TOXIC FRAGRANCES EXPOSURE

Try this shot when you've been exposed to toxic fragrances and scents through such circumstances as:

- Gatherings of people with fragrances coming off their persons
- Walking through department stores, grocery stores, other shops, or visiting doctors' offices where exposure to perfume, cologne, fabric softeners, scented candles, air fresheners, and other fragrances could be present
- Recently driving in a car where air fresheners are installed and/or family members saturated in perfume, cologne, laundry detergent, and other chemical toxic scents were in the car with you
- Close contact with others saturated in hair products, aftershave, cosmetics, body lotions, and body oils
- A neighbor's laundry sending dryer exhaust filled with perfumes, colognes, scented detergent, and fabric softener into the air

1 radish
1 cup roughly chopped green leaf lettuce, tightly packed
1 cup tightly packed fresh cilantro
½ apple

Run each ingredient through a juicer in the order listed from top to bottom.

Pour into a glass and serve.

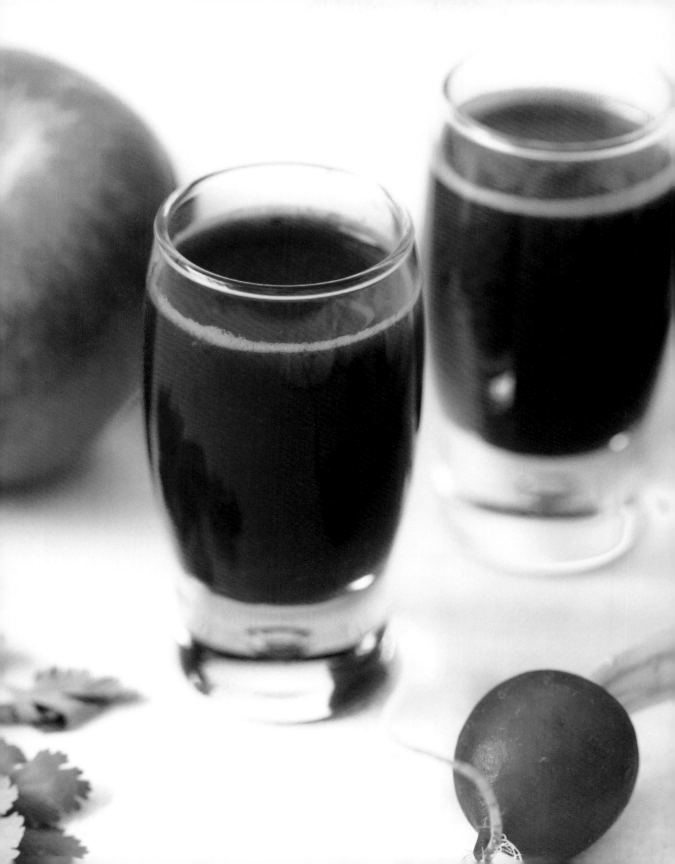

NEGATIVE ENERGY EXPOSURE

This is a helpful shot for those times when:

- You feel an unexplained sadness come over you
- You experience a confrontation or misunderstanding with another person
- Unexplained anger arises within you or even another person
- You're having a bad day
- Things in your life seem to be going wrong or you're feeling unlucky
- You're fearing something or someone and you can't shake it
- You're feeling dread after a bad dream
- You need to stay strong because you have no choice but to be around someone such as a friend or coworker who you feel has negative energy or a consistently negative attitude
- You're spending time around someone going through mental health challenges that may cause them to be angry or sad
- You're around someone who is struggling to the point of being suicidal
- You can't seem to break depressing, bad thoughts

¼ cup tightly packed fresh sage (approximately 30 leaves)
½ cup tightly packed sunflower sprouts
¼ cup tightly packed wheatgrass (or 2 teaspoons thawed frozen wheatgrass juice)
½ small garlic clove (optional)
½ to 1 orange or 1 to 2 tangerines, peeled

Run each ingredient through a juicer in the order listed from top to bottom.

Stir in the thawed wheatgrass juice (if using).

Pour into a glass and serve.

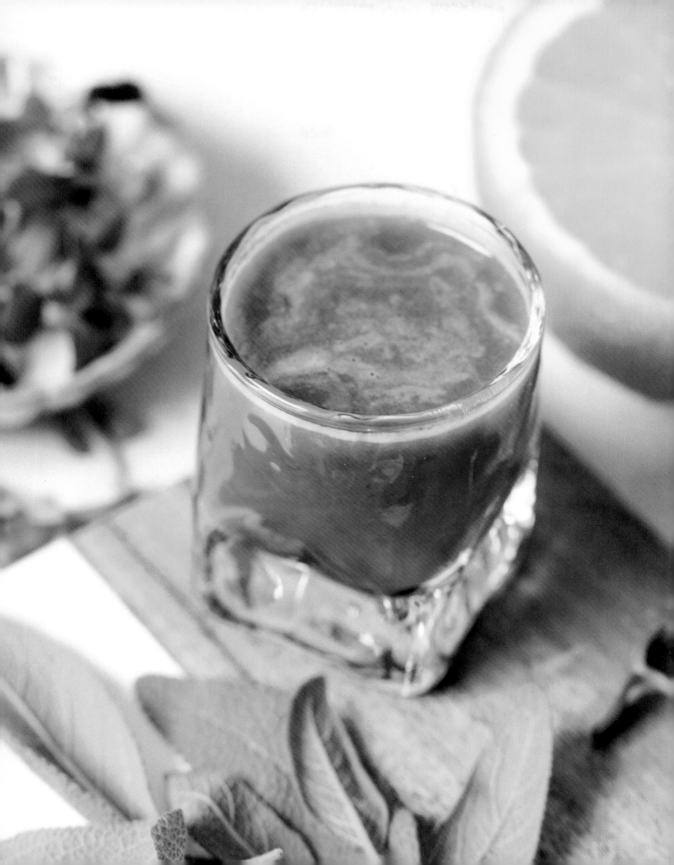

MOLD EXPOSURE

A helpful shot for any kind of mold or mildew exposure, including when you have been:

- Visiting or living in a moldy house or building
- Working in a moldy office or other workspace
- Inhaling mold off another person's clothing
- Consuming water contaminated with mildew or mold spores, or eating moldy food

½ cup tightly packed fresh basil
½ cup tightly packed fresh oregano
2 sprigs fresh rosemary
½-inch piece of fresh ginger
2 radishes
¼ bulb fennel (½ cup chopped)

Run each ingredient through a juicer in the order listed from top to bottom.

Pour into a glass and serve.

TIPS

- For the fresh rosemary, if the stems are woody, you can use just the leaves. If the stems are soft, you can juice them too.

- When juicing fennel for this recipe, you can use only the bulb itself or the bulb plus the lower-to-mid stalk (leaving out the leafy fronds in this case).

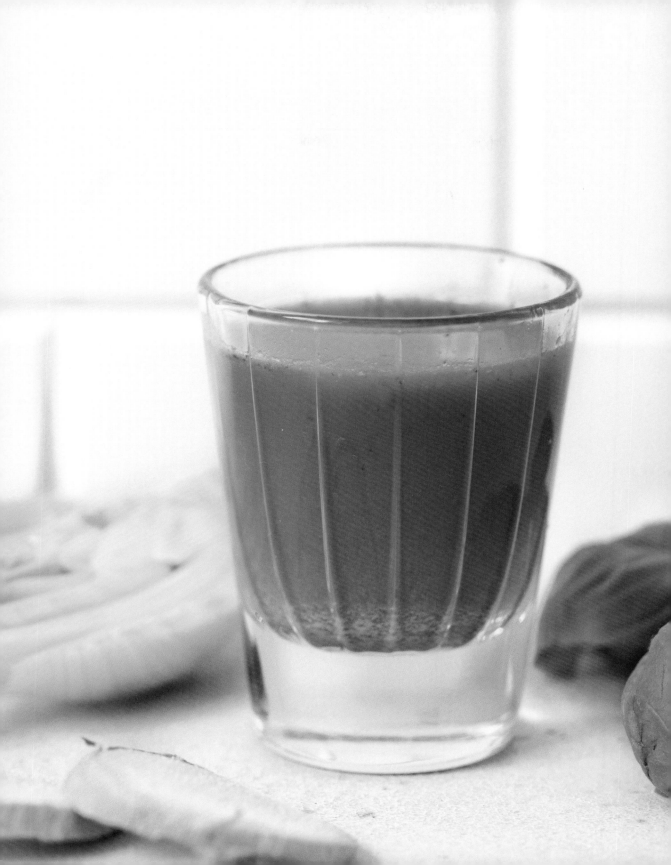

EMF AND 5G EXPOSURE

Makes 1 to 2 shots

Try this shot if you:

- Spend a lot of time on computers and computerized devices
- Live near a high-voltage area
- Spend time talking and texting on cell phones
- Travel by plane
- Live or work close to others while they're using devices
- Spend your day within several feet of a router
- Live near a cell tower

¼ cup tightly packed fresh parsley
½ cup peeled and cubed raw potatoes in a variety of your choosing, such as Yukon gold
1 to 2 stalks celery

Run each ingredient through a juicer in the order listed from top to bottom.

Pour into a glass and serve.

TIPS

- Before peeling, wash and scrub the potatoes well, discarding any that have green skins or are sprouting.

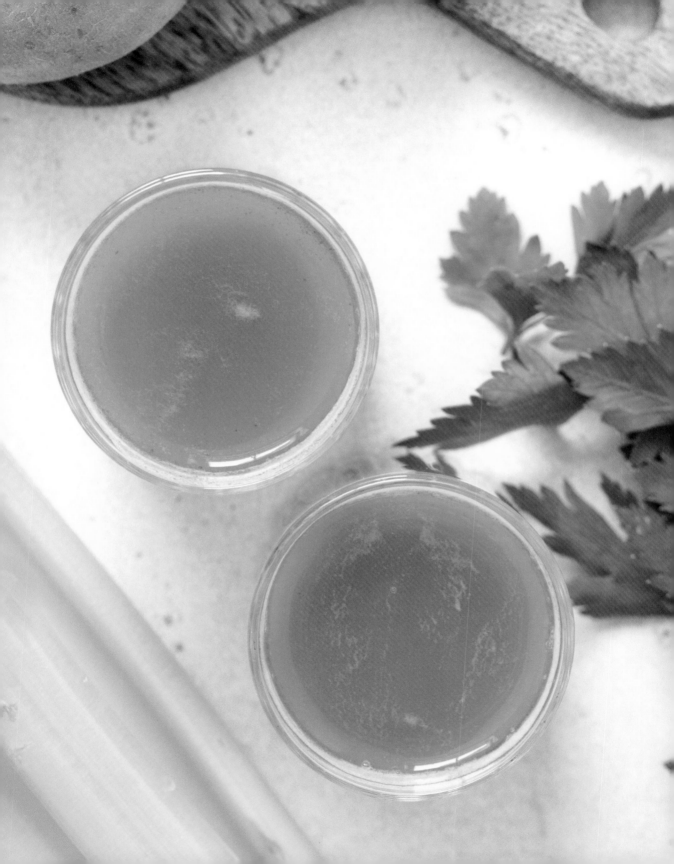

RADIATION EXPOSURE

Makes 1 to 2 shots

This is a supportive shot for circumstances such as:

- Airplane travel
- Walking through airports or being close to airport scanners or baggage scanners
- Being close to luggage that has gone through airport scanners
- Medical testing such as CT scans, X-rays, fluoroscopy, and even MRIs
- Being around others who have had medical testing such as CT scans, X-rays, fluoroscopy, and MRIs
- Exposure to computerized devices
- After a sunburn

½ cup tightly packed fresh cilantro
½ cup fresh or thawed frozen wild blueberries or 2 tablespoons pure wild blueberry juice or 1 tablespoon pure wild blueberry powder
4 raw medium asparagus spears (½ cup chopped)
1 stalk celery
½ teaspoon spirulina
½ teaspoon barley grass juice powder

Run the cilantro, wild blueberries, asparagus, and celery through a juicer in the order listed from top to bottom. If you are using the wild blueberry juice or wild blueberry powder, reserve for the next step.

Stir in the spirulina and barley grass juice powder. Stir in the wild blueberry juice or wild blueberry powder if using.

Pour into a glass and serve.

TIPS

- If you're in a part of the world where you can't access fresh or frozen wild blueberries, wild blueberry juice, or wild blueberry powder, you can substitute blackberries. Although a high-antioxidant alternative, blackberries do not have the potency to match how wild blueberries defend cells from metals, chemicals, radiation, and other toxins.

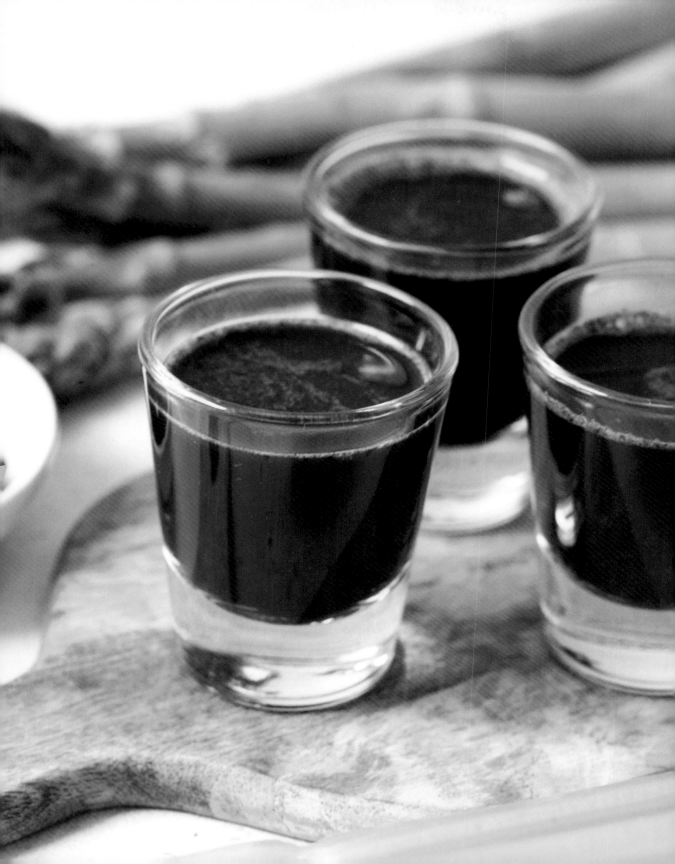

TOXIC HEAVY METALS EXPOSURE

This exposure shot is specially geared for recent exposure to toxic heavy metals, helping to stop toxic heavy metals from settling deep in the body. This shot can be used as an additional therapy to the Heavy Metal Detox Smoothies in Chapter 10, "Heavy Metal Detox," which are geared to extract toxic heavy metals that have already settled in the organs while providing ongoing support for toxic heavy metal exposure in the bloodstream, lymph, or intestinal tract.

Ideal times to use this toxic heavy metal exposure shot include when you:

- Have dental work done, such as getting mercury (amalgam) fillings removed or getting new fillings of any kind (including all composites)

- Have fluoride treatments, retainers, or braces

- Eat food cooked on a grill or from another type of cookout

- Consume restaurant food or beverages at coffee chains where town or city tap water is used in food and drink preparation

- Breathe in air fresheners, fragrances, perfumes, colognes, scented candles, detergents, or fabric softeners

- Smell smoke from something burning and do not know the smoke's origins or the purity of whatever is burning

- Get your hair done in a salon

- Are exposed to synthetic fragrances

- Spend time in or near an area recently treated with pesticide, herbicide, or insecticide spray

- Spend time outdoors during or after firework displays

TIPS

- If you're in a part of the world where you can't access fresh or frozen wild blueberries, wild blueberry juice, or wild blueberry powder, you can substitute blackberries. Blackberries do not uproot and attach themselves to toxic heavy metals like wild blueberries do, although the high antioxidant ratio in blackberries can at least slow down heavy metal oxidation, which is helpful.

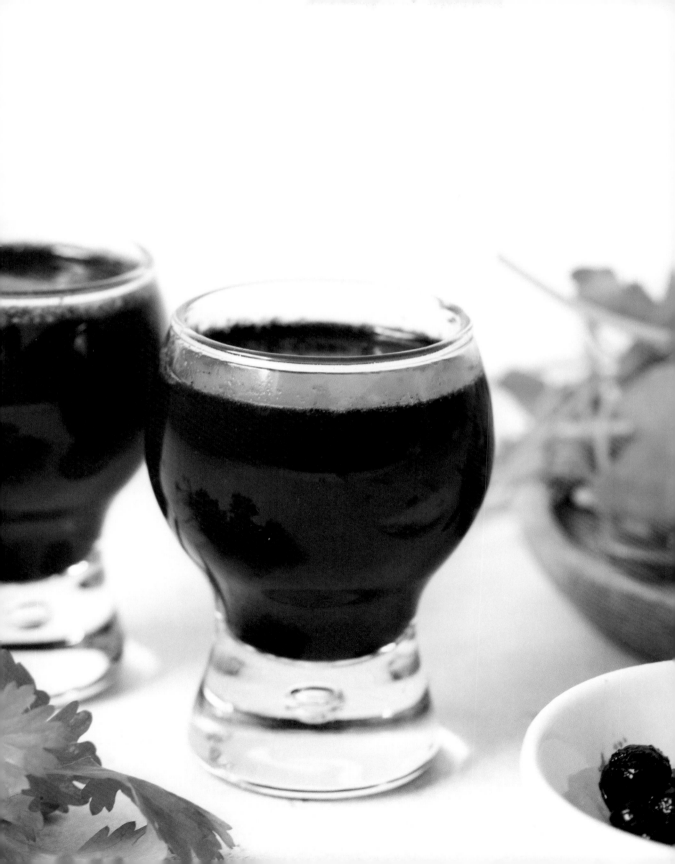

½ cup tightly packed fresh cilantro
⅓ cup tightly packed arugula
⅓ cup finely chopped cabbage
   (red or green), tightly packed
½ cup fresh or thawed frozen wild
   blueberries or 2 tablespoons pure
   wild blueberry juice or 1 tablespoon
   pure wild blueberry powder
1 to 2 stalks celery
½ to 1 orange or 1 to 2 tangerines, peeled
   (optional)
½ teaspoon spirulina

Run the cilantro, arugula, cabbage, wild blueberries, celery, and orange or tangerines through a juicer in the order listed from top to bottom. If you are using the wild blueberry juice or wild blueberry powder, reserve for the next step.

Stir in the spirulina. Stir in the wild blueberry juice or wild blueberry powder if using.

Pour into a glass and serve.

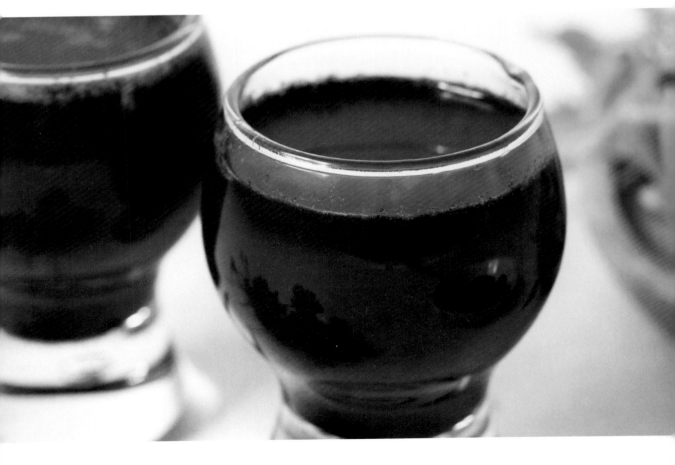

PESTICIDE, HERBICIDE, AND FUNGICIDE EXPOSURE

Makes 1 to 2 shots

This shot is an excellent tool when:

- You inhale an unfamiliar or strange odor
- You're exposed to recently delivered packages
- A neighbor sprays or treats their lawn with insecticide or chemical fertilizer treatments
- Chemical treatments are applied around an apartment building

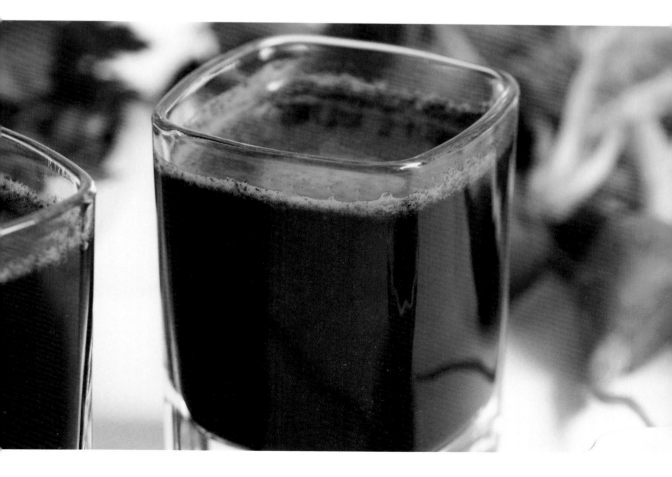

- You're exposed to a town or city treatment that's occurring on the side of the street

- You spot somebody with a tank on their back and a hose in their hand, spraying for weeds

- You see a small- to medium-sized truck with a large tank on the back and business signs on the side that say "lawn care," "bug control," or anything similar driving through your neighborhood (meaning that chances are they have recently sprayed someone's lawn or house)

- You're driving behind a truck that has a tank on the back with mysterious liquid leaking out of the tank

- You spend time sitting in or visiting parks, or you spend time on the golf course

- Insecticide treatments are sprayed in classrooms, from preschools to elementary schools to universities, and in dorm rooms, especially common at the beginning of the school year

- You live within 25 miles of a conventional fruit or vegetable farm during its growing season

¼ cup tightly packed fresh parsley
½ cup tightly packed fresh cilantro
2 large leaves kale
2 radishes
¼ cup fresh or thawed frozen blackberries
1 to 2 stalks celery
½ to 1 orange or 1 to 2 tangerines, peeled (optional)
¼ teaspoon spirulina

Run the parsley, cilantro, kale, radishes, blackberries, celery, orange or tangerines (if using) through a juicer in the order listed from top to bottom.

Stir in the spirulina.

Pour into a glass and serve.

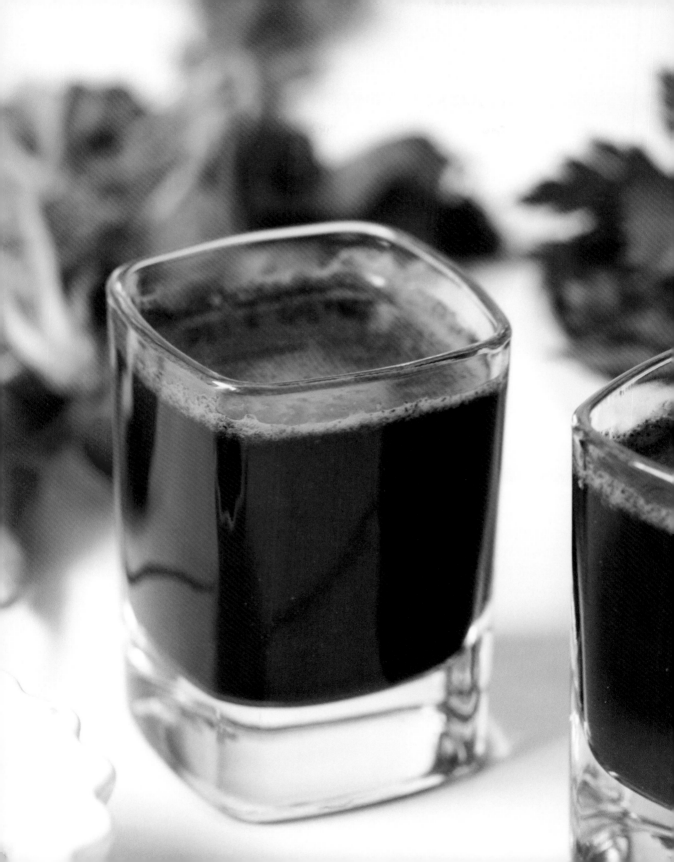

PHARMACEUTICAL EXPOSURE

This shot is formulated for exposure to prescribed or over-the-counter medications or other pharmaceuticals, whether on a one-time or continual basis. Examples of pharmaceutical exposure include:

- Antibiotic treatments for infections
- Numbing agents for dental work
- Birth control
- Painkillers
- Surgeries
- Cosmetic enhancements and procedures such as filler, botulinum toxin injections, or other applications
- Medical testing, which can include contrasts, sedatives, or numbing agents
- New medical treatments of any kind

¼ lemon, peeled
¼ lime, peeled
¼ cup chopped green onions
½ cup tightly packed fresh cilantro
2 raw medium asparagus spears
  (¼ cup chopped)
½ stalk celery
½ apple

Run each ingredient through a juicer in the order listed from top to bottom.

Pour into a glass and serve.

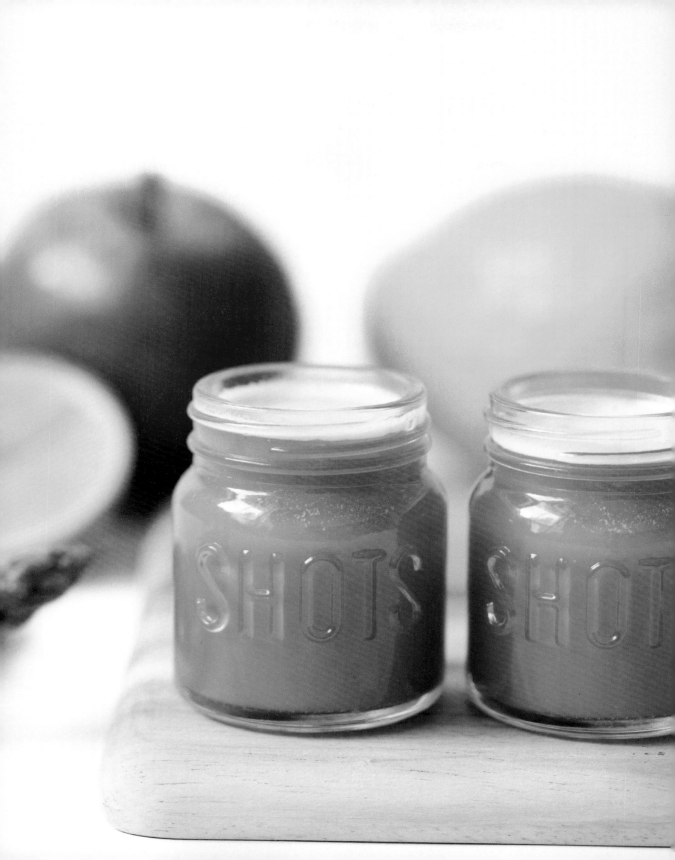

CHEM TRAILS EXPOSURE

Turn to this shot if:

- You're an avid outdoor runner or walker on public streets, parks, or trails
- You spend time at the beach or sitting outside at gatherings and spot several chem trails in the sky at one time
- You spend time outdoors during a holiday when the weather is nice (chem trails are purposely increased on holidays such as Easter and the Fourth of July)
- You spend time swimming in the ocean, lakes, rivers, or ponds
- You sleep with the windows open at night
- You get caught in the rain or otherwise get a substantial amount of rainwater on your head or skin

1 tablespoon fresh or thawed frozen wild blueberries or 1 teaspoon pure wild blueberry juice or 1 teaspoon pure wild blueberry powder
¼ cup tightly packed kale
¼ lemon, peeled
½ cup tightly packed fresh cilantro
¼ cup tightly packed fresh chives
2 raw brussels sprouts
2 raw medium asparagus spears (¼ cup chopped)
½ stalk celery

Run each ingredient through a juicer in the order listed from top to bottom. If you are using the wild blueberry juice or wild blueberry powder, mix it in after all the other ingredients have run through the juicer.

Pour into a glass and serve.

TIPS

- If you're in a part of the world where you can't access fresh or frozen wild blueberries, wild blueberry juice, or wild blueberry powder, you can substitute blackberries. Although a high-antioxidant alternative, blackberries do not have the potency to match how wild blueberries defend cells from metals, chemicals, radiation, and other toxins.

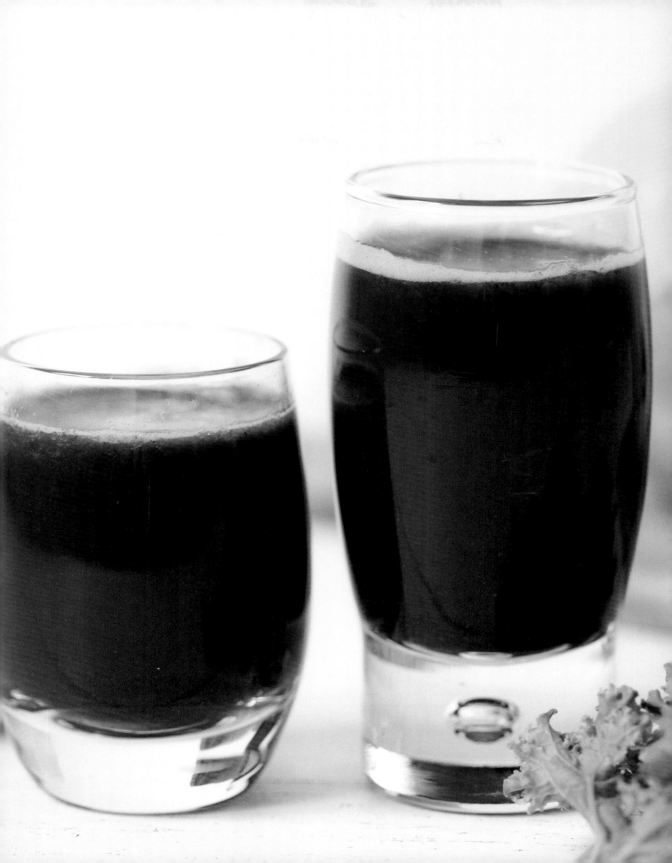

"Your soul does exist. Everyone has a soul. It is the voice of your entire existence. Your soul retains knowledge of all the events that have occurred in your life. Your soul is a record that contains the meaning of your physical existence. Your soul harnesses every journey you have chosen or experienced in a physical living form. Your soul sustains itself and lives forever, long after the physical part of you has perished."

— Anthony William, Medical Medium

Shifter Shots

The world is getting so complicated in so many ways, and we're being pushed in so many different directions, it's easy to get confused or stuck in a pattern that is not helpful to the healing process. These Brain Shots are designed to help shift our direction so our body can shift and heal and our emotional frame of mind can break a pattern or confinement that the complications of this world have created.

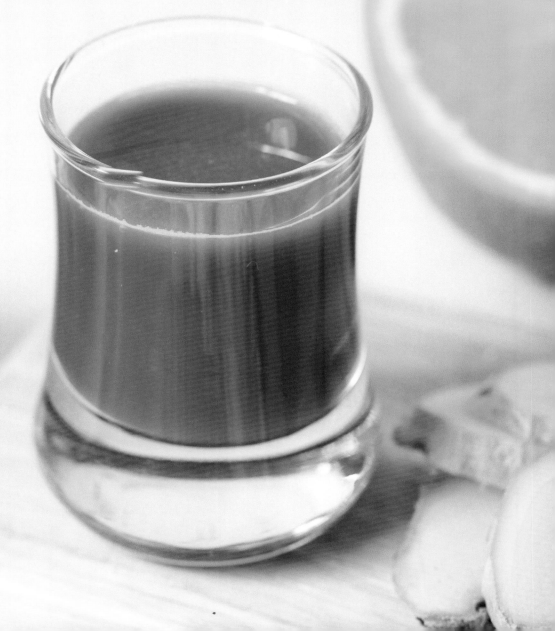

OBSESSIVE THOUGHTS SHIFTER

Try this shot when:

- You're trying to break repeated painful thought patterns resulting from a difficult situation or hardship

- You experience chronic OCD, or you're going through a relapse or heightening of OCD symptoms; this Brain Shot covers all forms and varieties of OCD

- A song you don't want to hear anymore keeps playing in your head

- Repetitive thoughts that are disturbing you continue to replay

- Repetitive thoughts are causing you to make repetitive actions

- You're hearing voices in your head or experiencing thoughts that are upsetting, unproductive, and/or highly questionable and may be telling you to do things that aren't good or smart

- A memory of a past experience keeps arising in your mind and it's not helpful to keep thinking about it

1 radish
⅛ cup loosely packed fresh sage
   (about 8 leaves)
½ to 1 apple
1 stalk celery

Run each ingredient through a juicer in the order listed from top to bottom.

Pour into a glass and serve.

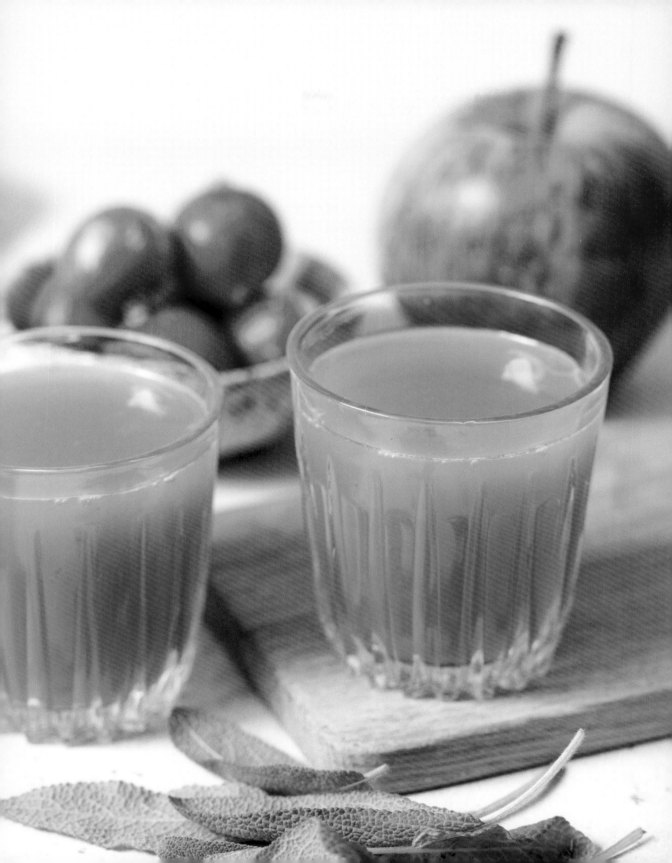

MOOD SHIFTER

Makes 1 to 2 shots

This is a great shot for:

- Irritability, chronic frustration, or crankiness
- Feelings of overwhelm and emotional exhaustion
- When someone you trust notices you're not yourself
- When you're feeling gloomy, downhearted, or low-spirited and need a lift
- When you're having a hard time keeping balanced emotionally, feeling like you're unsteady, getting triggered easily, or all over the place, up and down

1 tablespoon fresh or thawed frozen wild blueberries or 1 teaspoon pure wild blueberry juice or 1 teaspoon pure wild blueberry powder
¼ cup tightly packed fresh chives
¼ cup tightly packed fresh basil
½ cup tightly packed fresh alfalfa sprouts
½ lime, peeled
1 stalk celery
½ cup grapes (optional)

Run each ingredient through a juicer in the order listed from top to bottom. If you are using the wild blueberry juice or wild blueberry powder, mix it in after all the other ingredients have run through the juicer.

Pour into a glass and serve.

TIPS

- If you're in a part of the world where you can't access fresh or frozen wild blueberries, wild blueberry juice, or wild blueberry powder, you can substitute blackberries. Although a high-antioxidant alternative, blackberries do not have the potency to match how wild blueberries defend cells from metals, chemicals, radiation, and other toxins.

- If you can't find or don't like alfalfa sprouts, you can use any kind of sprouts or microgreens in this recipe, such as broccoli, clover, sunflower, or kale. Every sprout will bring a different flavor to the shot. If you choose to use radish or mustard sprouts, be aware that it will make the shot very spicy.

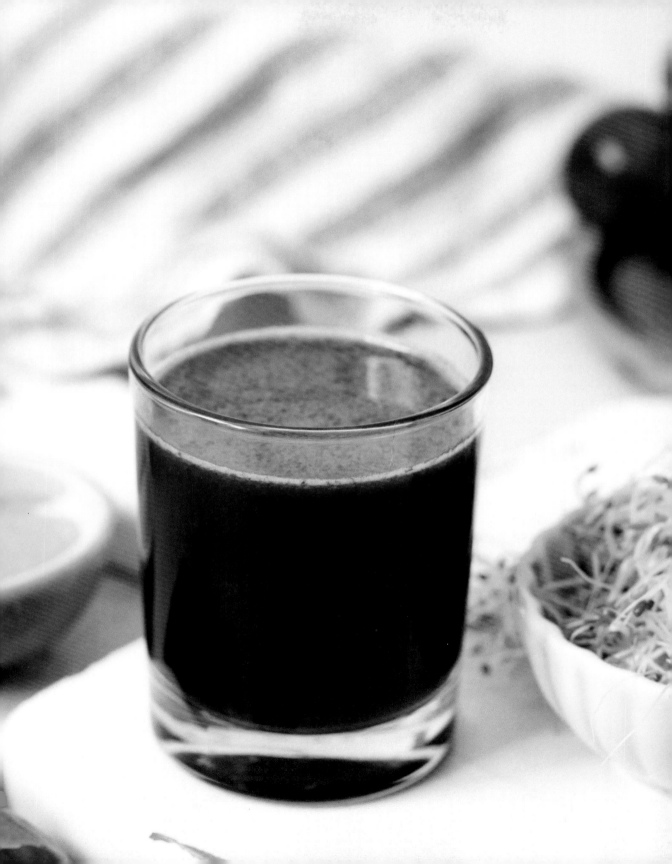

NERVE SHIFTER

This shot has a wide range of applications. Try it:

- When you're feeling shaky or anxious

- If you experience random spasms, twitches, tics, or shifting and moving pain throughout your body

- When struggling with any kind of neurological onset or episode

- To break a nervous feeling about the moment you're in, the future, or something that happened in the past

- To help calm restless legs syndrome

- Before flying or taking a trip

The Nerve Shifter is also an excellent tool to use for weddings and other events that have great meaning to you.

¼ lime, peeled
¼ cup tightly packed spinach
¼ cup roughly chopped kale, tightly
   packed
¼ cup roughly chopped lettuce, such as
   green leaf or butter leaf, tightly packed
¼ cup tightly packed fresh cilantro
¼ cup tightly packed fresh parsley
2 raw medium stalks asparagus (¼ cup
   chopped)
½ stalk celery

Run each ingredient through a juicer in the order listed from top to bottom.

Pour into a glass and serve.

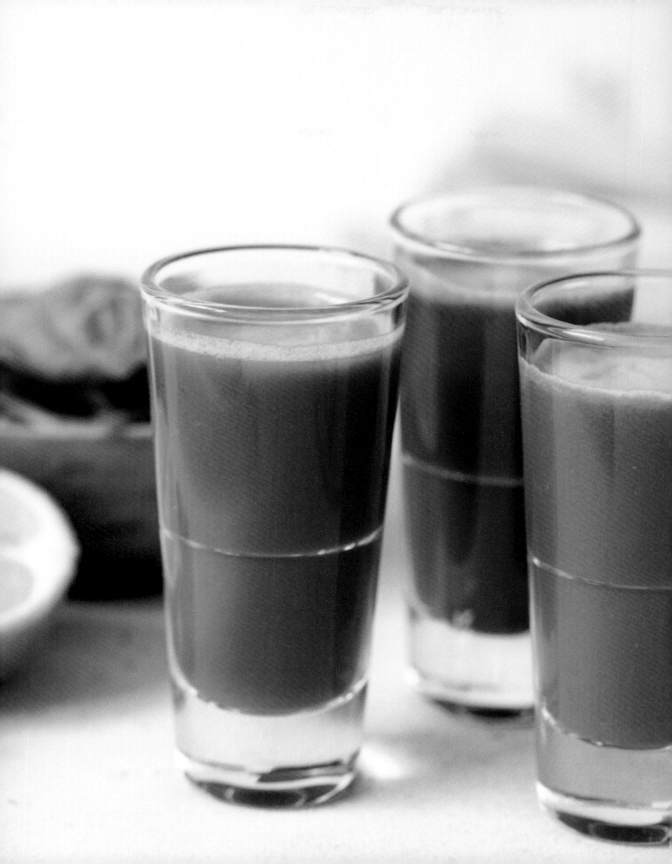

ENERGY SHIFTER

Use this shot when energetic strength is required. For example, you can try it:

- At the midpoint of a long day, when you're desperate for an energy boost
- When you feel unbalanced, as if you don't have enough energy
- If you're feeling that your energy is "off" and you're not on point
- If you feel like you have too much energy, and you're hoping to calm down an elevation of excitement
- When removing caffeine from your life
- When you want to wind down at the end of the day so you can recalibrate, rest, and retire for the night

The Energy Shifter is also ideal for:

- Overreactive or underreactive adrenals that are exhausted from excessive adrenal output
- Low blood sugar (hypoglycemia) sensations such as edginess, exhaustion, feeling emotional for unexplained reasons, or starting to get triggered easily

Try the Energy Shifter before going into a challenge or venture of any kind, whether beginning a new job, going on a retreat, starting a cleanse, or anything else shifting in your life.

¼ cup chopped carrots
½ cup chopped raw sweet potatoes
½ cup chopped red bell pepper
½ cup fresh or thawed frozen pineapple

Run each ingredient through a juicer in the order listed from top to bottom.

Pour into a glass and serve.

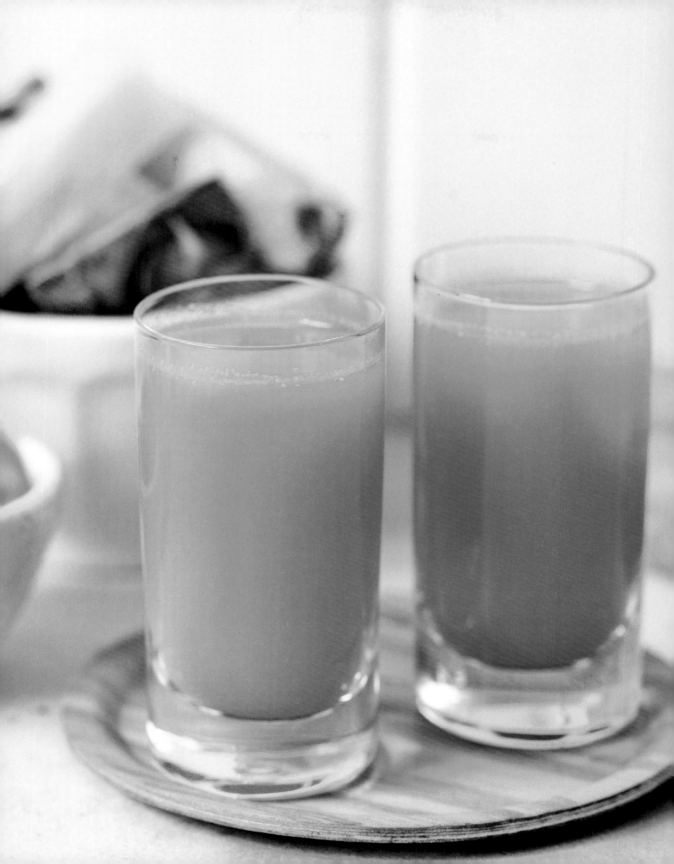

FOOD FEAR SHIFTER

Makes 1 to 2 shots

Food fear can take different shapes and forms. For example, apply this shot on a regular basis if you're living with an eating disorder. The Food Fear Shifter is also a useful tool when:

- Someone is pressuring you not to eat healthily
- You're upset about what you've been eating lately
- You're feeling locked up about food in general, afraid to eat because you're having trouble figuring out what foods you can eat comfortably without flaring up symptoms such as digestive discomfort
- You're experiencing other symptoms or conditions, and you're afraid of changing your diet to heal
- Someone wants you to eat healthily, yet you're afraid of fruits, herbs, leafy greens, wild foods, and vegetables
- You have an unexplained dislike or fear of certain foods that are healthy
- You have a fear of food that derives from misinformation about specific foods
- You're having a hard time letting go of a comfort food that's harming you

½ cup tightly packed fresh dill
½ cup tightly packed spinach
¾ cup fresh or thawed frozen mango
¼ stalk celery

Run each ingredient through a juicer in the order listed from top to bottom.

Pour into a glass and serve.

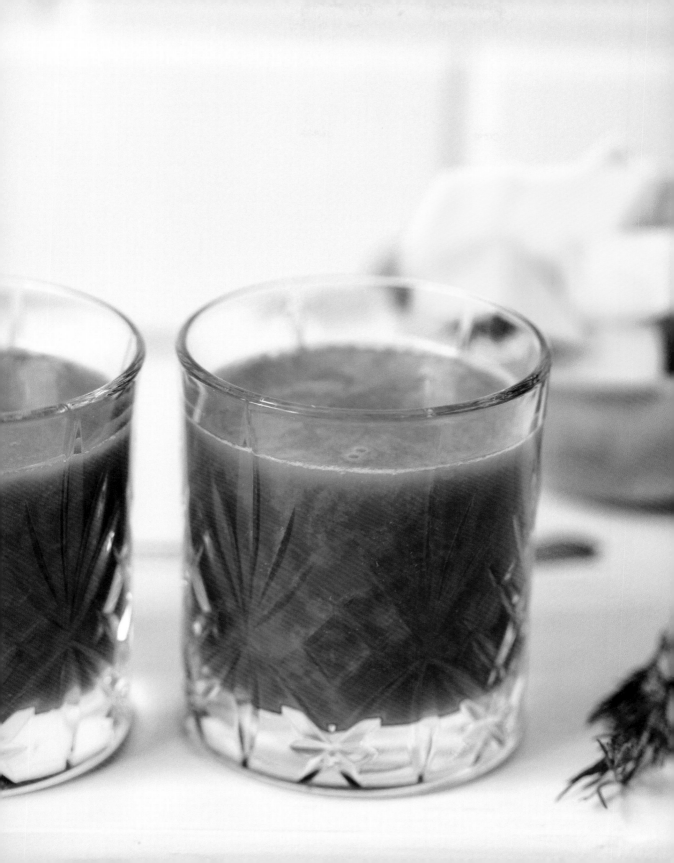

CRAVINGS SHIFTER

When cravings or addictive impulses are disrupting your life, this shot is a great tool. Try it:

- For hunger that feels insatiable or unstoppable
- As a craving buster
- As a hunger suppressant when you're trying to shift your diet
- If your diet is too high in fat and you're trying to reduce the amount of fat you're consuming
- To help break overeating patterns, food addictions, or even caffeine and salt addictions

If someone in your life is embarking on an unhealthy intermittent fasting diet, encourage them to incorporate this shot to help protect their adrenals and brain.

½-inch piece of fresh ginger
¼ cup tightly packed fresh basil
½ cup tightly packed spinach
½ cup chopped kale, tightly packed
½ cup chopped cabbage, any color, tightly packed
½ orange, peeled
½ stalk celery

Run each ingredient through a juicer in the order listed from top to bottom.

Pour into a glass and serve.

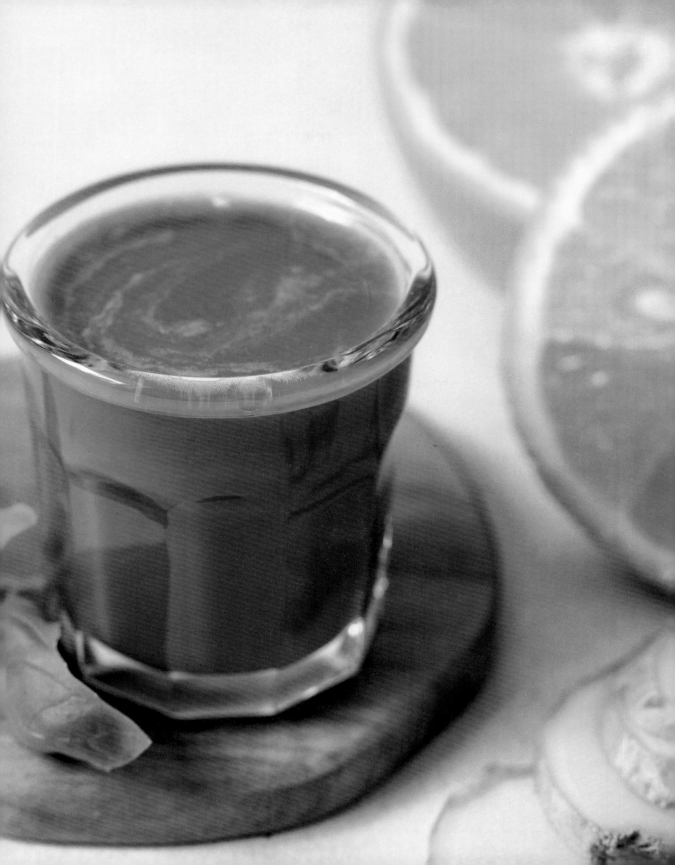

ANGER SHIFTER

Makes 1 to 2 shots

Use this shot for:

- Unexplained bouts of anger or anger surges that seem to arise without cause

- Anger surges that do have a cause

- Anger about being sick, injured, or dealing with health problems and chronic illness

- Moments of unhappiness, frustration, or irritability that bubble up from inside

- Anger that's triggered from being wronged in any way, such as from disappointment or betrayal

- Confrontations or disputes with others

- Anger about world events

- Anger at yourself

½ cup tightly packed fresh mint
¼ cup tightly packed fresh sage
½ cup fresh or thawed frozen mango
1 tablespoon fresh or thawed frozen wild blueberries or 1 teaspoon pure wild blueberry juice or 1 teaspoon pure wild blueberry powder
1 cup chopped carrots

Run each ingredient through a juicer in the order listed from top to bottom. If you are using the wild blueberry juice or wild blueberry powder, mix it in after all the other ingredients have run through the juicer.

Pour into a glass and serve.

TIPS

- If you're in a part of the world where you can't access fresh or frozen wild blueberries, wild blueberry juice, or wild blueberry powder, you can substitute blackberries. Although a high-antioxidant alternative, blackberries do not have the potency to match how wild blueberries defend cells from metals, chemicals, radiation, and other toxins.

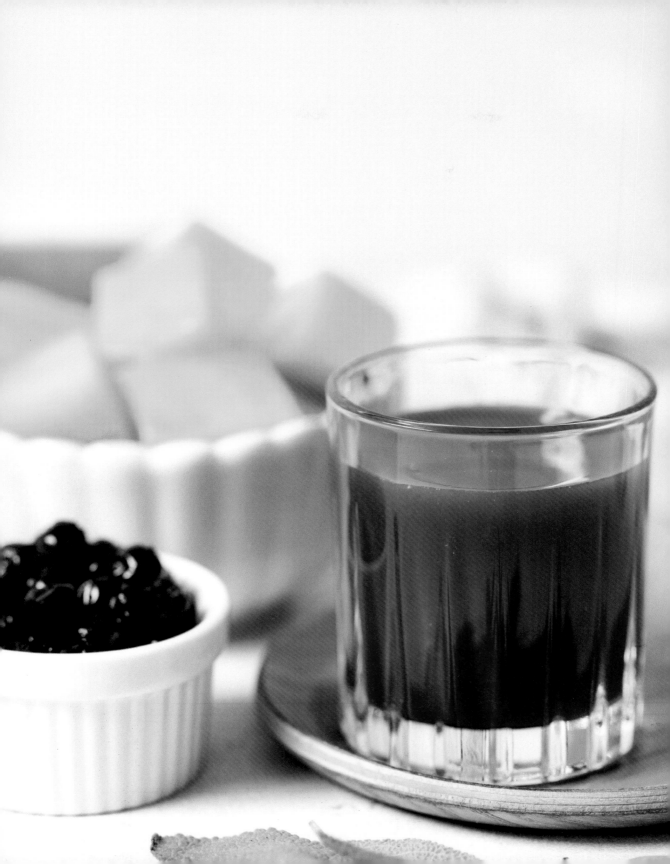

GUILT AND SHAME SHIFTER

Makes 1 to 2 shots

Try applying this shot when:

- You don't believe in yourself or you've lost confidence in yourself
- You're losing faith that you're a good person
- You're feeling guilt or shame about being sick
- You experience insecurity or loss of confidence due to chronic illness
- You're feeling less-than or like you are not good enough
- You can't forgive yourself for something you may believe was your fault
- You're feeling guilt or shame about something you said and can't unsay
- You're feeling guilt or shame about not being able to live your dream yet
- You're feeling guilt or shame about not being able to help a friend or family member in the present moment
- You're having difficulty forgiving someone else who has hurt you, upset you, or disappointed you
- You're feeling ashamed or guilty in any way—this shot can help you understand and release emotional wounds that are perpetuating guilt or shame

½-inch piece of fresh ginger
½ to 1 cup tightly packed spinach
½ to 1 orange, peeled

Run each ingredient through a juicer in the order listed from top to bottom.

Pour into a glass and serve.

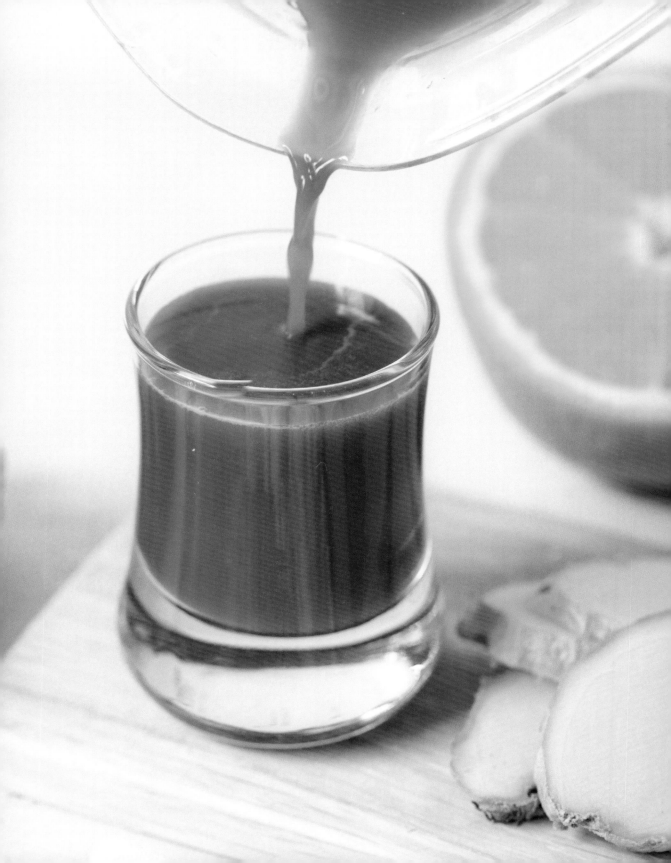

EGO SHIFTER

This shot is ideal in those moments when:

- You feel like your ego has taken over your senses, or your common sense and sensibility
- You feel like you're losing your true self, losing sight of what's truly important
- You feel like you may have been a little too self-absorbed
- You realize you've been completely self-consumed without caring for others
- You feel as if something inside of you is controlling your life and decisions while you watch from above
- You have a friend or loved one who has a very large ego and doesn't believe they do (make the Brain Shot for them)
- You feel you need to take control of your life and override the drive to harm yourself
- You need to free yourself so your authentic soul shines through and benefits you and the ones around you

½-inch piece of fresh turmeric
½ cup chopped peeled kiwi fruit
1 tablespoon fresh or thawed frozen wild blueberries or 1 teaspoon pure wild blueberry juice or 1 teaspoon pure wild blueberry powder
¼ cup chopped portobello mushroom*
¼ cup tightly packed, roughly chopped kale
½ cup tightly packed fresh parsley
½ stalk celery

Run each ingredient through a juicer in the order listed from top to bottom. If using the wild blueberry juice or wild blueberry powder, mix it in after all the other ingredients have run through the juicer.

Pour into a glass and serve.

*Wash and rinse the portobello mushroom thoroughly with warm to hot water before chopping. Do not use a slimy or decaying mushroom. That's a sign of the mushroom oxidizing and aging.

TIPS

- If you're in a part of the world where you can't access any form of wild blueberries, you can substitute blackberries. Although a high-antioxidant alternative, blackberries do not have the potency to match how wild blueberries defend cells from toxins.

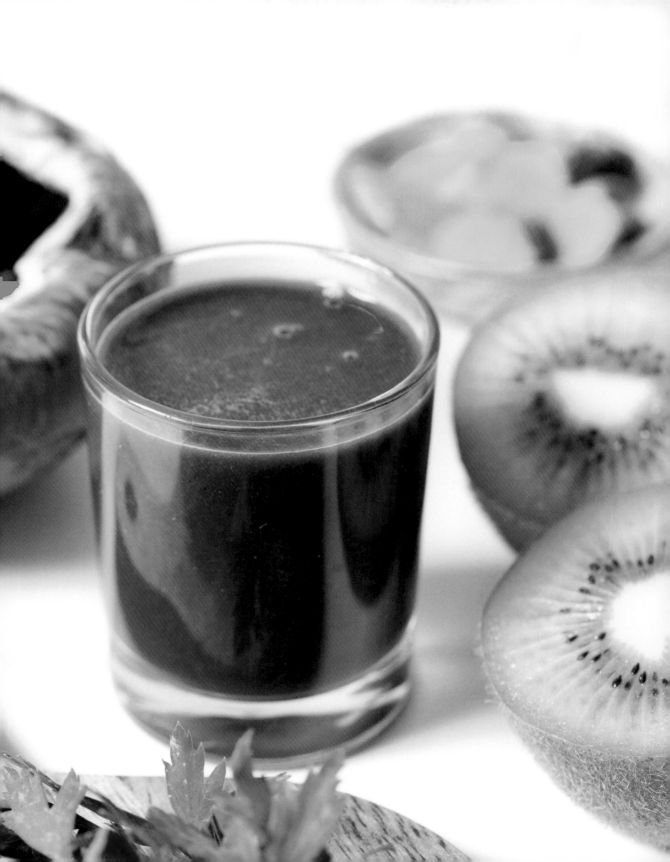

DREAMS SHIFTER

This shot can be taken at any time of day or evening. If you wish to take it before a nap or before bed, you're welcome to make the shot earlier in the day and save it in the refrigerator until you're ready. Examples of when to use it include when:

- You want to use your dreams as a gateway to understand your soul and your soul's past

- You're having difficulty dreaming and want to dream

- Your dreams are troubling, very stressful, or even frightening

- You want to decode the meaning of your dreams and gain more insight into your dreams

- Dreams are regularly waking you

- You're fearful of going to sleep

- You're trying to reach others through your dreams

- You're trying to enter other people's dreams

- You're not sleeping enough—this shot can help you heal through your dream process in the short amount of sleep you're getting

½-inch piece of fresh ginger
½ cup fresh or thawed frozen mango
½ cup fresh or thawed frozen cherries, pitted
½ cup chopped raw zucchini
¼ cup loosely packed fresh peppermint leaves (optional)

Run each ingredient through a juicer in the order listed from top to bottom.

Pour into a glass and serve.

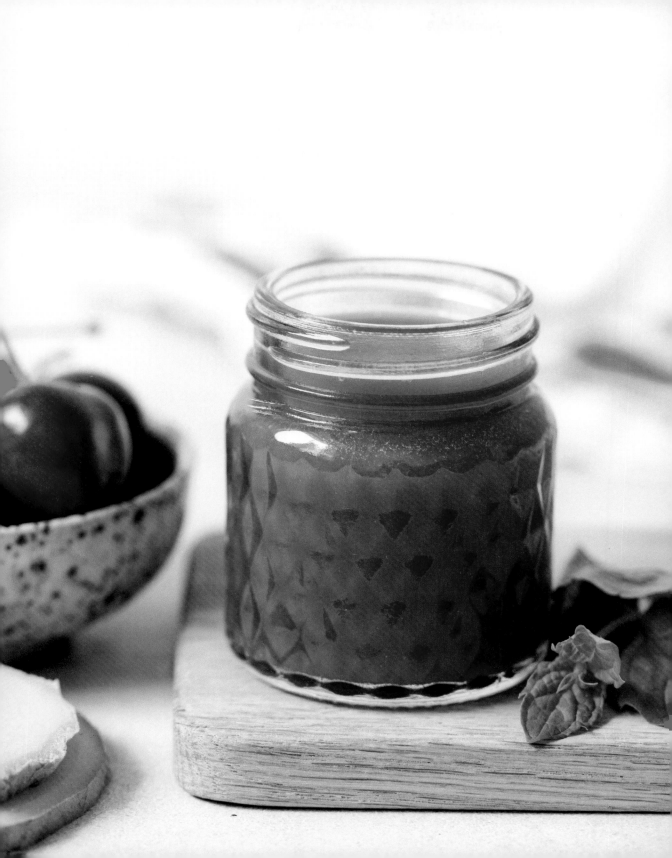

"Your soul is more than you. It is your light. A light that did not start here on earth but started above. Your soul is much older than your physical body and has memories and information from the past to which you don't have conscious access. Your soul has the power to lead you on your way even when it's underfed and broken by the people around you or the world we live in. Your soul's leftover fragments still hold the power and the glory that brighten the way on the darkest path."

— Anthony William, Medical Medium

Stabilizer Shots

These Brain Shots are designed to stabilize you in an increasingly destabilizing world.

NERVE-GUT ACID STABILIZER

Makes 1 to 2 shots

Use this stabilizing shot if:

- You're looking to strengthen your vagus nerves
- You're dealing with gastric spasms, flatulence, chronic gastritis, mild acid reflux, or other digestive disturbances (For acute acid reflux relief, see "Aloe Vera Shock Therapy" in Chapter 3, "Medical Medium Shock Therapies.")
- You feel your food is not digesting, breaking down, or assimilating
- You feel you have poor nutrient absorption
- You've been told you have a microbiome or gut microflora condition or problem
- You feel as if you're toxic, or your blood is toxic
- You feel that your liver and lymph are toxic, stagnant, and sluggish
- You're feeling an acidy stomach, acidy sensations in your throat or mouth, or acidy feelings throughout your body
- Your body odor is more noticeable than usual
- You're dealing with chronic nausea or chronic bloating
- You're trying to repair acidic body systems and make your body systems more alkaline

4 to 6 cups tightly packed fresh parsley or fresh cilantro*

Run the parsley or cilantro through the juicer.

Pour into a glass and serve immediately.

*Note: Select either parsley or cilantro (not both at once) to create either a pure parsley or pure cilantro shot.

TIPS

- You can use any variety of parsley for this recipe, flat-leaf Italian or curly parsley.
- Fresh cilantro is also known as coriander in some countries.

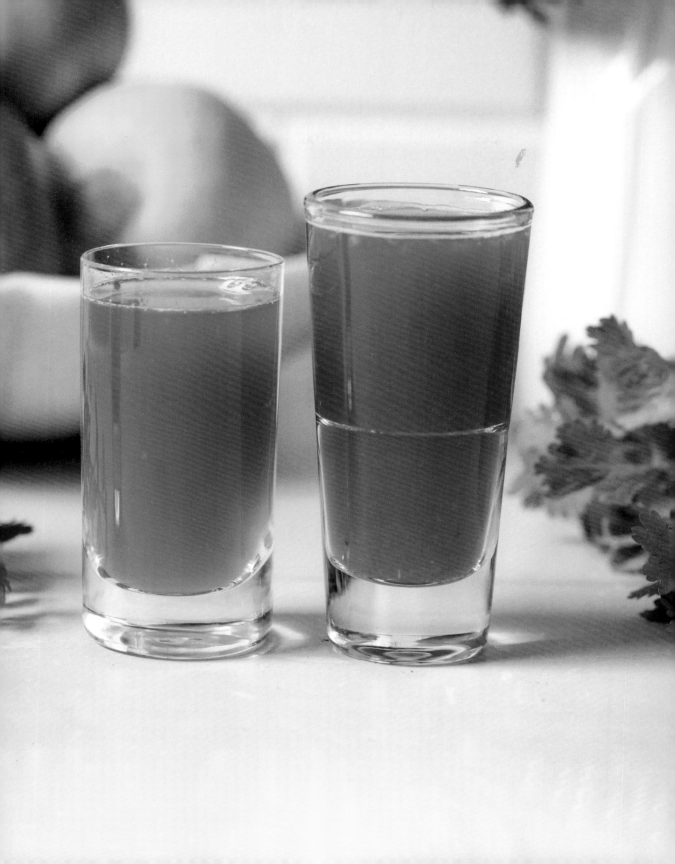

TRAUMA, SHOCK, AND LOSS STABILIZER

Makes 1 to 2 shots

This shot is a supportive tool for any kind of emotional upset, emotional challenge, or emotional stress. Consider using it when:

- You're given challenging news or you receive any emotional blows
- You're dealing with any kind of emotional upheaval
- You've lost a loved one or a pet
- You experience any kind of loss
- You've been diagnosed with a chronic illness or you learn something challenging about your health
- Local and world events are affecting your life
- You're going through emotional turmoil within your family or difficult friendships

½ cup fresh or thawed frozen cherries, pitted
1 cup tightly packed spinach
½ apple

Run each ingredient through a juicer in the order listed from top to bottom.

Pour into a glass and serve.

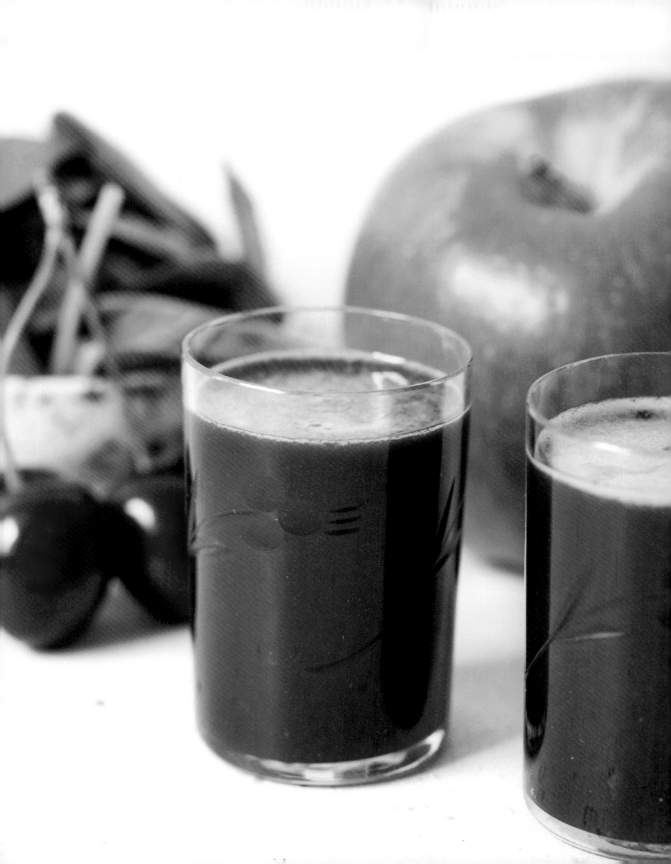

ADRENAL FIGHT OR FLIGHT STABILIZER

Makes 1 to 2 shots

Try this shot when:

- Stress is dominating your life and you're not getting a chance to have a break or reprieve from whatever you're up against
- Continual, chronic stress is occurring
- You feel involuntary reactions when receiving any kind of news or information from various people and sources
- You're experiencing any type of PTSD
- You feel like you're on a roller coaster ride and have lost control of your life
- You're addicted to adrenalized activities or drama
- You've been using sex as an escape
- You're living on adrenaline without realizing it, such as with intermittent fasting and/or caffeine use

1-inch piece of fresh ginger
1 small garlic clove
2 tablespoons fresh or thawed frozen wild blueberries or 2 teaspoons pure wild blueberry juice or 2 teaspoons pure wild blueberry powder
½ lemon, peeled
1 cup tightly packed fresh parsley
½ cup tightly packed kale
1 cup chopped watermelon rind (optional)

Run each ingredient through a juicer in the order listed from top to bottom. If using the wild blueberry juice or wild blueberry powder, mix it in after all the other ingredients have run through the juicer.

Pour into a glass and serve.

TIPS

- If you're in a part of the world where you can't access any form of wild blueberries, you can substitute blackberries. Although a high-antioxidant alternative, blackberries do not have the potency to match how wild blueberries defend cells from toxins.

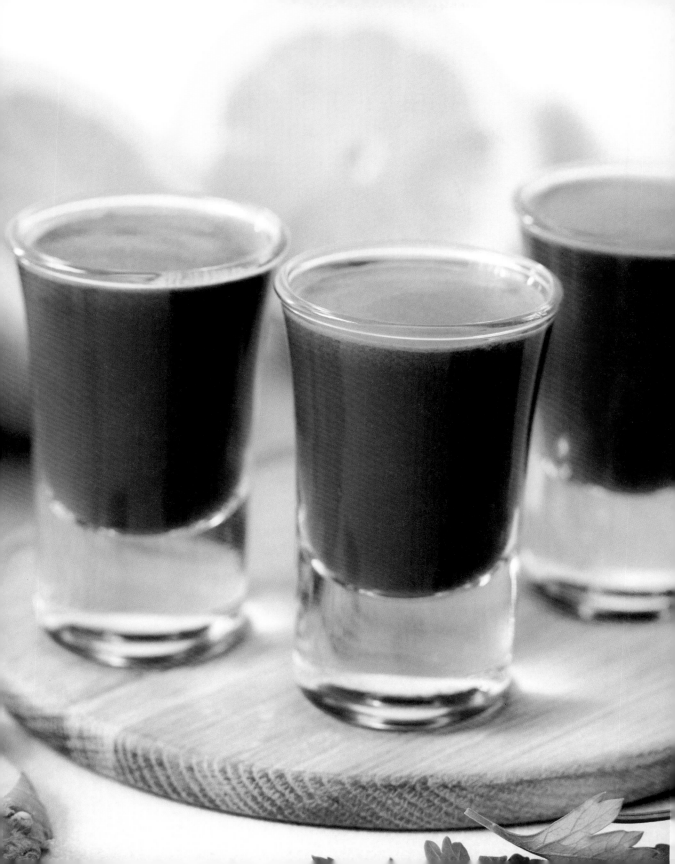

BURNOUT STABILIZER

Makes 1 to 2 shots

Use this shot when:

- You're feeling pushed past your limit
- You need a recharge
- You feel like you're missing something that your body needs, or you feel like you're running on empty
- You've given so much of yourself that you feel you have nothing more to give
- You're overworked
- You've been running on caffeine to gain focus and energy
- You feel you're short-circuiting or falling apart
- You're becoming allergic to work or allergic to others around you
- You feel like you're losing or missing a part of yourself
- You can't seem to focus because you feel exhausted on all levels

½-inch piece of fresh ginger
½ cup tightly packed pea shoots
½ cup tightly packed alfalfa sprouts
¼ cup fresh or thawed frozen pitaya
  (red dragon fruit) or ¼ cup peeled
  and chopped grapefruit
2 raw medium stalks asparagus
  (¼ cup chopped)
½ stalk celery

Run each ingredient through a juicer in the order listed from top to bottom.

Pour into a glass and serve.

TIPS

- If you can't find or don't like alfalfa sprouts or pea shoots, you can use any kind of sprouts or microgreens in this recipe, such as broccoli, clover, sunflower, and kale. Every sprout will bring a different flavor to the shot. If you choose to use radish or mustard sprouts, be aware that it will make the shot very spicy.

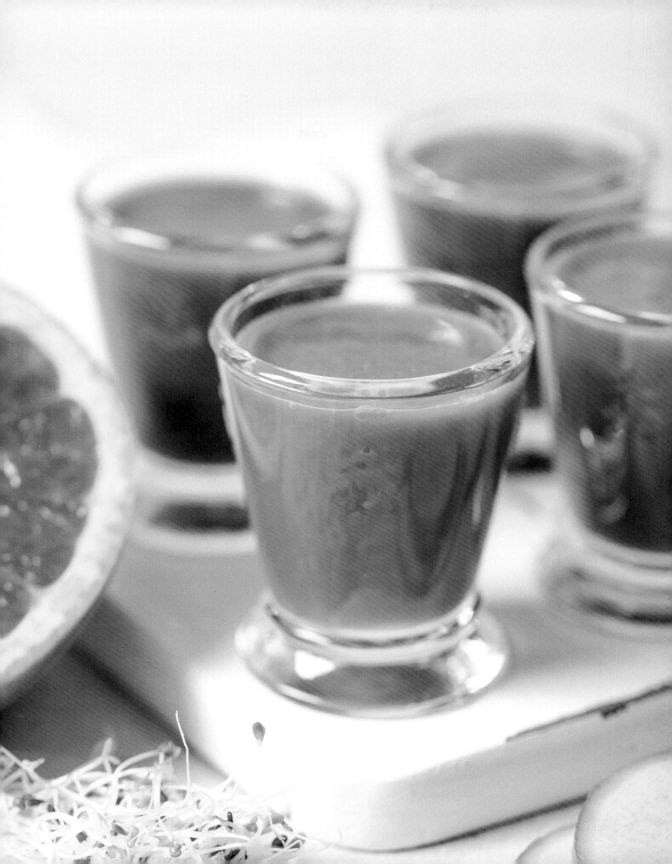

BETRAYAL AND BROKEN TRUST STABILIZER

Makes 1 to 2 shots

This tool provides support in situations where:

- You feel emotionally toyed with, played with, or not taken seriously
- You've been told your body has betrayed you
- You feel betrayed, let down, neglected, overlooked, used, or mistreated in any way
- You have been manipulated
- Someone or something you placed trust in falls through, lets you down, or disappoints you
- You feel you've let down someone you care about
- You have your heart set on something, and it doesn't come to fruition

½-inch piece of fresh turmeric
½ cup fresh or thawed frozen mango
½ lime, peeled
¼ cup tightly packed spinach
½ stalk celery
¹⁄₁₆ teaspoon cinnamon

Run the turmeric, mango, lime, spinach, and celery through a juicer in the order listed from top to bottom.

Sprinkle or mix in the cinnamon.

Pour into a glass and serve.

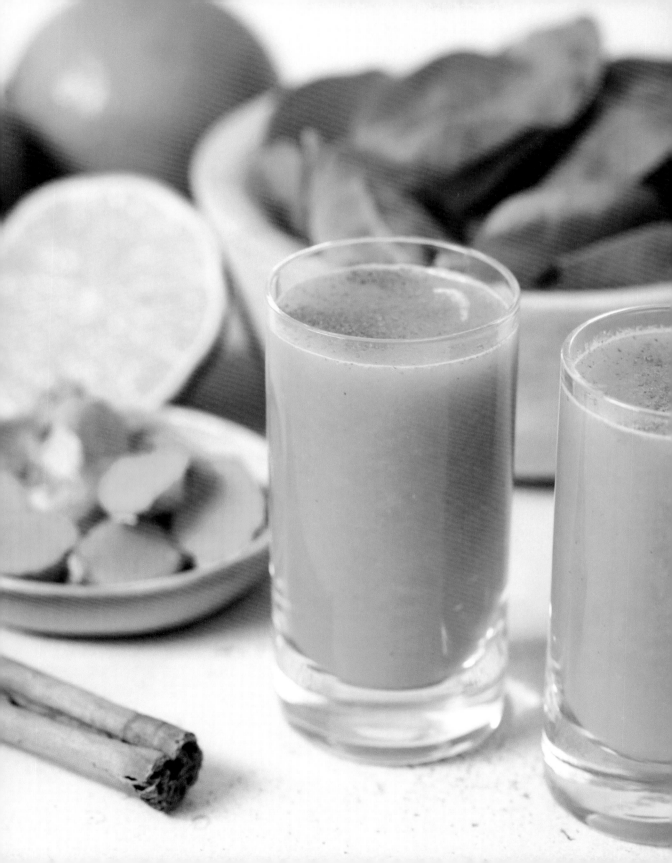

RELATIONSHIP BREAKUPS STABILIZER

Makes 1 to 2 shots

Try this Brain Shot if:

- You're going through any kind of relationship turmoil, whether or not it's reached a point of actual breakup or dismantling of a partnership
- You're having arguments, fights, or disagreements in any kind of relationship
- You feel there is no resolution to a situation or that there are unresolved issues with friends or family
- You're in a constant, vicious cycle of breaking up and making up
- There is deep-seated or growing resentment inside a relationship
- You're in an endless cycle of argument with a partner

½ cup fresh or thawed frozen strawberries
½ tomato or ¼ cup cherry tomatoes
¼ lemon, peeled
½ cup tightly packed fresh parsley
½ cup roughly chopped lettuce, such as green leaf or butter leaf, tightly packed
½ stalk celery

Run each ingredient through a juicer in the order listed from top to bottom.

Pour into a glass and serve.

TIPS

- If you select fresh strawberries for this recipe, remove the greens before using. Read why on page 287.

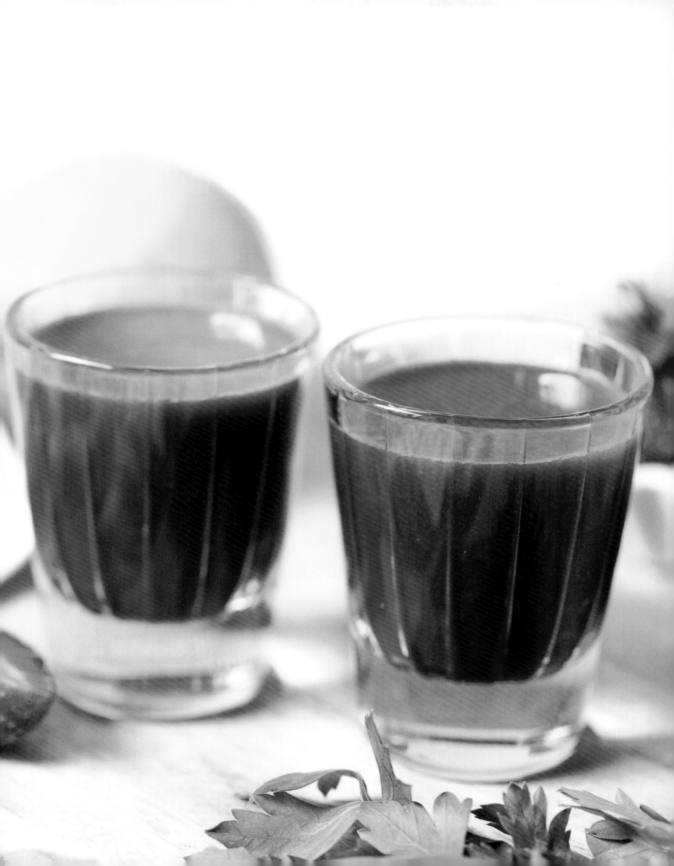

SLEEP AND RECHARGING STABILIZER

Turn to this shot:

- Before a nap

- When you want a quick recharge

- If you feel like your battery is constantly low

- If you are easily awakened during a night's sleep

- If you don't feel rejuvenated when you wake up from sleeping (You can drink the shot either after you've woken up or before you go to sleep.)

- When you've had a tremendous amount of output and want to regain strength

One healing technique is to drink this Brain Shot, place yourself in a resting position, and close your eyes. Even if you don't fall asleep while resting, the shot will deliver its benefits.

¾ cup fresh or thawed frozen mango

⅛ cup tightly packed fresh dill

¼ cup chopped cucumber

½ cup roughly chopped lettuce (preferably butter lettuce), tightly packed

½ teaspoon pure maple syrup (optional)

Run each ingredient through a juicer in the order listed from top to bottom.

Stir in the maple syrup (if using).

Pour into a glass and serve.

TIPS

- Look for pure maple syrup that is made only with 100 percent maple syrup. Avoid using maple-flavored syrups, which are not the same and often contain harmful ingredients.

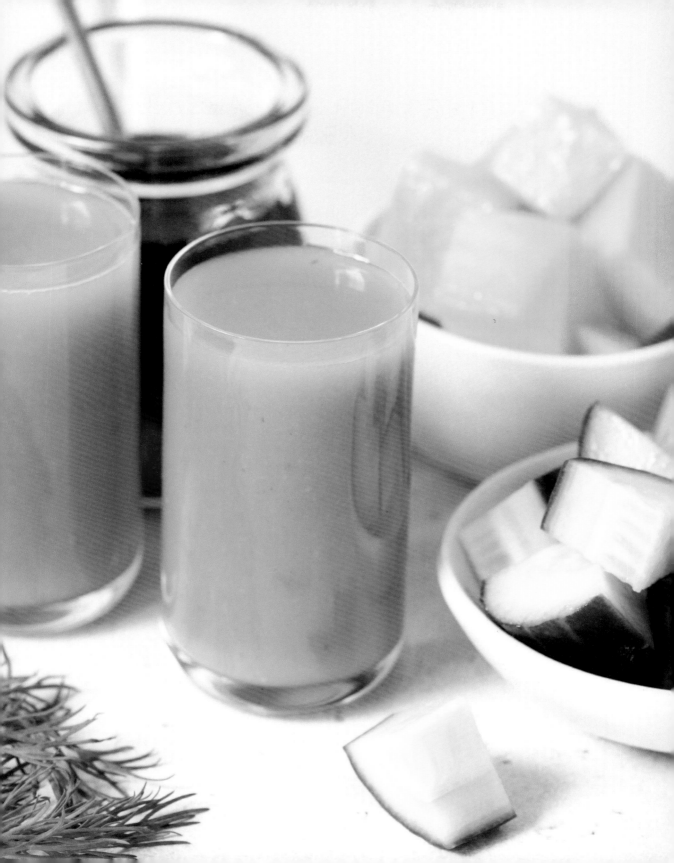

SPEAKING YOUR TRUTH STABILIZER

This shot provides support around three main areas of truth:

1. Getting in touch with and communicating your own truths. For example, when:
   - You're feeling stifled
   - You're not being heard
   - You aren't being taken seriously
   - You're afraid to speak up about something
   - You feel something you're doing isn't authentic to who you are

2. Receiving the truth. For example, when:
   - You're afraid to receive the truth about something
   - You want to know the truth about something
   - You've received the truth and you're having a difficult time accepting it

3. Learning about hidden truths. For example, when:
   - You want to expand your understanding and knowledge of what's happening with the world around you
   - You want to learn how to read between the lines and see what others are not seeing
   - You're seeking out hidden truths

1-inch piece of fresh ginger
2-inch piece of fresh turmeric
1 small garlic clove
½ cup tightly packed fresh basil
½ cup tightly packed arugula
1 cup roughly chopped lettuce, such as green leaf or butter leaf, tightly packed
1 orange, peeled

Run each ingredient through a juicer in the order listed from top to bottom.

Pour into a glass and serve.

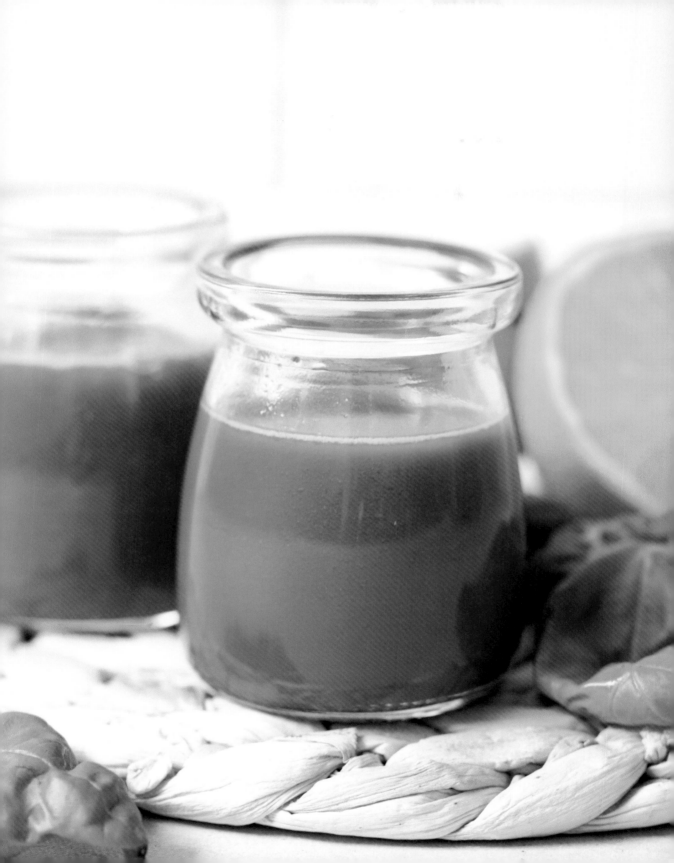

FINDING YOUR PURPOSE STABILIZER

Makes 1 to 2 shots

Try this shot if:

- You have the sense that you're missing out on something, and you don't know what it is
- You're feeling lost or out of place
- You have a sense of sadness
- You don't ever feel satisfied
- You feel you're not living the life you were meant to live or you're not fulfilling your destiny
- You feel like you've lost your free will, or you want to access your free will
- You're feeling unproductive
- You don't know where you're going in life
- You've lost meaning with anything or everything you're doing

¼ cup fresh or thawed frozen blackberries
¼ cup fresh or thawed frozen raspberries
¼ cup fresh or thawed frozen strawberries
1 tablespoon fresh or thawed frozen wild blueberries or 1 teaspoon pure wild blueberry juice or 1 teaspoon pure wild blueberry powder
¼ cup tightly packed fresh parsley

Run each ingredient through a juicer in the order listed from top to bottom. If using the wild blueberry juice or wild blueberry powder, mix it in after all the other ingredients have run through the juicer.

Pour into a glass and serve.

TIPS

- If you select fresh strawberries for this recipe, remove the greens before using. Read why on page 287.
- If you're in a part of the world where you can't access fresh or frozen wild blueberries, wild blueberry juice, or wild blueberry powder, you can add three or four more blackberries to the ¼ cup called for in the recipe.

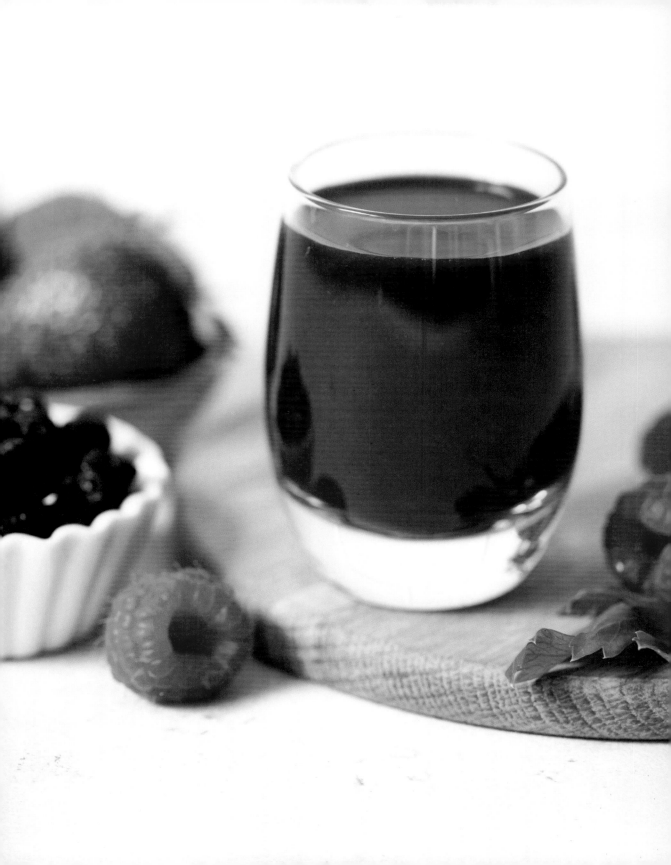

WISDOM AND INTUITION STABILIZER

Administer this powerful tool when:

- You're trying to improve your intuition
- You want to get the most out of your meditations
- You're trying to build up the strength of your psychic ability
- You're trying to gain sight and vision through your third eye, to see what others cannot see
- You want to strengthen your spiritual connection with above
- You feel you're lacking intuition or disconnected from your intuition
- You want to get the most out of a yoga session or spiritual training or gathering
- You're seeking wisdom about any topic, such as something occurring in your life
- You're seeking answers that pertain to you and the ones around you

1 tablespoon fresh or thawed frozen wild blueberries, or 1 teaspoon pure wild blueberry juice, or 1 teaspoon pure wild blueberry powder
¼ cup fresh or thawed frozen blackberries
¼ cup tightly packed fresh sage
¼ cup tightly packed fresh oregano
¼ cup tightly packed wheatgrass (or 2 teaspoons thawed frozen wheatgrass juice)
½ cup chopped raw yellow squash
¼ teaspoon spirulina

Run the wild blueberries, blackberries, sage, oregano, wheatgrass, and yellow squash through a juicer in the order listed from top to bottom. If you are using the wild blueberry juice, wild blueberry powder, or thawed wheatgrass juice, reserve for the next step.

Sprinkle or stir in the spirulina. Stir in the wild blueberry juice or wild blueberry powder. Stir in the thawed wheatgrass juice if using.

Pour into a glass and serve.

TIPS

- If you're in a part of the world where you can't access fresh or frozen wild blueberries, wild blueberry juice, or wild blueberry powder, you can add three or four more blackberries to the ¼ cup called for in the recipe.

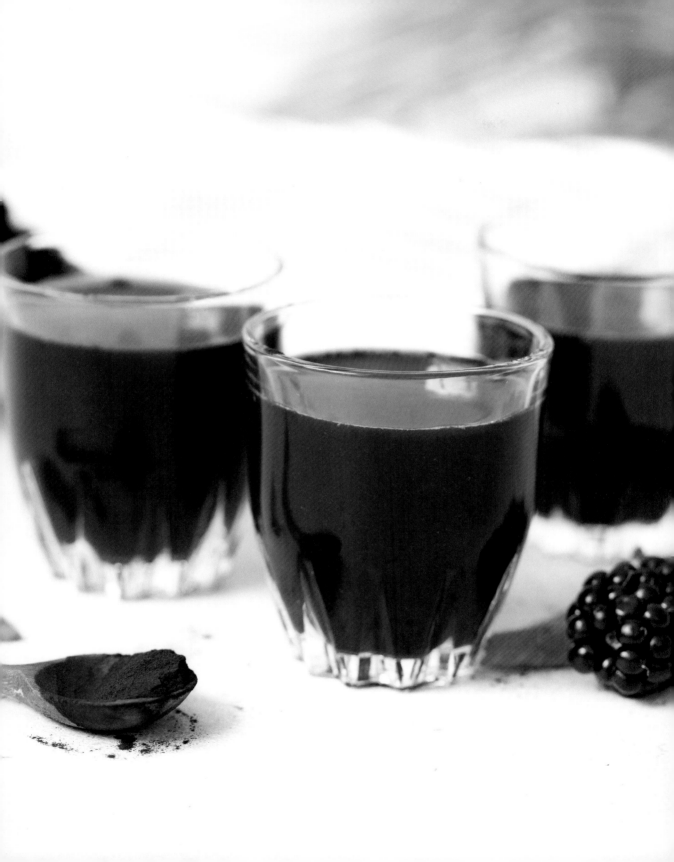

CHAPTER 9

Medical Medium Brain Shot Therapy Cleanses

These cleanses are imperative for what's to come in this world. The onslaught of domestic chemical warfare in our homes, in our schools, in our institutions, in our society today has reached cataclysmic proportions. When you embark on these cleanse options, you're using your free will and your intention to clean and protect the organ that harbors the knowledge of the past, present, and soon to be future of your life and harbors your soul. The Brain Shot Therapy Cleanses are beyond just physical. Removing poisons from the brain opens the door for your consciousness and subconsciousness to purify, allowing you to achieve enlightenment in a world of toxic corruption that keeps us from enlightenment.

Enlightenment is not about being all-knowing. Enlightenment is the freedom to be at peace because you have full control over what resides inside your brain—since we don't have control about what resides around us in the world. These cleanses purify your brain temple. You are removing the poisons from your brain that take away your clarity. Your intuitive, psychic, telepathic, clairvoyant skills will start to surface. You will be able to see truth easily and clearly and be able to express yourself, increase creativity, and experience joy in the simplest things that others would not realize are joyful. You will open your third eye and develop your skills as a seer when you rid yourself of poisons from the industries that were purposely placed in our brains to keep us in chains and keep us down. These are spiritual cleanses on top of being physical.

The physical benefits are truly special and powerful. With the Brain Shot Therapy Cleanses, you embark on removing toxins and poisonous chemicals from the brain that should never have been there to begin with—and helping restore what should be in your brain. These anti-pathogenic cleanses are designed for what we deal with on a daily basis—everything from deficiencies to burnout to brain acid to emotional brain injuries. These cleanses are designed to rid many different symptoms, conditions, and diseases. The Advanced and High-Powered options have the ability to get rid of 100 symptoms someone may have. (For long-term support, especially for pathogens, supplementation protocols are available in Part I, "Supplement Gospel.")

You can choose, at any given time, which of the seven cleanse options to select. You can also climb the ladder here. It's all part of how Medical Medium protocols are customizable to take you as far as you need to go. The higher up you go through the cleanse levels, the more symptoms and conditions can dissipate.

CLEANSE GUIDELINES

Choosing Brain Shot Therapies

- Most Brain Shot Therapy Cleanse levels offer the option to choose 10, 20, or 30 days for your cleanse. Each description will specify.

- Cleanse options will also specify whether you can decide from day to day which shot to try, or whether you should choose a new Brain Shot recipe each day.

- If the guidance says you can decide which shot to try each day, that means you have the option to move throughout the shots however you'd like. It's your choice. You're welcome to skip around or repeat shots from day to day.

- If the guidance says to choose a new Brain Shot recipe each day, move through the shots within one group at a time. For example, for a 10-day cleanse, choose either the Exposure shots, Shifter shots, or Stabilizer shots from Chapter 8, selecting one new shot recipe per day so that by the end of the 10 days, you've moved through all 10 shots in a group. For a 20-day or 30-day cleanse, you would choose two to three Brain Shot groups, moving through one group at a time. It's okay to go out of order within a group—you don't need to go through them in the exact order listed in Chapter 8—as long as you get to all the shots in a group within each segment of 10 days.

- For example, if you do a 30-day cleanse that instructs you to select a new shot each day, you could decide to work your way through the Shifters (in any order), then Stabilizers (in any order), then Exposures (in any order), until you've gotten through all 30 shots in 30 days.

Number of Shots

- When a cleanse option calls for 2 or more shots per day, the shots should all be the same type on any given day. That is, if you've chosen an option that calls for 3 shots per day, all 3 shots should be made from the same recipe.

Shot Timing

- Drink your shots at least 15 to 30 minutes apart from any food or drink. That is, wait a minimum of 15 to 30 minutes after consuming anything else before you have a shot, and then wait a minimum of 15 to 30 minutes after consuming a shot to consume anything else.

- This applies to every Brain Shot Therapy Cleanse level. You want to give yourself time to resonate with each shot, letting the therapy enter the bloodstream and allowing yourself to pick up the frequency of the shot metaphysically and physically. This is giving you a moment of time to take it in and experience what the shot is doing.

- For example, a morning sequence that incorporates other Medical Medium protocols could look like this: drink your lemon or lime water upon waking, then wait 15 to 30 minutes, drink your fresh celery juice, then wait another 15 to 30 minutes, drink your Brain Shot, then wait at least another 15 to 30 minutes, and then have your breakfast.

- When a cleanse option calls for multiple shots per day, space out the shots at least 4 hours apart throughout the day. (The brain starts to shift back to old patterns after 4 hours, so you want to wait until that has happened before having another shot.) For example, if you're doing 3 shots per day, don't have the shots any closer together than 8 A.M., 12 P.M., and 4 P.M. You have the option to space out the shots more than that minimum of 4 hours apart. For example, you could have your shots at 7 A.M., 1 P.M., and 7 P.M. How you'd like to customize the timing of the shots is up to you.

- If you're taking a Medical Medium supplement protocol, you can continue while you're on the Brain Shot Therapy Cleanse. Don't take your supplements *with* your shots. Space them out according to the guidance above.

Repeating the Cleanse

- You're welcome to do back-to-back Brain Shot Therapy Cleanses. You're also welcome to do the cleanse periodically, taking breaks in between rounds and then coming back to your cleanse level of choice. You could either repeat the same cleanse level however many times you'd like, or you could try moving from one level to another. Try whichever cleanse level you'd like at any time.

Missing Ingredients

- If you have difficulty sourcing ingredients in the Brain Shots—if you're missing an item or lacking one—use what you have and move forward.

- For questions about ingredient substitutions in recipes such as Lemon or Lime Water, Celery Juice, and the Heavy Metal Detox Smoothie, see the Tips that go with the individual recipes. If possible, try not to get into the habit of relying on substitutions, especially for celery juice. Keep trying to achieve the goal of using the proper ingredients for the cleanses.

Cleanse Interruptions

- If you miss Brain Shots (and/or the Heavy Metal Detox Smoothie, if specified) on any given day of a cleanse, still try to follow the rest of the cleanse guidance that day, and then add one day to the end of your cleanse.

- If you do something that breaks your cleanse, add three days to the end of your cleanse. "Breaking the cleanse" means consuming items your cleanse level specifies to avoid, whether radical fats such as nut butter in the morning or brain betrayer foods such as eggs, dairy, or gluten.

General Notes for All Cleanses

- If you're getting your blood drawn for some reason within the time period of your cleanse, ask if you can move your appointment to a time when you're not doing the cleanse, or learn how to ask for quarter or half tubes from the chapter "Blood Draining Agenda" in this book's companion title, *Brain Saver*. If you don't have the book on hand and you have an immediate need to apply that chapter's information due to a medical concern, listen to the "Blood Draw" episode of the *Medical Medium Podcast*. For food and supplement protocols to avoid weakening your immune system, refer to Chapter 4.

- For any general cleansing questions you have that are not addressed in this book, *Cleanse to Heal* is available to you as an additional resource.

Adjustments for Children

You can go ahead with the Brain Shot Therapy Cleanses for children, keeping the following in mind:

- It's fine to leave the lemon or lime water out for kids and also to reduce the amount of celery juice according to what feels right for your little one. See the table in Chapter 2 for more guidance on celery juice amounts for children.

- Depending on the age and size of your child, serve a small portion of a given Brain Shot, even if it means going as low as an ounce or down to a teaspoon.

- If the cleanse level you've chosen for your child includes the Heavy Metal Detox Smoothie, see "Adjustments

for Children" in Chapter 10, "Heavy Metal Detox," for guidance on the amount.

BRAIN SHOT THERAPY CLEANSE LEVELS

1. ENTRY LEVEL Brain Shot Therapy Cleanse

Add these steps to your normal eating routine:

- Drink 1 Brain Shot per day (recipes in Chapter 8).

- Your choice of 10, 20, or 30 days.

- Your choice of which Brain Shot option from day to day.

- Optional: Incorporate as many other Medical Medium tools and recipes as desired.

- Try to drink a minimum of 50 ounces of water throughout the day (that amount can include coconut water). Be mindful not to drink the water too close to drinking the Brain Shot—make sure you space them at least 15 to 30 minutes apart.

2. BASIC Brain Shot Therapy Cleanse

Add these steps to your normal eating routine:

- Drink 2 of the same Brain Shots per day (recipes in Chapter 8), spaced at least 4 hours apart.

- Your choice of 10, 20, or 30 days.

- Your choice of which Brain Shot option from day to day.

- Optional: Incorporate as many other Medical Medium tools and recipes as desired.

- Try to drink a minimum of 60 ounces of water throughout the day (that amount can include coconut water). Be mindful not to drink the water too close to drinking the Brain Shots—make sure you space them at least 15 to 30 minutes apart.

3. SIMPLIFIED Brain Shot Therapy Cleanse

Add these steps to your normal eating routine:

- Drink 2 of the same Brain Shots per day (recipes in Chapter 8), spaced at least 4 hours apart.

- Your choice of 10, 20, or 30 days.

- Your choice of which Brain Shot option from day to day.

- Start each day with 16 to 32 ounces of fresh lemon or lime water upon waking (recipe with the proper ratio of lemon or lime to water in Chapter 12).

- At least 15 to 30 minutes later, drink 16 to 32 ounces of fresh celery juice on an empty stomach (then wait another 15 to 30 minutes before you have your first Brain Shot or breakfast).

- Optional: Heavy Metal Detox Smoothie anytime (recipe in Chapter 10); should not be consumed directly after a fat-based meal.

- Stay fat-free until at least lunchtime.

- Optional: For even better results, take a look at the brain betrayer foods and food chemicals in Chapters 5 and 7. Start chipping away at the lists, seeing what foods you'd like to avoid while cleansing. The fewer brain betrayers such as eggs, dairy, gluten, corn, soy, tuna, lamb, and pork in your diet, the more effective the Brain Shots can be.

- Try to incorporate as many Medical Medium recipes from this book (and/or *Cleanse to Heal* and the expanded edition of *Medical Medium*) into your snacks and meals as you can.

- Try to drink a minimum of 60 ounces of water throughout

the day (that amount can include coconut water and your morning lemon water). Be mindful not to drink the water too close to drinking the celery juice or Brain Shots—make sure you space them at least 15 to 30 minutes apart.

4. INTERMEDIATE Brain Shot Therapy Cleanse

Make these steps your complete eating routine:

- Drink 3 of the same Brain Shots per day (recipes in Chapter 8), spaced at least 4 hours apart.

- Your choice of 10, 20, or 30 days.

- Your choice of which Brain Shot option from day to day.

- Start each day with 16 to 32 ounces of fresh lemon or lime water upon waking (recipe with the proper ratio of lemon or lime to water in Chapter 12).

- At least 15 to 30 minutes later, drink 16 to 32 ounces of fresh celery juice on an empty stomach (then wait another 15 to 30 minutes before you have your first Brain Shot or breakfast).

- Optional: Heavy Metal Detox Smoothie anytime (recipe in Chapter 10); should not be consumed directly after a fat-based meal.

- Avoid eggs, dairy, gluten, corn, soy, tuna, lamb, and pork.

- Use exclusively Medical Medium recipes from this book (and/or *Cleanse to Heal* and the expanded edition of *Medical Medium*).

- Stay fat-free until at least lunchtime.

- Keep fats limited to one serving (if at all) from lunchtime on, preferably at the end of the day. If you're plant-based, it's okay to incorporate one serving of plant fat, such as avocado, nuts or nut butters, seeds, coconut, coconut oil, olives, or olive oil, in a Medical Medium recipe. If you eat animal products, it's okay to incorporate one serving of animal fat, such as chicken, grass-fed beef, turkey, salmon, or sardines, in a Medical Medium recipe.

- Try to drink a minimum of 60 ounces of water throughout the day (that amount can include coconut water and your morning lemon water). Be mindful not to drink the water too close to drinking the celery juice or Brain Shots—make sure you space them at least 15 to 30 minutes apart.

5. PERFORMANCE Brain Shot Therapy Cleanse

Make these steps your complete eating routine:

- Drink 3 of the same Brain Shots per day (recipes in Chapter 8), spaced at least 4 hours apart.

- Your choice of 10, 20, or 30 days.

- Select a new Brain Shot every day, working methodically through one group (Exposures, Shifters, or Stabilizers) at a time (okay to go out of order within a group).

- Start each day with 32 ounces of fresh lemon or lime water upon waking (recipe with the proper ratio of lemon or lime to water in Chapter 12).

- At least 15 to 30 minutes later, drink 32 ounces of fresh celery juice on an empty stomach (then wait another 15 to 30 minutes before you have your first Brain Shot or breakfast).

- Optional: Heavy Metal Detox Smoothie anytime (recipe in Chapter 10); should not be consumed directly after a fat-based meal.

- Avoid all foods and food chemicals from Chapters 5 and 7, including caffeine.

- Use exclusively Medical Medium recipes from this book (and/or *Cleanse to Heal* and the expanded edition of *Medical Medium*).

- Stay fat-free until at least lunchtime.

- Keep fats limited to one serving (if at all) from lunchtime on, preferably at the end of the day. If you're plant-based, it's okay to incorporate one serving of plant fat, such as avocado, nuts or nut butters, seeds, coconut, coconut oil, olives, or olive oil, in a Medical Medium recipe. If you eat animal products, it's okay to incorporate one serving of animal fat, such as chicken, grass-fed beef, turkey, salmon, or sardines, in a Medical Medium recipe.

- Try to drink a minimum of 60 ounces of water throughout the day (that amount can include coconut water and your morning lemon water). Be mindful not to drink the water too close to drinking the celery juice or Brain Shots—make sure you space them at least 15 to 30 minutes apart.

6. ADVANCED Brain Shot Therapy Cleanse

Make these steps your complete eating routine:

- Drink 3 of the same Brain Shots per day (recipes in Chapter 8), spaced at least 4 hours apart.

- Your choice of 20 or 30 days.

- Select a new Brain Shot every day, working methodically through one group (Exposures, Shifters, or Stabilizers) at a time (okay to go out of order within a group).

- Start each day with 32 ounces of fresh lemon or lime water upon waking (recipe with the proper ratio of lemon or lime to water in Chapter 12).

- At least 15 to 30 minutes later, drink 32 ounces of fresh celery juice on an empty stomach (then wait another 15 to 30 minutes before you have your first Brain Shot or breakfast).

- Drink the Heavy Metal Detox Smoothie daily (recipe in Chapter 10). (Optional: okay to take one day off from the smoothie every 10 days.)

- Avoid all foods and food chemicals from Chapters 5 and 7, including caffeine.

- Use exclusively fat-free Medical Medium recipes from this book (and/or *Cleanse to Heal* and the expanded edition of *Medical Medium*).

- Stay off all fat-based foods, both plant fats (e.g., nuts, seeds, avocado) and animal fats (e.g., chicken, fish, meat).

- Try to drink a minimum of 60 ounces of water throughout the day (that amount can include coconut water and your morning lemon water). As ever, be mindful not to drink the water too close to drinking the celery juice or Brain Shots— make sure you space them at least 15 to 30 minutes apart.

7. HIGH-POWERED Brain Shot Therapy Cleanse

Make these steps your complete eating routine:

- Drink 3 of the same Brain Shots per day (recipes in Chapter 8), spaced at least 4 hours apart.

- Continue for 30 days.

- Select a new Brain Shot every day, working methodically through one group (Exposures, Shifters, or Stabilizers) at a time (okay to go out of order within a group).

- Start each day with 32 ounces of fresh lemon or lime water upon waking (recipe with the proper ratio of lemon or lime to water in Chapter 12).

- At least 15 to 30 minutes later, drink 32 ounces of fresh celery juice on an empty stomach (then wait another 15 to 30 minutes before you have your first Brain Shot or breakfast).

- Drink the Heavy Metal Detox Smoothie daily (recipe in Chapter 10). (Optional: okay to take one day off from the smoothie every 10 days.)

- Avoid all foods and food chemicals from Chapters 5 and 7, including caffeine.

- Use exclusively fat-free Medical Medium recipes from this book (and/or *Cleanse to Heal* and the expanded edition of *Medical Medium*).

- Stay off all fat-based foods, both plant fats (e.g., nuts, seeds, avocado) and animal fats (e.g., chicken, fish, meat).

- Remove scented candles, colognes, perfumes, scented laundry detergents, fabric softeners, air fresheners, fragrances, scented aftershaves, scented deodorants, scented soaps, scented body sprays, scented body lotions, scented body oils, scented hair products, incense, and car fresheners.

- Try to drink a minimum of 60 ounces of water throughout the day (that amount can include coconut water and your morning lemon water). As ever, be mindful not to drink the water too close to drinking the celery juice or Brain Shots— make sure you space them at least 15 to 30 minutes apart.

"These are special configurations synergistically combined just right to crack the code of how fruits, herbs, leafy greens, wild foods, and vegetables work as medicine."

— Anthony William, Medical Medium

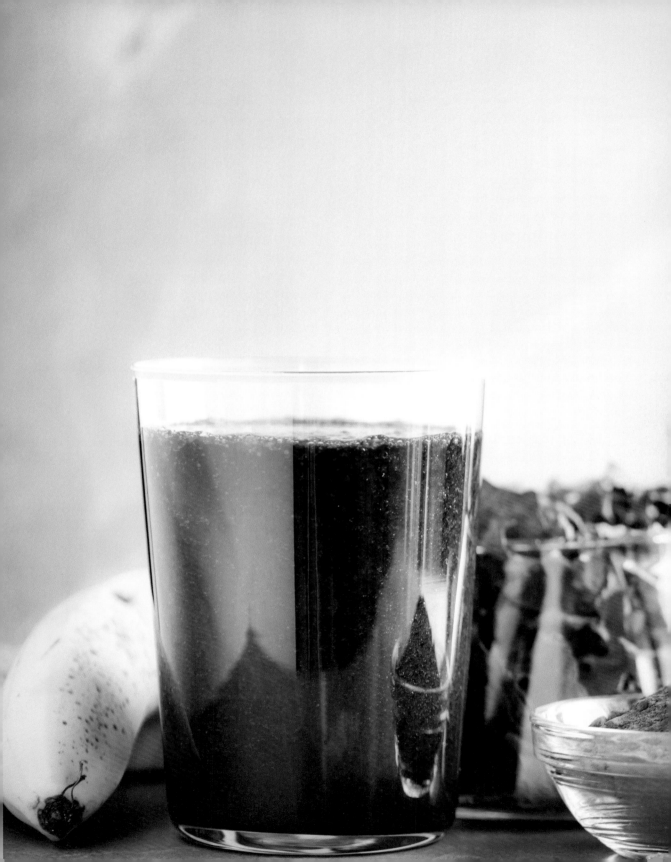

PART IV

HEAVY METAL DETOX

"Your brain has abilities to heal beyond what medical research and science are aware of today. Hold on to that knowledge, and you'll become a beacon of light for others who need answers."

— Anthony William, Medical Medium

CHAPTER 10

Medical Medium Heavy Metal Detox

Beyond the damage that toxic heavy metals themselves can do, there's the truth that they act as viral fuel—which supports viruses in their mission to elevate inflammation throughout the body and cause auto-immune conditions—and so taking metals away helps lower a viral load. Viral loads create neurological symptoms. Extracting heavy metals also addresses mental and emotional struggles and well-being by allowing the electricity and energetic frequencies of the brain to flow freely. When you break down and dismantle the alloys that have interfered with your brain, you minimize viral invasion, allow for emotional injuries to heal faster, reduce inflammation of the brain and cranial nerves, address burnout and deficiencies, and help relieve an addicted, acid brain.

(Read much more about toxic heavy metals, viruses, and the brain in this book's companion title, *Brain Saver.*)

OLD METALS VERSUS NEW METALS

Heavy metals that we inherit have age to them. They're old, many times going back as far as 2,000 to 3,000 years, depending on what part of the world someone's bloodline stems from. Older heavy metals also have a higher oxidative rate than heavy metals from newer exposures. The aging process of toxic heavy metals that were mined many generations ago started when the metals were removed from the earth. An oxidative countdown occurred as the metals aged. Those metals became highly unstable when they entered and sat inside human bodies, where metals are exposed to oxygen, acids, heat, blood gases, electricity, outside chemicals, and more.

New metals differ greatly from old metals. Newer metals recently mined and taken out of the earth are still highly toxic, although they are more stable, making them less destructive than older metals. Newer metals don't break down inside the body as quickly. It all depends on how many generations the metals have been passed down through and how much metal is in each individual. Most people have a mix of older metals and newer metals being passed down from generation to generation. The newest metal exposure is when a child gets a medical treatment at the pediatrician's office that contains mercury, aluminum, and copper. Most likely the mercury and aluminum were unearthed in the last 50 to 70 years, saved in storage, and eventually purchased by the medical industry and placed inside a pharmaceutical. Many medications have toxic heavy metals in them, and at the same time, a child could have inherited toxic heavy metals that have been in the family line for hundreds to thousands of years from periodic exposures that our ancestors encountered. For example, we can inherit metals from 2,000 to 3,000 years ago, plus metals from 300 to 400 years ago that our ancestors were exposed to in, for example, quicksilver treatments, plus metals from more recent exposure in our family line. Older metals' faster oxidation rate makes viruses more interested in these aging metals, because they are easier to access and consume due to their instability.

One reason heavy metals are passed down from generation to generation is that their presence in the body isn't recognized by medical research and science, unless it's an obvious poisoning such as from a lead tank filled with water. So heavy metals aren't identified as a destructive, dangerous threat to health, and the metals aren't cleaned out of the bodies of parents before a new generation is born. Toxic heavy metals are a big part of why human health is not prospering at this time—why it's even declining.

ALLOY FUEL

Normally, the viruses that cause autoimmune disorders feed on one metal or maybe two. In difficult neurological autoimmune cases, either one virus is feeding on three, four, or more metals, or two or more viruses are each feeding on multiple metals. A virus or viruses feeding on multiple metals leads to metals mixing and creating highly potent waste. Once this waste matter is excreted from the virus, it can cause many neurological and physical reactions, especially if the metals are aged. When more than two metals are consumed by a virus, the resulting neurotoxins become muscle-damaging, nerve-damaging, bone-damaging, and organ-damaging because this toxic waste is suffocating cells, not allowing cells to receive critically needed nutrients to survive on an optimum level. The cell walls break down from exposure to the highly acidic and denaturing toxic waste matter.

Different toxic heavy metals have different weights to them. Copper, mercury, and lead are a few of the heavier metals, and so the neurotoxins and dermatoxins excreted by viruses feeding on these metals are heavier in weight. Neurotoxins and dermatoxins can be a mix of heavy and lighter metals, and the heavier metals will mix with the lighter metals and weigh the lighter metals down, causing neurotoxins and dermatoxins to settle in lower extremities. This is why some people only get eczema on their hands and feet or legs (heavier dermatoxins) while others get eczema on their chest (when the dermatoxins are mostly composed of lighter metals). Restless legs syndrome and Raynaud's syndrome are examples of neurotoxins settling in feet, hands, arms, and legs.

HEAVY METAL DETOX AT WORK

For the best way to get rid of heavy metals from the brain and body, look no further than the Heavy Metal Detox Smoothie and cleanses. These protocols are the most effective methods on the planet for removing heavy metals and repairing the damage they've left behind. There are countless stories worldwide of people getting results from the original Heavy Metal Detox Smoothie and the original Heavy Metal Detox Cleanse. Now you have even more options.

The Power of the Heavy Metal Detox Smoothie

Let's start with the basics. The Heavy Metal Detox Smoothie (full recipe at the end of this chapter) incorporates five key ingredients:

- Wild blueberries (available frozen or as pure wild blueberry powder or juice)
- Spirulina (find the most potent and productive kind in my supplement directory at www.medicalmedium.com)
- Barley grass juice powder (find the correct kind in my supplement directory)
- Fresh cilantro
- Atlantic dulse

Together, these medicinals extract both deep-rooted and free-floating metals and carry them all the way out of your body, rather than dropping them along the way or not working at all. This makes the Heavy Metal Detox Smoothie totally unique—it's responsible. It doesn't simply pick up metals and then let them go again, causing additional stress and harm on someone's nervous system or digestive system. This is one reason it doesn't cause side effects. The Heavy Metal Detox Smoothie also helps heal brain tissue with its nourishing composition.

(If there is a mild reaction, it's not a sign of harm. It's common for that person to react to any protocols they try from any other sources, and it means the person is highly toxic. The difference between the Heavy Metal Detox Smoothie and other protocols is that the smoothie can eventually clear up those toxins so the person can stop having reactions.)

If you're familiar with the Medical Medium series, you'll recall that consuming these five foods within 24 hours of each other is sufficient for them to do their work together. That holds true for generally removing heavy metals in various places throughout the body. When you're specifically targeting toxic heavy metals in the brain, it's best to consume these five foods blended together.

The process of removing heavy metals from the brain is something like mining precious metals from the earth. Although in mining, earth and ore must usually be removed or displaced to extract the metals, with this extraction method from the brain, the phytochemical compounds in the five key foods collectively and carefully loosen and gather the metals through a chemical reaction. Chemical compounds from these five ingredients join together and align with supernatural abilities of the brain. The chemical compounds from the smoothie ingredients drive information into the brain's electrical grid, activating the electrical grid to work alongside other chemical compounds that the brain possesses, jolting the electrical grid to project the metals and waste out of the brain tissue to then be gathered up by the chemical compounds of the five ingredients. This process keeps brain tissue safe. It's the power of the chemical compounds in the Heavy Metal Detox Smoothie's five medicinal ingredients working together. If someone doesn't have one or two ingredients, the ingredients that are present still work together in harmony.

Here's a simpler way to view it: the brain, filled with toxic brain betrayers, as a dirty sponge, and the phytochemicals in this Heavy Metal Detox Smoothie almost acting as a squeezing method for cells to draw out heavy metals. Or see the smoothie like an expectorant for brain tissue, helping the brain cough up what's holding it back.

A bonus of the Heavy Metal Detox Smoothie is that it doesn't only remove toxic heavy metals from the brain. While getting rid of toxic heavy metals is your number one goal with this recipe, it will also help purge solvents, pesticides, radiation, and other brain betrayers.

Any makeshift or trendy way of trying to remove metals out of the body really falls short. For example, chlorella, if it even picks up metal, will drop it, creating another, possibly bigger problem in another area of the brain. Charcoal and zeolite also don't measure up to claims. Read more in Chapter 6, "Brain Betrayer Supplements."

Removing all the metals from the brain takes time. One big part of the detox process is reaching and purging actual fragments of nested metal, which can be clusters of truly small, nano-sized and tinier metals. That's not an overnight process. Even if some symptoms start to relieve and subside quickly, it still may take time to get to the finish line of removing all of the toxic heavy metals and getting past your most persistent symptoms. Those metal fragments have built up over the years, forming larger deposits with even bigger effects that this Heavy Metal Detox can address too. As brain tissue starts to purge the metals, not all of the metals will come out at once. Instead the metals begin to surface from deep within the brain. That's one reason why keeping up with this Heavy Metal Detox protocol for a long duration is critical: we can have older metals from generations and generations ago that are deeper, unstable, and fragile, and they won't project out of the brain quickly because it takes time for them to migrate closer to various surfaces in the brain. Newer metals that are more stable project out more easily. If they are deeper inside the brain, it does still take time to migrate those newer metals to the surface.

Metals travel through oxidation: when they corrode and expand, their debris run-off spreads and they react with each other. Heavy metal contamination bleeding into adjacent brain tissue is what's behind so many of the diseases and symptoms in this book. To address that, another big part of what the Heavy Metal Detox Smoothie does is deal with that corrosive metal debris. Chemical compounds in the Heavy Metal Detox Smoothie's five key ingredients bind on to the corrosion and contamination from decaying metal alloys. This, too, takes time and patience; stabilizing and safely dispersing corrosive debris that's formed from heavy metal alloys such as aluminum plus mercury or copper interacting in the brain is an extra level of cleanup.

People's toxic heavy metal situations are different. One person may have metals in their early phase of oxidation, forms that haven't yet interacted much with each other, which means there's not a lot of oxidative debris. Those metals can be faster and easier to cleanse. Another person could have a lot of heavy metal interactions transpiring—a lot of aluminum, mercury, and copper, for example, reacting with each other over a long period of time, creating pockets of oxidative discharge. In that case the Heavy Metal Detox Smoothie must start pulling away at this debris and then packaging it up and moving it out to

keep it from spreading and causing more problems—before the Heavy Metal Detox Smoothie's chemical compounds can get down to the root metals. Brain fog, depression, OCD, memory loss, and anxiety could take a longer time to heal until repeated use of the Heavy Metal Detox Smoothie allows heavy metal extraction to go deeper into the brain.

Everyone's alloy brain is unique. What particular metal blend it is, how many years the different metals have been sitting there, what quantity they're present in, how they're distributed in the brain, and how quickly they've been oxidizing differ from person to person. Because the Heavy Metal Detox Smoothie contains five key elements that address various aspects of healing, it covers everyone.

If you don't have all five ingredients, don't let that hold you back from making the Heavy Metal Detox Smoothie. Unlike chlorella and other sources, these ingredients hold the power to capture metals properly. They have individual qualities and abilities to remove metals. Keep in mind, using three or four out of the five smoothie ingredients could mean it takes longer to see results or completely heal. The ingredients still work best together. All five ingredients put together as a group uproot metals most effectively.

Wild Blueberries and the Other Key Ingredients

Understanding a little more about the Heavy Metal Detox Smoothie's ingredients helps us appreciate even more how hard the formula is working for us. In addition to the collective uprooting power of the ingredients' chemical compounds, the individual ingredients benefit us profoundly.

To begin with, wild blueberries ignite a purging effect in the brain. Wild blueberries contain dozens of unique and many undiscovered antioxidant phytochemical compounds. These antioxidant compounds break up debris pockets that have formed as a byproduct of heavy metals interacting and aging in the brain—it's like the dentist breaking up plaque on your teeth. Wild blueberries also go after the metals themselves.

We have to remember that heavy metals sitting in the brain take up space. Even if they're not oxidizing yet, even if they're on a nano or smaller scale, they have a physical presence in a place that's not supposed to have any toxic physical substances in it. Sometimes that can be a larger physical presence. For example, mercury tends to find more mercury, so if you were exposed to mercury early on, perhaps as a baby, additional mercury that you were exposed to throughout life, perhaps even on a monthly basis, could have rolled into that early mercury, creating bigger deposits. Sometimes metals' physical presence in the brain is compact, as in the case of the tiniest specks and micro-pockets of metals. No matter their size, heavy metal deposits create divots and pits in the brain. Once those heavy metals are purged, brain tissue needs to be repaired. Not only do wild blueberries' antioxidant phytochemical compounds extract the metals, they excel at healing the damage the metals have left behind by restoring the brain cells that are lining the walls of a divot or pit so that new brain cell growth is stimulated.

With heavy metals gone, your brain can create new cells in the space, although they need wild blueberries' help to do it well, clearing the area of contamination so that healthy growth can occur. When the damage is on a small scale, that healing can happen faster. If it's an older deposit of metals, where oxidative waste has accumulated too, it takes long-term commitment to the Heavy Metal Detox Smoothie to decontaminate the area. Brain cells die off because of heavy metals and their runoff, and not until it's all cleaned up will the body recognize that new growth can occur safely so the area can start to come back to life. While this extraction and remediation process is still happening, some symptoms can stick around for a while because even after heavy metals are removed, there is still brain tissue repair. Wild blueberries' antioxidant phytochemical compounds have the ability to increase healthy brain cell growth on a rapid scale to help spur healing—these antioxidants purify the brain tissue enough to freely repair.

Once wild blueberries have expelled and carried out heavy metals and their debris into the bloodstream, other chemical compounds from spirulina, barley grass juice powder, and cilantro can help navigate this debris safely out of the body. Thanks to the wild blueberries, the heavy metals won't re-disperse and cause trouble in the brain. The key five ingredients' chemical compounds are all working together to carry toxic heavy metals out of the body safely;

all the Heavy Metal Detox foods have the ability to harness radical, destabilized, corroded, oxidized metal debris as well as new metals that would otherwise aggressively injure tissue as they traveled.

Cilantro, barley grass juice powder, and spirulina work together specially, each playing unique and critical roles in removing toxic heavy metals. To begin with, some of cilantro's responsibility is to assist in removing metals from the brain, while another responsibility for cilantro is to remove heavy metals from the liver, other organs, and the intestinal tract—catching toxic heavy metals that are oxidizing and corroding early on, before the metals' oxidative byproduct and waste find their way to the brain. Cilantro's chemical compounds aren't going to attach themselves to heavy metals still being held by wild blueberries' compounds, only to rogue metals.

It's a long journey from where metals are nested in the brain to the point of being excreted out of the body because there are many obstacles along the route. High blood fat, acids, blood gases, pharmaceuticals, chemical toxins, chronic dehydration, and adrenaline are some of the obstacles. The metals themselves are highly toxic. We can't rely solely on wild blueberries and cilantro when we're trying to uproot and remove alloys from the brain and body. Bringing in barley grass juice powder at the same time is imperative. It works similarly to cilantro, although it travels farther and wider, even to the outer reaches of the skin, and also possesses a strong absorption mechanism for oxidized, destabilized metals.

Spirulina has similar abilities, more so for the brain and liver. Its profound ability to round up heavy metals in the brain, liver, and intestinal tract is one of its great virtues. The pigment in spirulina, which gives it its deep blue-green color, reaches the metaphysical part of the brain at the same time as the physical part, helping restore brain tissue that connects between the physical and metaphysical. Spirulina is so versatile that it can clean up metals that the other smoothie ingredients have unearthed from the brain, *and* spirulina can clean up metals from the liver and intestinal tract that would otherwise travel up to the brain.

Having all three—cilantro, barley grass juice powder, and spirulina—in your system at once provides exactly the formula you need to go along with wild blueberries, because everyone has a different toxic load, and that affects how the different medicinals perform. Atlantic dulse, a type of sea vegetable, acts as a safety net as metals expel out of the liver, gallbladder, and bile duct into the intestinal tract. Dulse also aids the kidneys by helping safely absorb metals leaving the body that could otherwise get trapped in the kidneys. Dulse is insurance to assist in escorting out of the body any metals that are hosted by (meaning captured by and attached to) other key ingredients, or metals that are on their own.

The key ingredients in the Heavy Metal Detox Smoothie also have some ability to remove other chemical toxins and poisons, which include radiation, insecticides, and fragrances.

Your Healing Goals

Some people respond immediately to the Heavy Metal Detox Smoothie because oxidative debris was saturating easy-to-reach hot spots of brain tissue, causing life-disrupting symptoms, and clearing some of that up gives a person an instant boost. Someone else might have been experiencing heavy metal oxidative runoff for years or decades, or have experienced much more aggressive alloy interactions, leading to more intense symptoms. The necessary cleanup in that case can mean that a person only sees some immediate results.

Some people have metals in the brain that aren't reacting with other metals yet, so pulling those out can mean they see a difference quickly. Other people have metals deep in different areas of the brain, and that means a longer process of extracting them.

Whatever situation someone is in, it's best to stick with all five ingredients to get someone to that place where they start feeling a difference. Whatever your timeline is, know that with every Heavy Metal Detox Smoothie you give yourself, you're getting closer and closer to your goals of healing.

Here's one more important point: when the brain is purging metals and oxidative debris from brain tissue, there are no rules for where this process starts to happen first in the brain. It's not systematic. It all depends on where the Heavy Metal Detox Smoothie's phytochemical compounds land first and how many metals are there.

Considerations include: Are the metals old or new? Are they from generations ago? How deep are they inside the brain? Are there larger deposits? Smaller deposits? And what kinds of metals are they?

If the first area of the brain the phytochemicals reach has a smaller amount of metals, those little specks and pockets of metal and debris will be purged to begin with. It won't be until later on, with more and more Heavy Metal Detox Smoothies, that the compounds of the ingredients get a chance to reach the larger pockets to start breaking down, absorbing, and uprooting the metals. It's yet one more reason to keep up with the smoothie regularly—ideally, daily—to make sure those critical heavy metal–extracting nutrients get where they need to go.

ADJUSTMENTS FOR CHILDREN

A child usually doesn't have the appetite for the full amount that the Heavy Metal Detox Smoothie recipe yields. To figure out the right portion for your child, think about when they're drinking a glass of apple juice—how much will they usually drink? Eight ounces? Ten or 12 ounces? Wherever you land, that's an appropriate amount of Heavy Metal Detox Smoothie to give your child. You can either reduce the recipe accordingly—for example, cutting it by half or two-thirds (making sure to keep the five key ingredients in there, in proportionate amounts)—or make the full recipe and drink the leftover that your child doesn't want.

Heavy Metal
Detox Recipes

HEAVY METAL DETOX SMOOTHIE

Makes 1 serving

This smoothie is a perfect and powerful combination of the five key ingredients for safely detoxifying toxic heavy metals from your brain and body. It's an honorable, life-giving blessing to help reverse so many symptoms.

2 bananas

2 cups frozen or fresh wild blueberries, or 2 ounces pure wild blueberry juice, or 2 tablespoons pure wild blueberry powder

1 cup tightly packed fresh cilantro

1 teaspoon barley grass juice powder

1 teaspoon spirulina

1 tablespoon Atlantic dulse or 2 dropperfuls Atlantic dulse liquid

1 orange, juiced

½ to 1 cup water, coconut water, or additional fresh-squeezed orange juice (optional)

Combine the bananas, wild blueberries, cilantro, barley grass juice powder, spirulina, and Atlantic dulse with the juice of 1 orange in a high-speed blender and blend until smooth.

Add up to 1 cup of water, coconut water, or orange juice if a thinner consistency is desired. Serve and enjoy!

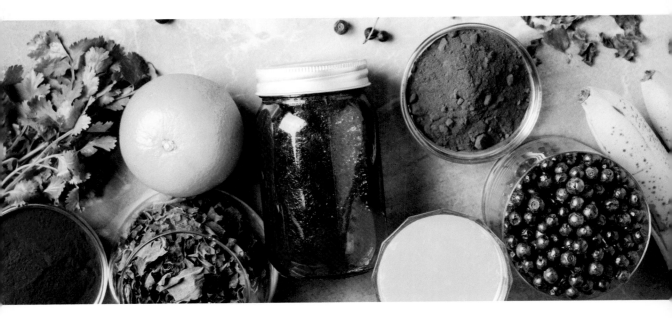

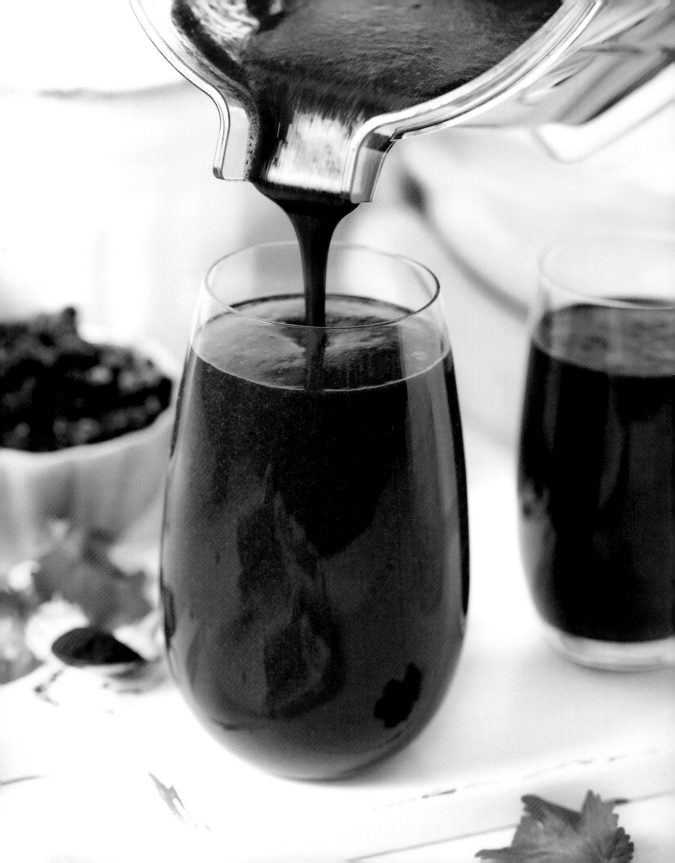

Heavy Metal Detox Smoothie continued

TIPS

- If the barley grass juice powder and spirulina taste is too strong for you, start with a smaller amount of each and work your way up.

- Seek out wild blueberries (whether fresh, frozen, powdered, or as pure juice). Wild blueberries are not to be confused with cultivated blueberries.

- If you're in a part of the world where you can't access fresh or frozen wild blueberries, wild blueberry juice, or wild blueberry powder, you can substitute blackberries. Blackberries do not uproot and attach themselves to toxic heavy metals like wild blueberries do, although the high antioxidant ratio in blackberries can at least slow down heavy metal oxidation, which is helpful.

- As an alternative to adding the juice from 1 orange to the smoothie, you have the option to peel the orange, remove its seeds, and blend it whole in the smoothie.

- If you're using coconut water in this smoothie, make sure the coconut water doesn't contain natural flavors and isn't pink or red.

- If you're not a fan of banana, you can substitute Maradol papaya or mango.

- On days when you can't access every smoothie ingredient, don't skip your Heavy Metal Detox Smoothie. Make it with whichever ingredients you do have. Keep aiming to make the smoothie with all five key ingredients.

ADVANCED HEAVY
METAL DETOX SMOOTHIE

Makes 1 serving

This smoothie uses the five key ingredients to take you to a faster pace of removing toxic heavy metals.

2 bananas

2 cups frozen or fresh wild blueberries, or 2 ounces pure wild blueberry juice, or 2 tablespoons pure wild blueberry powder

2 cups tightly packed fresh cilantro

2 teaspoons barley grass juice powder

2 teaspoons spirulina

1 tablespoon Atlantic dulse or 2 dropperfuls Atlantic dulse liquid

2 oranges, juiced

½ to 1 cup or more of water, coconut water, or additional fresh-squeezed orange juice (optional)

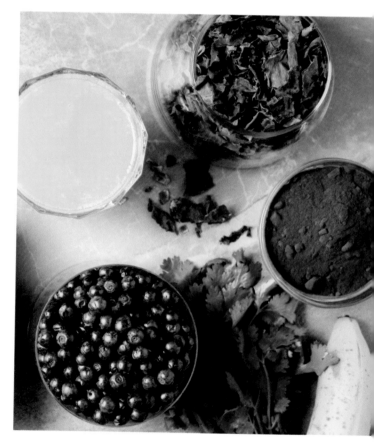

Combine the bananas, wild blueberries, cilantro, barley grass juice powder, spirulina, and Atlantic dulse with the juice of 2 oranges in a high-speed blender and blend until smooth. Add up to 1 cup or more of water, coconut water, or orange juice if a thinner consistency is desired.

Serve and enjoy!

TIPS

- This smoothie contains more spirulina, barley grass juice powder, and cilantro than the regular Heavy Metal Detox Smoothie. If you wish to do this Advanced version yet you find the taste of the greens too strong, you can add another banana, juice from one additional orange, or up to 2 teaspoons of raw honey as needed.

- Seek out wild blueberries (whether fresh, frozen, powdered, or as pure juice). Wild blueberries are not to be confused with cultivated blueberries.

- If you're in a part of the world where you can't access fresh or frozen wild blueberries, wild blueberry juice, or wild blueberry powder, you can substitute blackberries. Blackberries do not uproot and attach themselves to toxic heavy metals like wild blueberries do, although the high antioxidant ratio in blackberries can at least slow down heavy metal oxidation, which is helpful.

- As an alternative to adding the juice from 2 oranges to the smoothie, you have the option to peel the oranges, remove their seeds, and blend the oranges whole in the smoothie.

- If you're using coconut water in this smoothie, make sure the coconut water doesn't contain natural flavors and isn't pink or red.

- If you're not a fan of banana, you can substitute Maradol papaya or mango.

- On days when you can't access every smoothie ingredient, don't skip your Advanced Heavy Metal Detox Smoothie. Make it with whichever ingredients you do have. Keep aiming to make the smoothie with all five key ingredients.

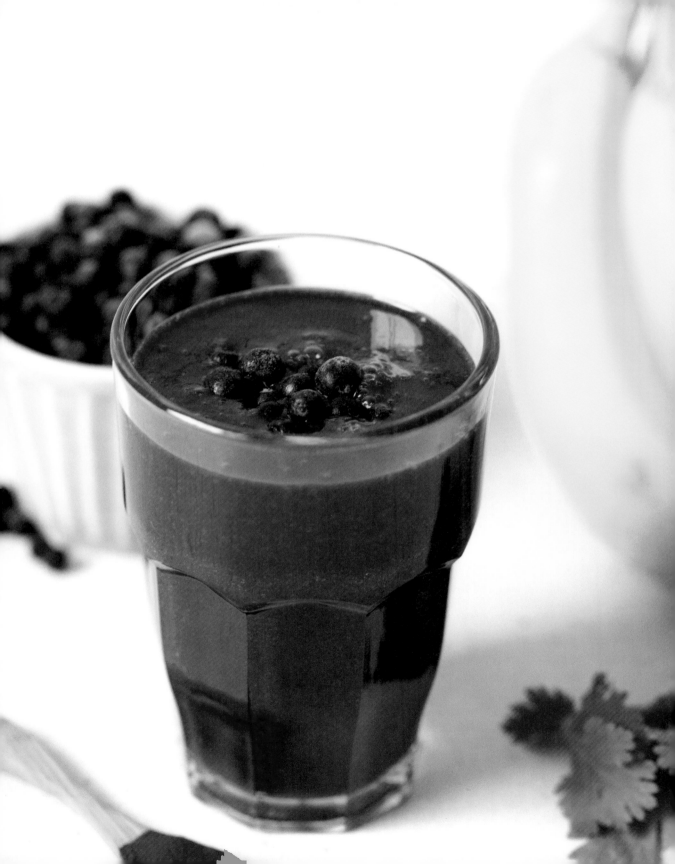

EXTRACTOR SMOOTHIE

The Extractor aids in removing different varieties of chemical toxicity, also freeing the path for toxic heavy metals to uproot and exit the body more quickly.

1 apple, chopped

1 cup frozen or fresh wild blueberries, or 1 ounce pure wild blueberry juice, or 1 tablespoon pure wild blueberry powder

1 cup fresh or frozen mango or 1 fresh or frozen banana

1 cup tightly packed fresh parsley

1 radish root

1 teaspoon mustard seed powder

1 cup of water, coconut water, fresh apple juice, or bottled organic and additive-free 100 percent apple juice

Blend the ingredients together until smooth. Add up to 1 cup of water, coconut water, fresh apple juice, or bottled organic and additive-free 100 percent apple juice if a thinner consistency is desired. Serve and enjoy!

TIPS

- Choose red-skinned apples when possible, as they have the most nutrients.

- Mango is the first preference for this smoothie. If you can't get fresh or frozen mango, banana is a great replacement.

- You can use any color radish root, including red radish, black radish, and purple radish. Avoid using daikon radish.

- If you're using coconut water in this smoothie, make sure the coconut water doesn't contain natural flavors and isn't pink or red.

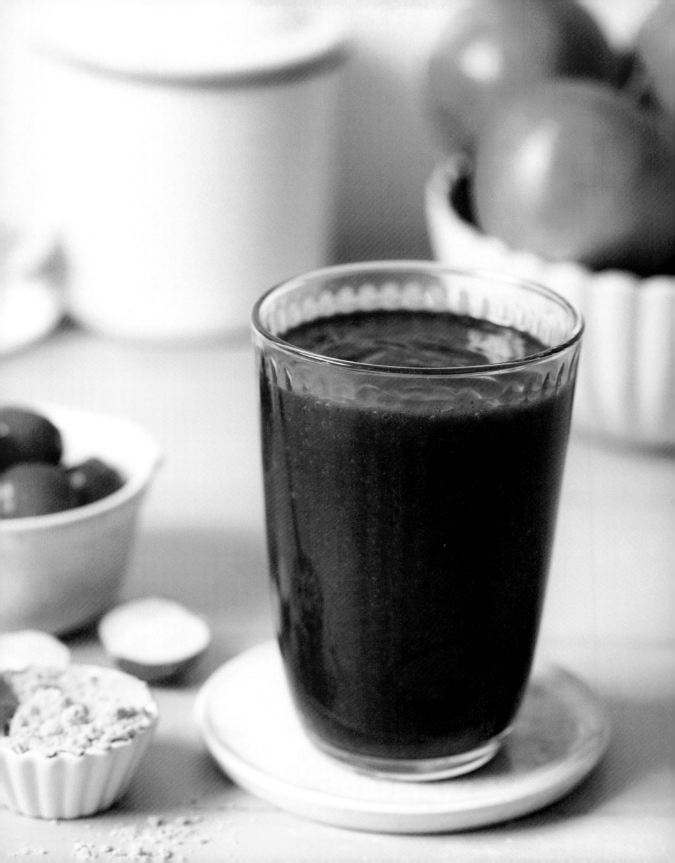

- If you are using a bottled, pasteurized apple juice, look for one that contains 100 percent organic apple juice with nothing else added such as sugar, citric acid, or preservatives.

- If you're having difficulty with the mustard seed flavor, you have the option to cut the amount of mustard in half, to ½ teaspoon, or even less if desired, with the goal of working your way back up to the recommended dosage of 1 teaspoon over time.

- If you're having difficulty with the parsley flavor, you have the option to cut the amount of parsley in half, to ½ cup, with the goal of working your way back up to the recommended dosage of 1 cup over time.

- If you're in a part of the world where you can't access fresh or frozen wild blueberries, wild blueberry juice, or wild blueberry powder, you can substitute blackberries. Although a high-antioxidant alternative, blackberries do not have the potency to match how wild blueberries defend cells from metals, chemicals, radiation, and other toxins.

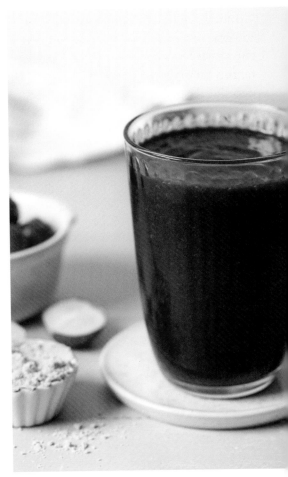

- If you can't get apples, ripe pears can be substituted in this recipe. If you can't access apples or pears, look for oranges as a substitute. If you can't find oranges, look for papayas. If you can't get papayas, look for bananas. And if you can't get bananas, you can use mangoes in place of apples or pears.

- See the next chapter, "Medical Medium Heavy Metal Detox Cleanses," for advice on how to integrate the Extractor into your day and time it with the Heavy Metal Detox Smoothie for optimal results.

ADVANCED
EXTRACTOR SMOOTHIE

Makes 1 serving

The Advanced Extractor works faster than the regular Extractor, also grabbing additional chemicals that the Extractor may not grab. Normally the Heavy Metal Detox Smoothie has the responsibility of removing other toxins in addition to toxic heavy metals. The Advanced Extractor's power at escorting those other chemical toxins out of the brain and body frees up the Heavy Metal Detox Smoothie to access and remove metals more quickly and easily.

1 apple, chopped

1 cup frozen or fresh wild blueberries, or 1 ounce pure wild blueberry juice, or 1 tablespoon pure wild blueberry powder

1 cup fresh or frozen mango or 1 fresh or frozen banana

1 cup tightly packed fresh parsley

1 radish root

2 cups roughly chopped radish greens, loosely packed

2 teaspoons mustard seed powder

1 cup of water, coconut water, fresh apple juice, or bottled organic and additive-free 100 percent apple juice

Blend the ingredients together until smooth. Add up to 1 cup of water, coconut water, fresh apple juice, or bottled organic and additive-free 100 percent apple juice if a thinner consistency is desired. Serve and enjoy!

TIPS

- Choose red-skinned apples when possible, as they have the most nutrients.

- Mango is the first preference for this smoothie. If you can't get fresh or frozen mango, banana is a great replacement.

- If you find the taste of this smoothie isn't to your liking, you can add an additional cup of fresh or frozen mango or an extra fresh or frozen banana to make it sweeter.

- You can use any color radish root, including red radish, black radish, and purple radish. Avoid using daikon radish.

- For best results look for fresh radish greens that are not wilted or yellowing. If you are unable to find radish greens, the next best choice is mustard greens. While they won't perform the same function as radish greens, they will still offer many benefits.

- If you're using coconut water in this smoothie, make sure the coconut water doesn't contain natural flavors and isn't pink or red.

- If you are using a bottled, pasteurized apple juice, look for one that contains 100 percent organic apple juice with nothing else added such as sugar, citric acid, or preservatives.

- If you're having difficulty with the mustard seed flavor, you have the option to cut the amount of mustard in half, to 1 teaspoon, or even less if desired, with the goal of working your way back up to the recommended dosage of 2 teaspoons over time.

- If you're having difficulty with the parsley flavor, you have the option to cut the amount of parsley in half, to ½ cup, with the goal of working your way back up to the recommended dosage of 1 cup over time.

- If you're in a part of the world where you can't access fresh or frozen wild blueberries, wild blueberry juice, or wild blueberry powder, you can substitute blackberries. Although a high-antioxidant alternative, blackberries do not have the potency to match how wild blueberries defend cells from metals, chemicals, radiation, and other toxins.

- If you can't get apples, ripe pears can be substituted in this recipe. If you can't access apples or pears, look for oranges as a substitute. If you can't find oranges, look for papayas. If you can't get papayas, look for bananas. And if you can't get bananas, you can use mangoes in place of apples or pears.

- See the next chapter, "Medical Medium Heavy Metal Detox Cleanses," for advice on how to integrate the Advanced Extractor into your day and time it with the Advanced Heavy Metal Detox Smoothie for optimal results.

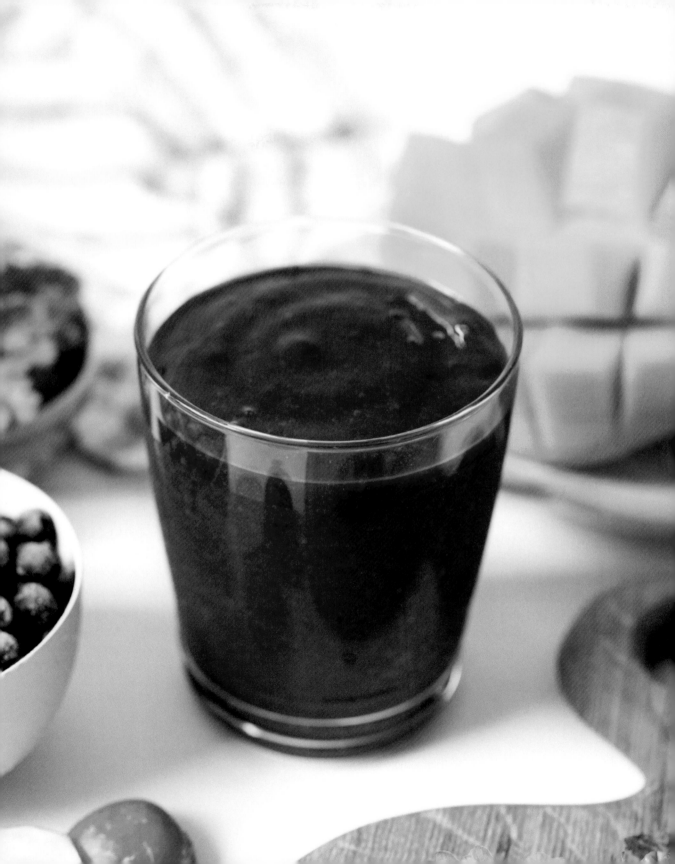

CHAPTER 11

Medical Medium Heavy Metal Detox Cleanses

Empowerment is knowing there's something you can do that can change your life and bring your health into a direction that you dream about. As you're venturing into this cleanse, you're venturing in with the knowledge of why you've been struggling all along. No longer are your hands tied when it comes to finding answers about how to move forward with your health.

If you're knocking on the door of these cleanses, it means you have struggled in some way. Maybe you've struggled so much that no one else could even know what it's been like unless they've struggled in a similar way. Spiritual forces of the light help us find our way when we've been walking down such a difficult path. It's not just a chance that you're here. There were powers at work all along in your journey that brought you to this place.

Removing toxic heavy metals isn't just a physical experience. It's a spiritual experience, because having toxic heavy metals inside the brain harms us spiritually. All

along, you've been taking notice of your symptoms and conditions and your struggles and hardships. It's time to take notice of the tangible recovery you have set before you.

As you venture into a Heavy Metal Detox Cleanse, there are some different sensations that you may experience. The feeling of metals leaving the brain can bring about nostalgia, déjà vu, a temporary sense of sadness, or a sense of feeling more complete, as well as increased and more vivid dreams, especially dreams that make no sense whatsoever, eventually leading to more euphoric dreams that feel peaceful and good. As metals are removed, a sense of clarity, a sense of peace, a sense of excitement, and the feeling of joy can come from out of nowhere for no apparent reason. Everybody experiences different sensations, depending on how many metals, what kind of metals, where in the brain those metals are, and how toxic someone is with a variety of different chemicals.

HEAVY METAL DETOX CLEANSE GUIDELINES

15-Day or 30-Day Options

- For each of these cleanse options, select a period of either 15 days or 30 days.

Repeating the Cleanse

- You're welcome to do any of these cleanse levels continually and long term by repeating cleanses back-to-back.

- When you're repeating a Heavy Metal Detox Cleanse back-to-back, you could either repeat the same level or switch to a milder or more advanced level once you've made it through any 15- or 30-day cleanse period.

- You can also take breaks between cleanses. When you're not on a Heavy Metal Detox Cleanse, you can keep up with doing the Heavy Metal Detox Smoothie every day.

Smoothie Timing

- If you've selected a cleanse option that includes both a version of the Heavy Metal Detox Smoothie and a version of the Extractor Smoothie, keep in mind: don't reverse their order. When consuming them on the same day, you want to have the Heavy Metal Detox Smoothie (regular or Advanced) in the first half of your day, and the Extractor Smoothie (regular or Advanced) in the second half of your day.

Substitutions

- Many of these cleanses incorporate the option of daily apples as a snack. You can chop or blend those apples, substitute with ripe pears, enjoy the "Applesauce or Pear Sauce" recipe in Chapter 12, or have cooked applesauce (as long as it doesn't contain additives) if needed. If you can't access apples or pears, look for oranges as a substitute. If you can't find oranges, look for papayas. If you can't get papayas, look for bananas. And if you can't get bananas, you can use mangoes in place of apples or pears.

- For more questions about ingredient substitutions, see the Tips that go along with individual recipes. If possible, try not to get into the habit of relying on substitutions. Keep trying to achieve the goal of using the proper ingredients for the cleanses.

Cleanse Interruptions

- If you miss the Heavy Metal Detox Smoothie and/or Extractor Smoothie (regular or Advanced) on any given day of a cleanse, still try to follow the rest of the cleanse guidance that day, and then add one day to the end of your cleanse.

- If you do something that breaks your cleanse, add three days to the end of your cleanse. "Breaking the cleanse" means consuming items your cleanse level specifies to avoid, whether radical fats such as nut butter in the morning or brain betrayer foods such as eggs, dairy, or gluten.

General Notes for All Cleanses

- If you're getting your blood drawn for some reason within the time period of your cleanse, ask if you can move your appointment to a time when you're not doing the cleanse, or learn how to ask for quarter or half tubes from the "Blood Draining Agenda" chapter in this book's companion title, *Brain Saver.* If you don't have the book on hand and you have an immediate need to apply that chapter's information due to a medical concern, listen

to the "Blood Draw" episode of the *Medical Medium Podcast.* For protocols to avoid weakening your immune system, refer to Chapter 4.

- For any general cleansing questions you have that are not addressed in this book, *Cleanse to Heal* is available to you as an additional resource.

Adjustments for Children

You can go ahead with the Heavy Metal Detox Cleanses for children, keeping the following in mind:

- It's fine to leave the lemon or lime water out for kids and also to reduce the amount of celery juice according to what feels right for your little one. See the table in Chapter 2 for more guidance on celery juice amounts for children.

- See "Adjustments for Children" in Chapter 10, "Heavy Metal Detox," for guidance on Heavy Metal Detox Smoothie amounts for children.

- The amounts of the Advanced Heavy Metal Detox Smoothie, Extractor Smoothie, and Advanced Extractor Smoothie are up to your discretion as parent or caregiver. Children can have these recipes in small portions, with serving sizes depending on the age and size of the child. You can go as low as 4 ounces or down to a tablespoon or even less.

HEAVY METAL DETOX CLEANSE LEVELS

1. ENTRY LEVEL Heavy Metal Detox Cleanse

Add these steps to your normal eating routine:

- Drink the original Heavy Metal Detox Smoothie daily (recipe in Chapter 10); it should not be consumed directly after a fat-based meal.

- Optional: Incorporate as many other Medical Medium tools and recipes as desired.

- Try to drink a minimum of 50 ounces of water throughout the day (that amount can include coconut water).

- If you're sensitive or believe you're extra toxic, Entry Level is a good place to begin. You have the option of making the Heavy Metal Detox Smoothie with the amounts of the five key ingredients reduced by 50 percent. Once you've gotten comfortable with those smaller

dosages, you can work your way up to the full recipe.

2. BASIC Heavy Metal Detox Cleanse

Add these steps to your normal eating routine:

- Drink the Advanced Heavy Metal Detox Smoothie daily (recipe in Chapter 10); it should not be consumed directly after a fat-based meal.

- Optional: Incorporate as many other Medical Medium tools and recipes as desired.

- Try to drink a minimum of 60 ounces of water throughout the day (that amount can include coconut water).

3. SIMPLIFIED Heavy Metal Detox Cleanse (same as the original Heavy Metal Detox Cleanse from *Cleanse to Heal*)

Add these steps to your normal eating routine:

- Start each day with 16 to 32 ounces of fresh lemon or lime water upon waking (recipe with the proper ratio of lemon or lime to water in Chapter 12).

- At least 15 to 30 minutes later, drink 16 to 32 ounces of fresh celery juice on an empty stomach (then wait another 15 to 30 minutes before you have your smoothie).

- Drink the original Heavy Metal Detox Smoothie (recipe in Chapter 10) for breakfast.

- If you get hungry again before lunchtime, stick to snacking on apples (have more than one if you want). You're welcome to chop or blend your apples, enjoy the "Applesauce or Pear Sauce" recipe in Chapter 12, go with cooked applesauce (as long as it doesn't contain additives), or opt for ripe pears if apples don't work for you.

- Stay fat-free until at least lunchtime.

- Optional: For even better results, take a look at the brain betrayer foods and food chemicals in Chapters 5 and 7. Start chipping away at the lists, seeing what foods you'd like to avoid while cleansing. The fewer brain betrayers such as eggs, dairy, gluten, corn, soy, tuna, lamb, and pork in your diet, the more effective the Heavy Metal Detox Smoothie can be.

- Try to drink a minimum of 60 ounces of water throughout the day (that amount can include coconut water and your morning lemon or lime water).

Be mindful not to drink the water too close to drinking the celery juice—make sure you space them at least 15 to 30 minutes apart.

4. INTERMEDIATE Heavy Metal Detox Cleanse

Add these steps to your normal eating routine:

- Start each day with 16 to 32 ounces of fresh lemon or lime water upon waking (recipe with the proper ratio of lemon or lime to water in Chapter 12).

- At least 15 to 30 minutes later, drink 16 to 32 ounces of fresh celery juice on an empty stomach (then wait another 15 to 30 minutes before you have your smoothie).

- Drink the Advanced Heavy Metal Detox Smoothie (recipe in Chapter 10) for breakfast.

- If you get hungry again before lunchtime, stick to snacking on apples (have more than one if you want). You're welcome to chop or blend your apples, enjoy the "Applesauce or Pear Sauce" recipe in Chapter 12, go with cooked applesauce (as long as it doesn't contain additives), or opt for ripe pears if apples don't work for you.

- Stay fat-free until at least lunchtime.

- Optional: For even better results, take a look at the brain betrayer foods and food chemicals in Chapters 5 and 7. Start chipping away at the lists, seeing what foods you'd like to avoid while cleansing. The fewer brain betrayers such as eggs, dairy, gluten, corn, soy, tuna, lamb, and pork in your diet, the more effective the Advanced Heavy Metal Detox Smoothie can be.

- Try to drink a minimum of 60 ounces of water throughout the day (that amount can include coconut water and your morning lemon or lime water). Be mindful not to drink the water too close to drinking the celery juice—make sure you space them at least 15 to 30 minutes apart.

5. PERFORMANCE Heavy Metal Detox Cleanse

Add these steps to your normal eating routine:

- Start each day with 16 to 32 ounces of fresh lemon or lime water upon waking (recipe with the proper ratio of lemon or lime to water in Chapter 12).

- At least 15 to 30 minutes later, drink 16 to 32 ounces of fresh celery juice on an empty stomach (then wait another 15 to 30 minutes before you have your smoothie).

- Drink the original Heavy Metal Detox Smoothie (recipe in Chapter 10) for breakfast.

- If you get hungry again before lunchtime, stick to snacking on apples (have more than one if you want). You're welcome to chop or blend your apples, enjoy the "Applesauce or Pear Sauce" recipe in Chapter 12, go with cooked applesauce (as long as it doesn't contain additives), or opt for ripe pears if apples don't work for you.

- Stay fat-free until at least lunchtime.

- Drink the Extractor Smoothie (recipe in Chapter 10) anytime in the second half of your day, as long as it's not after a fat-based snack or meal.

- Try to incorporate as many fat-free Medical Medium recipes from this book (and/or *Cleanse to Heal* and the expanded edition of *Medical Medium*) into your snacks and meals as you can.

- Avoid all foods and food chemicals from Chapters 5 and 7, including caffeine.

- Keep fats limited to one serving (if at all) from lunchtime on, preferably at the end of the day. If you're plant-based, it's okay to incorporate one serving of plant fat such as avocado, nuts or nut butters, seeds, coconut, coconut oil, olives, or olive oil in a Medical Medium recipe. If you eat animal products, it's okay to incorporate one serving of animal fat such as chicken, grass-fed beef, turkey, salmon, or sardines in a Medical Medium recipe.

- Try to drink a minimum of 60 ounces of water throughout the day (that amount can include coconut water and your morning lemon or lime water). Be mindful not to drink the water too close to drinking the celery juice—make sure you space them at least 15 to 30 minutes apart.

6. ADVANCED Heavy Metal Detox Cleanse

Make these steps your complete eating routine:

- Start each day with 16 to 32 ounces of fresh lemon or lime water upon waking (recipe with the proper ratio of lemon or lime to water in Chapter 12).

- At least 15 to 30 minutes later, drink 16 to 32 ounces of fresh celery juice on an empty stomach (then wait another 15 to 30 minutes before you have your smoothie).

- Drink the original Heavy Metal Detox Smoothie (recipe in Chapter 10) for breakfast.

- If you get hungry again before lunchtime, stick to snacking on apples (have more than one if you want). You're welcome to chop or blend your apples, enjoy the "Applesauce or Pear Sauce" recipe in Chapter 12, go with cooked applesauce (as long as it doesn't contain additives), or opt for ripe pears if apples don't work for you.

- Stay off all fat-based foods, both plant fats (e.g., nuts, seeds, avocado) and animal fats (e.g., chicken, fish, meat).

- Drink the Extractor Smoothie (recipe in Chapter 10) anytime in the second half of your day.

- Use exclusively fat-free Medical Medium recipes from this book (and/or *Cleanse to Heal* and the expanded edition of *Medical Medium*).

- Avoid all foods and food chemicals from Chapters 5 and 7, including caffeine.

- Try to drink a minimum of 60 ounces of water throughout the day (that amount can include coconut water and your morning lemon or lime water). Be mindful not to drink the water too close to drinking the celery juice—make sure you space them at least 15 to 30 minutes apart.

7. HIGH-POWERED Heavy Metal Detox Cleanse

Make these steps your complete eating routine:

- Start each day with 32 ounces of fresh lemon or lime water upon waking (recipe with the proper ratio of lemon or lime to water in Chapter 12).

- At least 15 to 30 minutes later, drink 32 ounces of fresh celery juice on an empty stomach (then wait another 15 to 30 minutes before you have your smoothie).

- Drink the Advanced Heavy Metal Detox Smoothie (recipe in Chapter 10) for breakfast.

- If you get hungry again before lunchtime, stick to snacking on apples (have more than one if you want). You're welcome to chop or blend your apples, enjoy the "Applesauce or Pear Sauce" recipe in Chapter 12, go with cooked applesauce (as long as it doesn't contain additives), or opt for ripe pears if apples don't work for you.

- Stay off all fat-based foods, both plant fats (e.g., nuts, seeds, avocado) and animal fats (e.g., chicken, fish, meat).

- Drink the Advanced Extractor Smoothie (recipe in Chapter 10) anytime in the second half of your day.

- Use exclusively fat-free Medical Medium recipes from this book (and/or *Cleanse to Heal* and the expanded edition of *Medical Medium*).

- Avoid all foods and food chemicals from Chapters 5 and 7, including caffeine.

- Remove fragrances, colognes, perfumes, air fresheners, incense, and **scented** candles, laundry detergents, fabric softeners, aftershaves, deodorants, soaps, body sprays, body lotions, body oils, hair products, and car fresheners.

- Try to drink a minimum of 60 ounces of water throughout the day (that amount can include coconut water and your morning lemon or lime water). Be mindful not to drink the water too close to drinking the celery juice—make sure you space them at least 15 to 30 minutes apart.

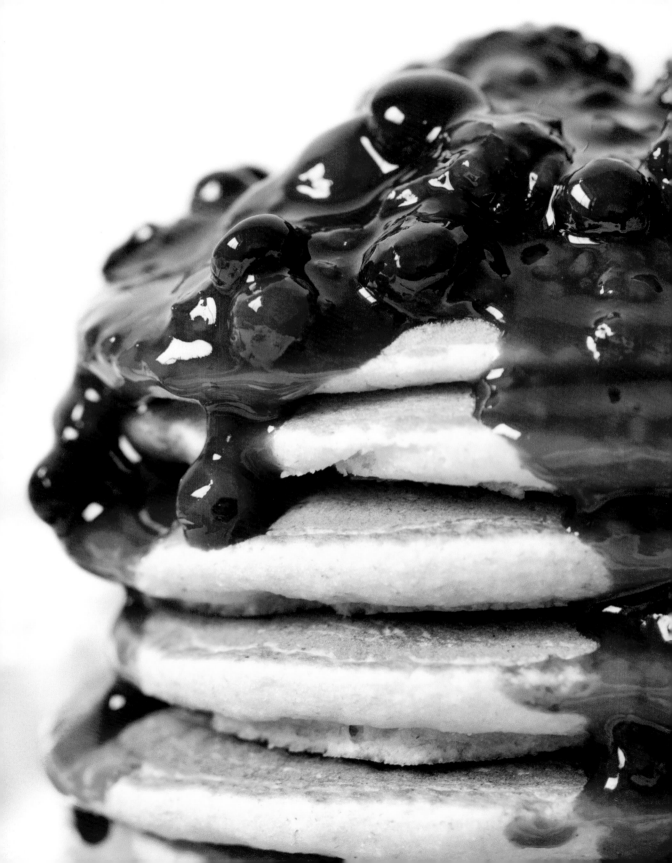

PART V

BRAIN SAVER RECIPES

"The healing process is not just the passive process of waiting for the body to heal. The healing process is the steps you take so your body can heal. Healing is an active combination of your free will, learning the information, your body's ability to heal on its own, the tools you're using, what you give your body so it can heal, and the details within it all."

— Anthony William, Medical Medium

CHAPTER 12

Medical Medium Brain Saver Recipes

NOTES:

- When preparing juices and other recipes with apples, cucumbers, and other fruits and vegetables that have edible skins, you can keep the skins on if a recipe does not specify and the items are organic, or you're welcome to peel them. If they're conventionally grown, peel and discard the skins—or if you can't peel the conventional fruit or vegetable for any reason, wash it with vigor before using.

- In recipes that call for bananas, select ripe bananas that have small brown dots on the skin yet are still mostly yellow and have some firmness. Try not to consume bananas that are overripe, where the skin is completely brown, or underripe, where the skin is green or doesn't have any spots yet. Bananas in different parts of the world have variability in appearance when ripe. If a banana gives you a fuzzy feeling on your tongue, is too hard or firm, or is difficult to peel, to the point that the skin starts to break, these are all signs that the fruit is underripe.

- For recipes that call for fresh strawberries, you'll see a note to remove the green leaves before using. While the greens on top of strawberries are edible, they may also harbor bacteria from farm water that got trapped between the strawberries and the leaves. This is why the advice is to remove the strawberry greens altogether.

BRAIN SAVER RECIPE LIST

1. Lemon, Ginger, and Honey Water
2. Lemon or Lime Water
3. Thyme Tea and Thyme Water
4. Aloe Water
5. Cucumber Juice
6. Pomegranate Juice
7. Brain Soother Juice
8. Brain Detox Bitters
9. Brain Builder
10. Watermelon, Orange, Turmeric, and Ginger Juice
11. Celery Juice
12. Heavy Metal Detox Smoothie
13. Heavy Metal Detox Smoothie Bowl
14. Heavy Metal Detox Smoothie Pops
15. Brain Detox Tonic
16. Brain Fueler Smoothie
17. Wild Blueberry "Yogurt"
18. Applesauce or Pear Sauce
19. Peaches and Cream
20. Banana, Mango, and Wild Blueberry Trifle
21. Brain Saver Salad
22. Brain Armor Salad
23. Spinach Soup
24. Brain Saver Wraps
25. Asparagus-Spinach Dip
26. Stuffed Tomatoes with Herbed Cauliflower Rice
27. Raw "Stir-Fry"
28. Mango Nori Wraps
29. Leafy Green and Berry Salad
30. Raw Chili
31. Raw Portobello Mushroom Burgers
32. Green Salad with French Dressing
33. Strawberry Salsa
34. Cobb Salad
35. Raw Cilantro Chutney
36. Cauliflower Ceviche
37. Greek Salad
38. Sesame Cucumber Noodles
39. Healing Broth
40. Roasted Tomato Soup with Potato Croutons
41. Pot Pie Soup
42. Chickpea Dumpling Soup
43. Sweet Potato Nacho Cheese Soup
44. Zucchini Lasagna Soup
45. Curry Potato Samosas
46. Spiced Squash Soup
47. Baba Ganoush
48. Cauliflower and Squash Bowl
49. Potato Lettuce Sandwiches
50. Sweet Potato Nori Wraps
51. Zucchini Noodles with Marinara Sauce
52. Asian-Inspired Potato Skillet
53. Steamed Cabbage Rolls

1. LEMON, GINGER, AND HONEY WATER

Makes 1 serving

This Lemon, Ginger, and Honey Water is refreshing and hydrating. It's the perfect drink to begin your day, enjoy as an afternoon pick-me-up, or sip over the course of the day. (If you're starting your day with it, try it 15 to 30 minutes or more before or after your celery juice.) When you drink this healing tonic upon waking, it will help your liver flush out toxins it's collected for release throughout the night while giving your liver and body the critical hydration and glucose they need to begin your day.

1- to 2-inch piece of fresh ginger
16 ounces (2 cups) water (room temperature or cooler, not hot)
½ lemon, juiced
1 teaspoon raw honey

Grate the ginger into the 2 cups of water. Allow the ginger to steep for at least 15 minutes or, ideally, longer. You can even let it steep in the fridge overnight if you wish.

When you're ready to drink it, strain the ginger out of the water, add the lemon juice and raw honey, and stir well.

TIPS

- As an alternative to grating the ginger, chop it into a few small pieces and squeeze them in a garlic press—it will act like a mini juicer.

- It can be helpful to prepare a big batch of ginger water in advance to sip as desired. For best results, add the raw honey and lemon just prior to consuming.

- This recipe should not be made with hot water.

- It's important to use raw honey for this recipe. You won't receive the same healing benefits from heated processed honey.

- For greater hydrating and healing benefits, try drinking 32 ounces upon waking of Lemon, Ginger, and Honey Water instead of 16 ounces. Just double the recipe.

- For a powerful morning cleanse that includes lemon water or this Lemon, Ginger, and Honey Water, then celery juice, and specific foods to allow cleansing and healing to happen in the body every day, try making the Morning Cleanse that's outlined in the Medical Medium series book *Cleanse to Heal* part of your everyday life.

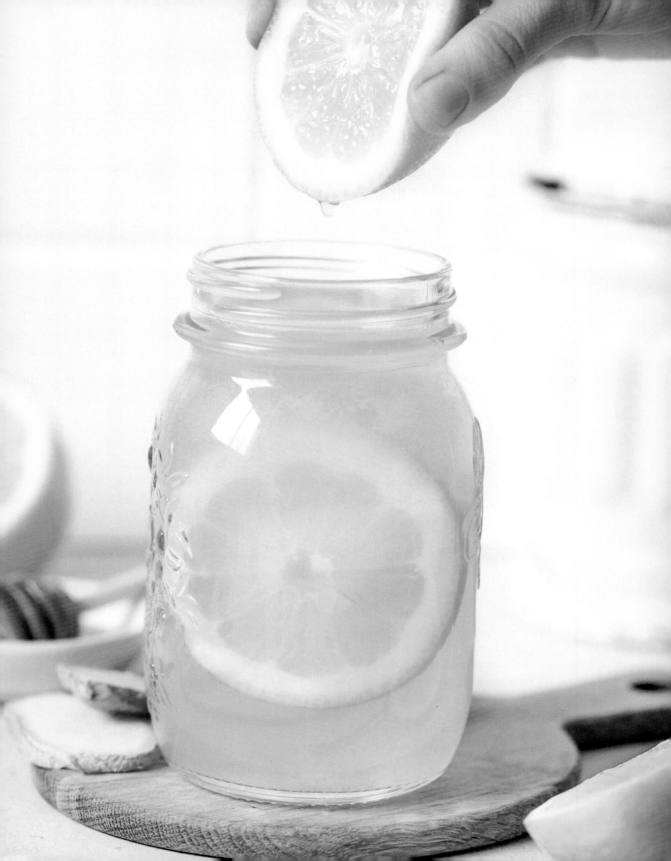

2. LEMON OR LIME WATER

This simple recipe brings your water to life, priming toxic heavy metals and toxic chemicals to be more easily removed from your brain and body. Making lemon or lime water a part of your daily routine helps you stay hydrated enough to flush out the toxins and metals you're uprooting with the Heavy Metal Detox Smoothie and other tools and protocols in this book.

½ lemon or 2 limes, freshly cut
16 ounces (2 cups) water (room
   temperature or cooler, not hot)

Squeeze the juice from the freshly cut lemon or limes into the water, straining seeds if necessary.

Wait at least 15 to 20 minutes and ideally 30 minutes after you finish drinking your lemon or lime water before you consume your celery juice or anything else.

TIPS

- If you prefer 32 ounces (4 cups) of lemon or lime water upon rising, that's a great way to give yourself extra hydration and cleansing support. Simply double the recipe and enjoy.

- This recipe should not be made with hot water. Use room temperature or cold water.

- In your daily life, it's best to drink at least two or more 16-ounce lemon or lime waters over the course of a day. A great routine is to drink one upon rising, a second in the afternoon, and a third one hour before bed.

- Limes vary in size and juiciness. If your limes are dry, use 2 limes per 16 ounces of water, as the recipe calls for, to get enough juice. If your limes are big and juicy, you may only need half a lime.

- If you'd like, you're welcome to add a teaspoon of raw honey to your morning lemon or lime water.

- If for some reason lemons or limes don't work for you or you can't access them, you can make ginger water instead or opt for plain water.

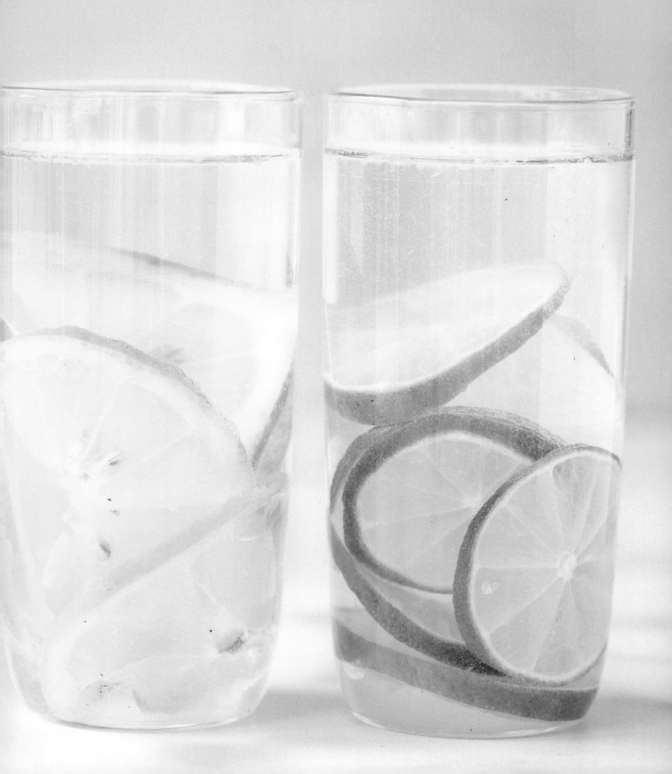

3. THYME TEA AND THYME WATER

Thyme Tea and Thyme Water are both powerful antiviral drinks you can incorporate daily or as often as possible to receive their healing benefits.

THYME TEA

Makes 1 serving

2 sprigs fresh thyme or 2 teaspoons dried thyme
1 cup hot water
Juice of ½ lemon and/or 1 teaspoon raw honey (optional)

Place the thyme in a mug and pour hot water over the herb, allowing it to steep for 15 minutes or more. Remove the thyme sprigs or strain the tea, especially if you're using dried thyme. Sweeten with lemon juice and/or raw honey.

THYME WATER

Makes 4 to 8 cups

4 to 8 cups water
8 sprigs fresh thyme or 1 tablespoon dried thyme
Optional additions: fresh lemon slices or freshly squeezed lemon juice, raw honey, berries, cucumber slices, mint

Fill a jug or pitcher with room temperature water and add the thyme. Steep at room temperature on the counter overnight. In the morning, remove or strain out the thyme and add lemon juice or raw honey or any optional ingredients you'd like.

TIPS

- Fresh thyme can be found in the produce section of your local supermarket or health food store. Thyme is also very easy to grow and can produce abundantly in both containers and home gardens.

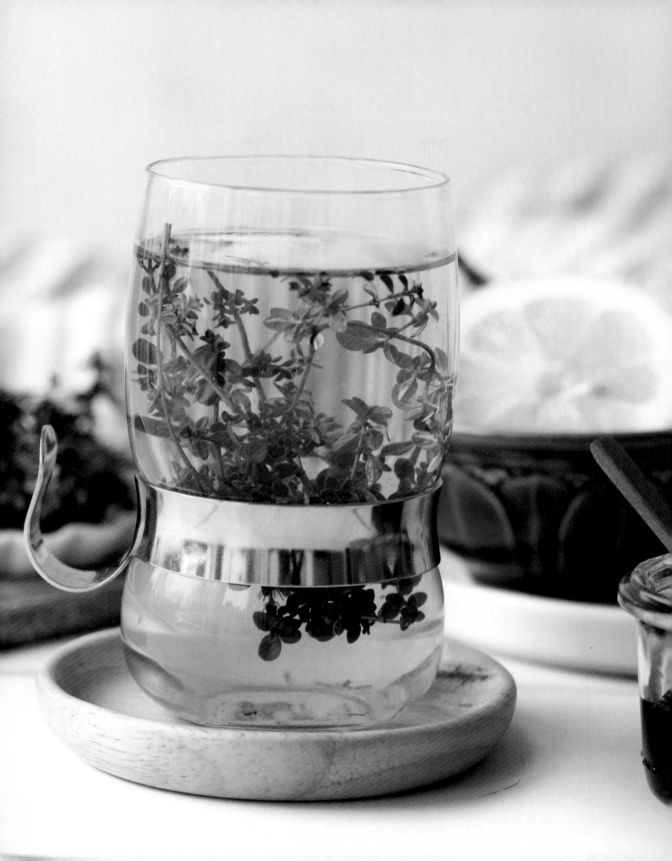

4. ALOE WATER

As you drink this soothing beverage, think about aloe vera's profound ability to neutralize acid, calm nerves in the intestinal tract linings, inhibit the growth of unproductive bacteria, yeast, mold, and viruses in the gut, and alleviate pressure on the vagus nerves.

2- to 4-inch piece of fresh aloe vera leaf
2 cups (16 ounces) water

This recipe is based on using a large, store-bought aloe vera leaf, which you can find in the produce section of many grocery stores. If you're using a homegrown aloe vera plant, make sure it's an edible source. Either way, avoid using the bitter base of the leaf—cut off 1 inch from the very end of the leaf and discard.

Carefully slice your section of aloe leaf open, filleting it as if it were a fish and trimming away the green skin and spikes. Scoop out the clear gel and place it in the blender.

Add the water to the blender and blend for 10 to 20 seconds, until the aloe is thoroughly liquefied.

Drink immediately, on an empty stomach, for best results.

TIPS

- Save the remainder of the aloe leaf by wrapping the cut end in a damp towel or plastic wrap and storing it in the refrigerator for up to two weeks.

- Make sure you do not use the aloe leaf skin. As you're scooping out the aloe gel, try not to scrape the skin. The chemical compound in the green skin can be irritating for some people.

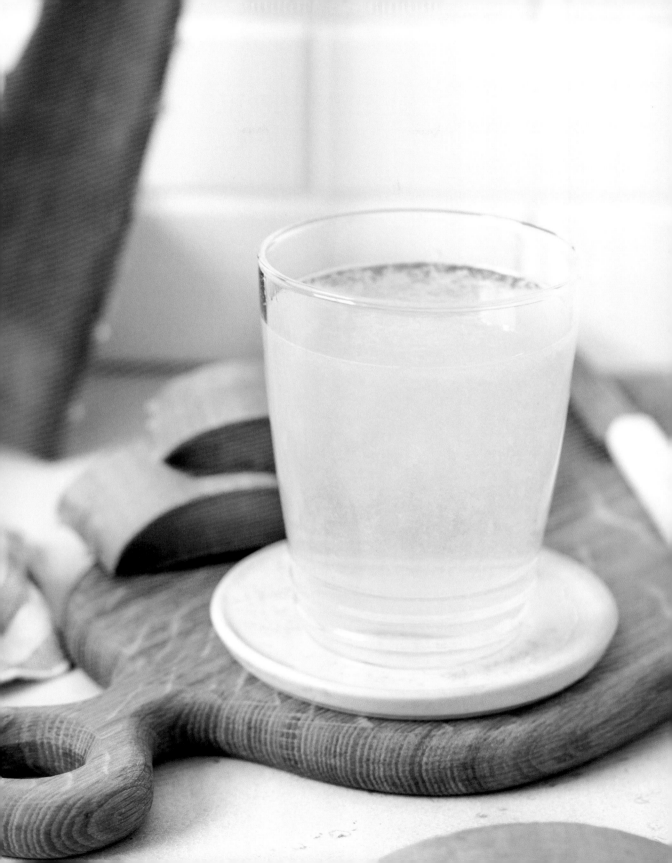

5. CUCUMBER JUICE

Makes 1 serving

Fresh cucumber juice is an incredible rejuvenation tonic. Highly alkalizing and hydrating, cucumber juice has the ability to cleanse and detox the entire body. Its mildly sweet flavor makes it easy to drink.

2 large cucumbers

Rinse the cucumbers and run them through the juicer of your choice. Drink immediately on an empty stomach for best results.

If you don't have access to a juicer, here's how to make it in a blender:

Rinse the cucumbers, chop them, and blend them in a high-speed blender until smooth. (Don't add water.) Strain the liquefied cucumber well; a nut milk bag is handy for this. Drink immediately on an empty stomach for best results.

TIPS

- Fresh cucumber juice is a good alternative to celery juice if you're not able to find celery or you really struggle with the flavor of celery juice. While cucumber juice is an incredible healing drink, it does not offer the same healing benefits as celery juice, so it's important to include celery juice daily as much as possible. For most people, the taste of celery juice becomes more enjoyable with consistent consumption.

- Steer clear of putting additional ingredients such as lemon, apple, ginger, or leafy greens in your cucumber juice. While these are healing foods, cucumber juice offers the most benefits when consumed as pure cucumber juice. Instead, enjoy a mixed green juice at another time of day if you wish, such as the Brain Soother Juice in a few pages. Also avoid adding ice, water, or any supplements or powders to your cucumber juice.

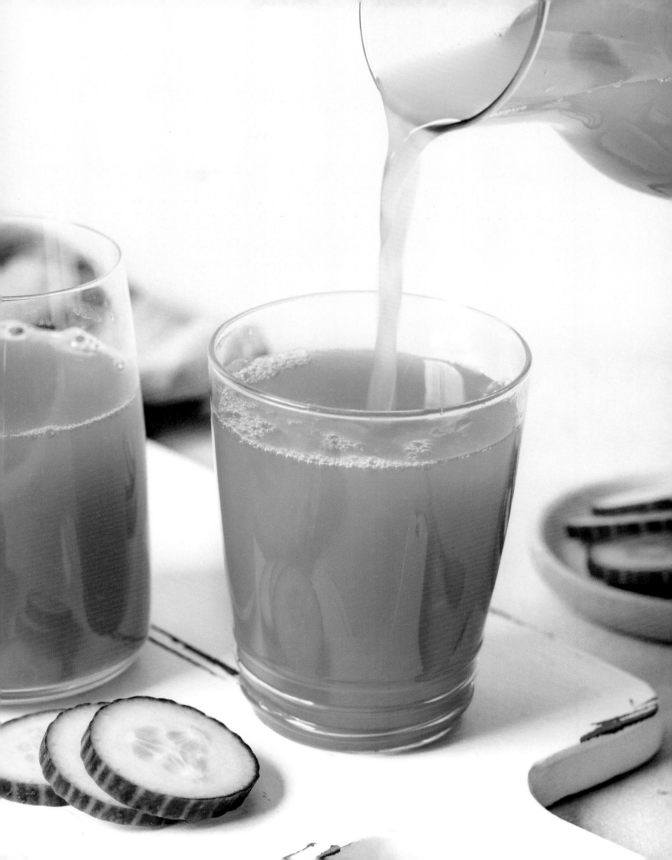

6. POMEGRANATE JUICE

Pomegranate juice is at its most beneficial when freshly juiced with a juicer and not store bought. When the inner core of the pomegranate seed is pulverized, powerful undiscovered phytochemical compounds are released into the juice that comes from the outer part of the seed, the jewel-like, juicy pulp called an aril. This combination brings pomegranate juice to a higher medicinal level. Nutrients extracted from the inner core of the seeds are detoxifying for the liver, gallbladder, lungs, lymphatic system, and the kidneys. These phytochemical compounds and nutrients are antiviral, antibacterial, anti-yeast, anti-mold, and contribute to feeding immune cells needed to consume toxic waste in the bloodstream, becoming a helpful blood purifier that helps to keep the brain clean.

2 medium-sized pomegranates, seeded (about 3 cups pomegranate seeds)

Run the pomegranate seeds through a juicer. Serve immediately.

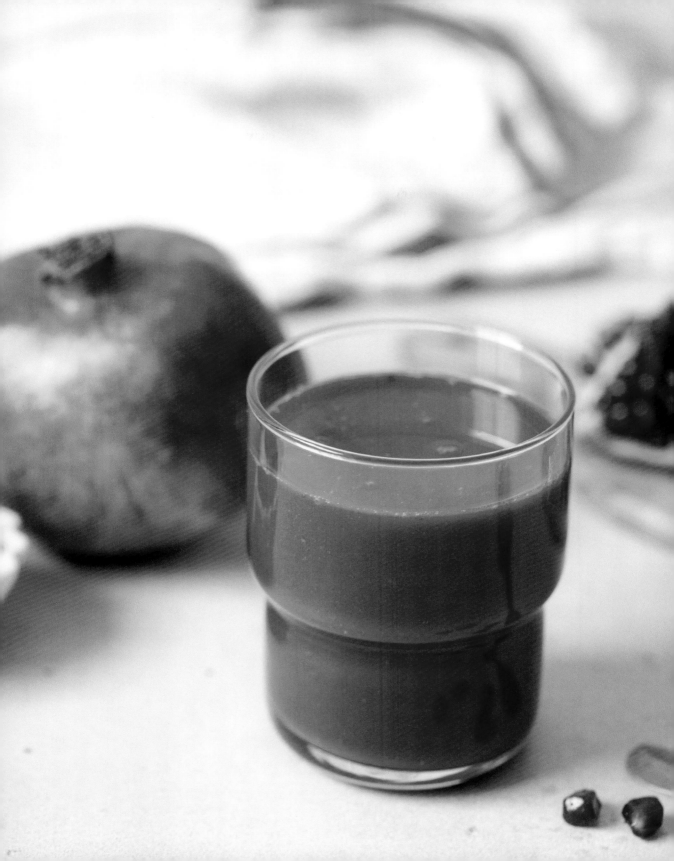

7. BRAIN SOOTHER JUICE

Makes 1 serving

When life surprises us with high stress and intense moments, our brain can overheat, and we can lose precious electrolyte and glucose reserves. This tonic helps calm the mind and cool the brain down from overheating while replenishing reserves.

2 medium cucumbers
6 stalks celery
2 medium apples
1 whole bulb fennel

Run all the ingredients through the juicer of your choice.

Serve immediately.

TIPS

- When juicing fennel for this recipe, you can use only the bulb or the bulb plus the lower part of the stalks.

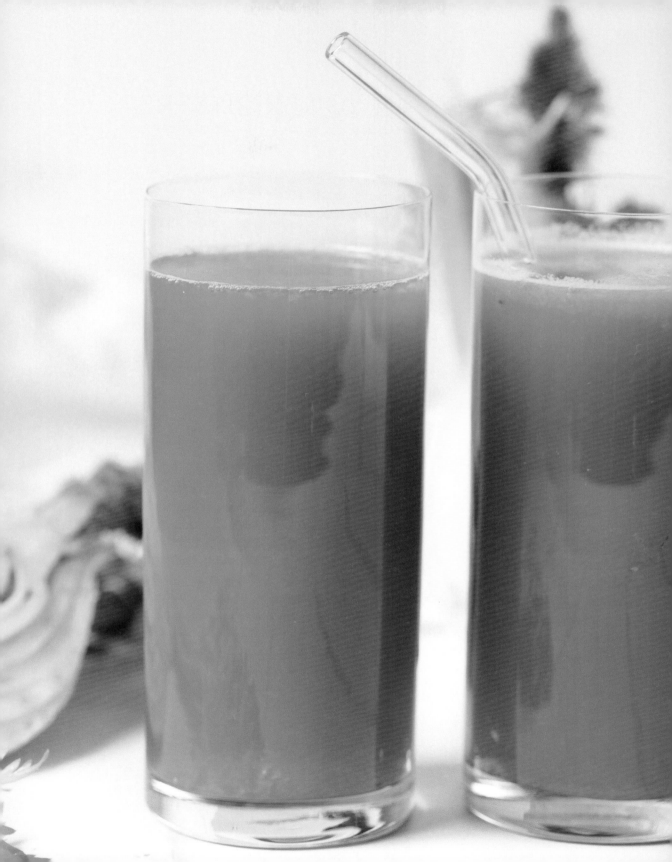

8. BRAIN DETOX BITTERS

Makes 1 serving

This special recipe helps remove various toxic chemicals from the brain that cloud the mind.

3 to 5 apples
2 cups loosely packed dandelion greens
2 cups loosely packed kale
2 cups loosely packed spinach

Run all the ingredients through the juicer of your choice.

Serve immediately.

TIPS

- A cold press, masticating juicer will be more effective at juicing and extracting all the nutrients from leafy greens such as spinach and dandelion than a centrifugal juicer; however, any juicer can be used. If you are using a centrifugal juicer, you may have better success wrapping your leafy greens around pieces of apple or firmer ingredients instead of dropping a whole handful of the leafy greens into the juicer chute separately.

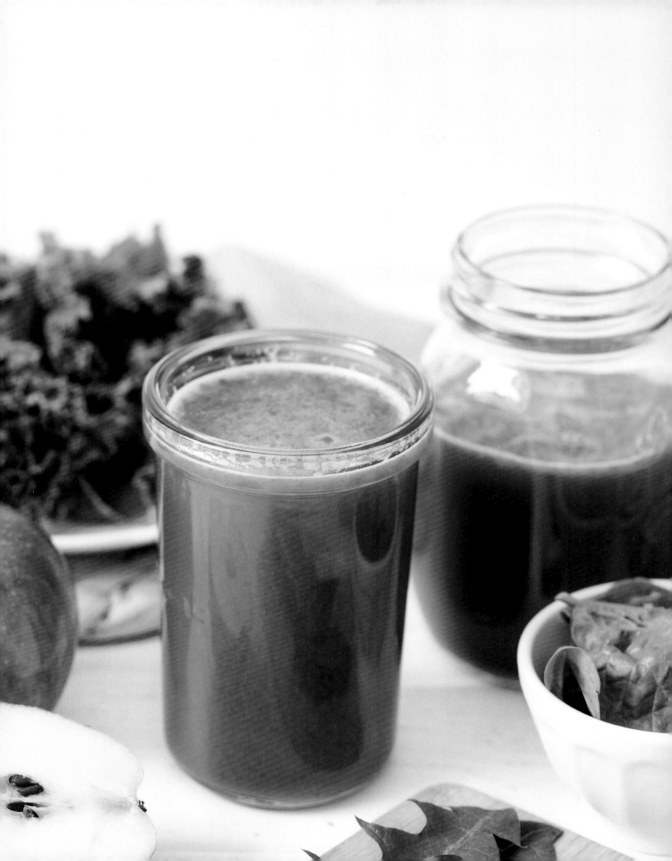

9. BRAIN BUILDER

This healing tonic helps to strengthen the brain quickly in stressful situations, providing a burst of glucose and electrolytes.

2 medium cucumbers
6 stalks celery
2 medium apples
1 cup fresh or thawed frozen wild blueberries, or 1 ounce pure wild blueberry juice, or 1 tablespoon pure wild blueberry powder

Run the cucumber, celery, and apples through the juicer of your choice.

Pour the juice into a blender and add the wild blueberries or pure wild blueberry juice or wild blueberry powder. Blend until smooth.

Serve immediately or strain if desired.

TIPS

- If you're in a part of the world where you can't access fresh or frozen wild blueberries, wild blueberry juice, or wild blueberry powder, you can substitute blackberries. Although a high-antioxidant alternative, blackberries do not have the potency to match how wild blueberries defend cells from metals, chemicals, radiation, and other toxins.

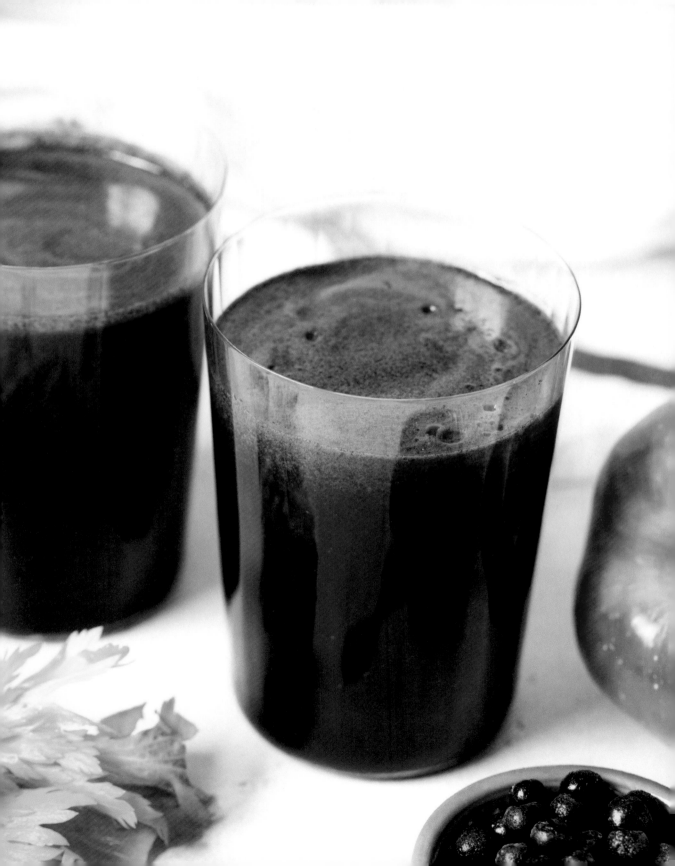

10. WATERMELON, ORANGE, TURMERIC, AND GINGER JUICE

Makes 1 to 2 servings

Hydrating and refreshing, this juice will uplift the body and soul and strengthen the immune system while providing critical glucose and healing to the body and brain.

1½ cups freshly squeezed orange juice
   (from 3 to 5 oranges, peeled)
5 cups (about 2 pounds) diced watermelon
2-inch piece of fresh ginger, peeled
1-inch piece of fresh turmeric, peeled

Juice all the ingredients in a juicer of your choice or place all the ingredients in a high-speed blender and blend until smooth.

Strain through a fine-mesh sieve, cheese-cloth, or nut milk bag to remove any pulp.

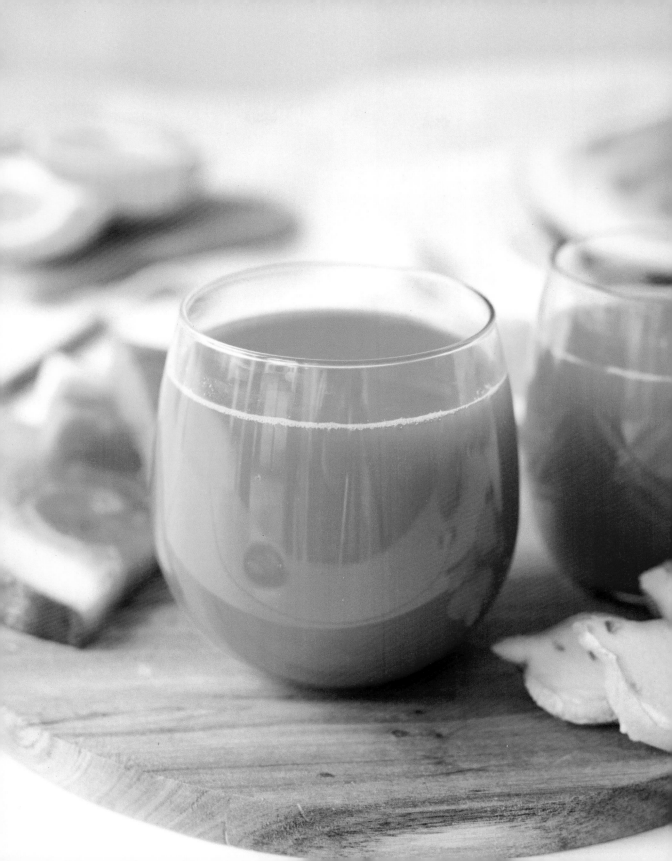

11. CELERY JUICE

Makes 1 serving

This simple herbal extraction has an incredible ability to create sweeping improvements for all kinds of health issues when consumed in the right way. That's why celery juice is such an important Medical Medium healing tool. It's an ideal way to start your day whether you want to heal a symptom or condition or protect your health for the future.

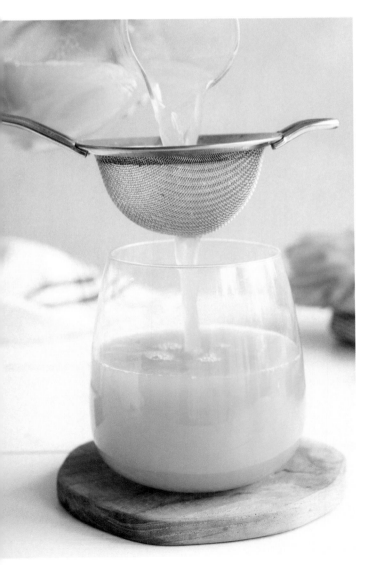

1 bunch of celery

Trim about a quarter inch off the base of the celery bunch to break apart the stalks.

Rinse the celery.

Run the celery through the juicer of your choice. Strain the juice to remove any grit or stray pieces of pulp. Drink immediately on an empty stomach for best results. Wait at least 15 to 30 minutes before consuming anything else.

If you don't have a juicer, you can make celery juice in a blender. Here's how:

Trim about a quarter inch off the base of the celery bunch, if desired, to break apart the stalks.

Rinse the celery. Place the celery on a clean cutting board and chop into roughly 1-inch pieces. Place the chopped celery in a high-speed blender and blend until smooth. (Don't add water.) Use your blender's tamping tool if needed. Strain the liquefied celery well; a nut milk bag is handy for this. Drink immediately on an empty stomach for best results. Wait at least 15 to 30 minutes before consuming anything else.

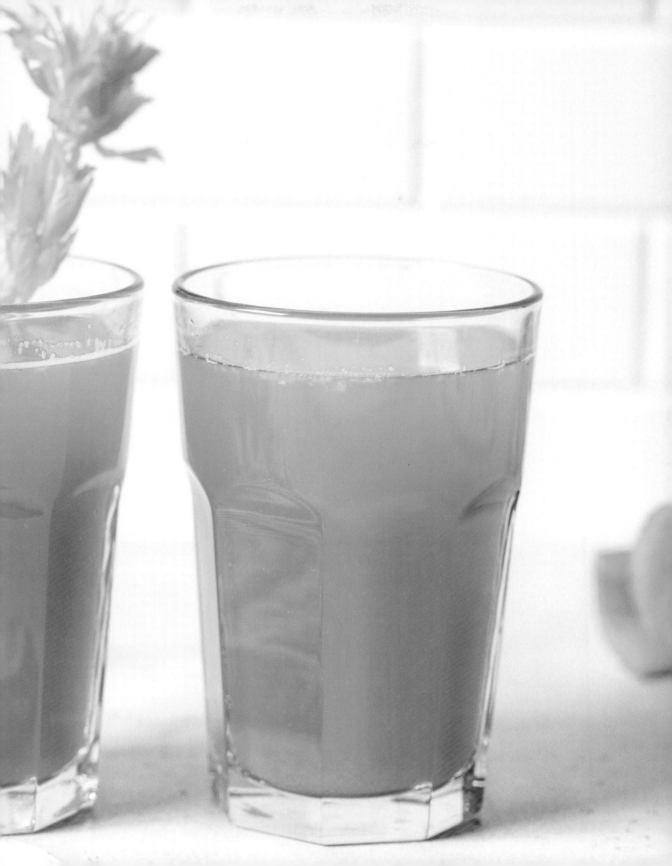

TIPS

- Steer clear of putting additional ingredients such as lemon, apple, ginger, or leafy greens in your celery juice. While these are wonderful foods, celery juice only offers its full benefits when consumed as pure celery juice by itself. Also avoid adding ice, water, or any supplements or powders to your celery juice.

- If you're not going to be able to drink your full batch of celery juice right away, the best way to store it is in an airtight glass jar or bottle in the fridge. Freshly juiced celery retains its healing benefits for about 24 hours, but it does lose potency by the hour, so it's best to drink it as soon after making it as possible. If you have no choice but to keep it for longer than 24 hours, it's still worth juicing ahead and consuming it when you can.

- If you can't access celery to make celery juice and you can't get fresh, pure celery juice from your local juice bar, don't despair. Cucumber juice is the ideal substitute in this case. While it can't offer the specific healing benefits that celery juice does, it does have unique benefits such as cell hydration to support your health. Treat it the same way you would celery juice—make it pure (cucumber only) and drink it on an empty stomach, apart from other food and drink. Ginger water, aloe water, and lemon or lime water are alternatives if you can get neither celery juice nor cucumber juice. That said, try not to make a habit of substituting anything for celery juice.

- For more on celery juice, including children's amounts, please see Chapter 2, "Golden Rules of Supplements."

12. HEAVY METAL DETOX SMOOTHIE

Makes 1 serving

This smoothie is a perfect and powerful combination of the five key ingredients for safely detoxifying toxic heavy metals from your brain and body. It's an honorable, life-giving blessing to help reverse so many symptoms.

2 bananas
2 cups frozen or fresh wild blueberries, or 2 ounces pure wild blueberry juice, or 2 tablespoons pure wild blueberry powder
1 cup tightly packed fresh cilantro
1 teaspoon barley grass juice powder
1 teaspoon spirulina
1 tablespoon Atlantic dulse or 2 dropperfuls Atlantic dulse liquid
1 orange, juiced
½ to 1 cup water, coconut water, or additional fresh-squeezed orange juice (optional)

Combine the bananas, wild blueberries, cilantro, barley grass juice powder, spirulina, and Atlantic dulse with the juice of 1 orange in a high-speed blender and blend until smooth.

Add up to 1 cup of water, coconut water, or additional orange juice if a thinner consistency is desired. Serve and enjoy!

TIPS

- If the barley grass juice powder and spirulina taste is too strong for you, start with a smaller amount of each and work your way up.

- Seek out wild blueberries (whether fresh, frozen, powdered, or as pure juice). Wild blueberries are not to be confused with cultivated blueberries.

- If you're in a part of the world where you can't access fresh or frozen wild blueberries, wild blueberry juice, or wild blueberry powder, you can substitute blackberries. Blackberries do not uproot and attach themselves to toxic heavy metals like wild blueberries do, although the high antioxidant ratio in blackberries can at least slow down heavy metal oxidation, which is helpful.

- As an alternative to adding the juice from 1 orange to the smoothie, you have the option to peel the orange, remove its seeds, and blend it whole in the smoothie.

313

- If you're using coconut water in this smoothie, make sure the coconut water doesn't contain natural flavors and isn't pink or red.

- If you're not a fan of banana, you can substitute Maradol papaya or mango.

- On days when you can't access every smoothie ingredient, don't skip your Heavy Metal Detox Smoothie. Make it with whichever ingredients you do have. Keep aiming to make the smoothie with all five key ingredients.

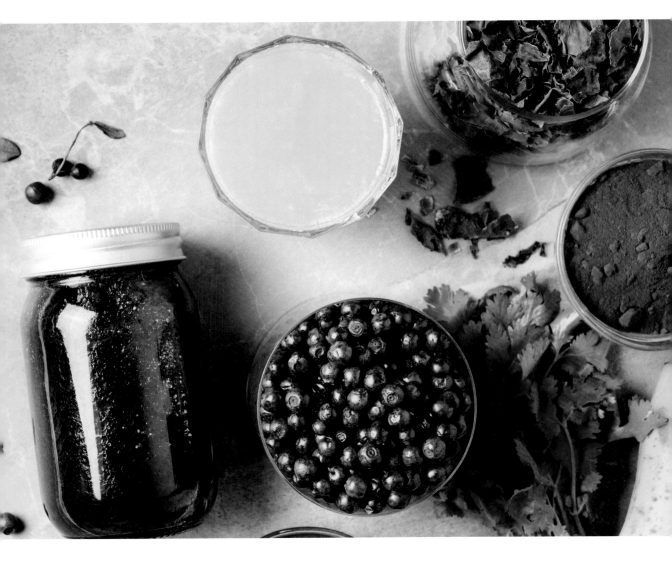

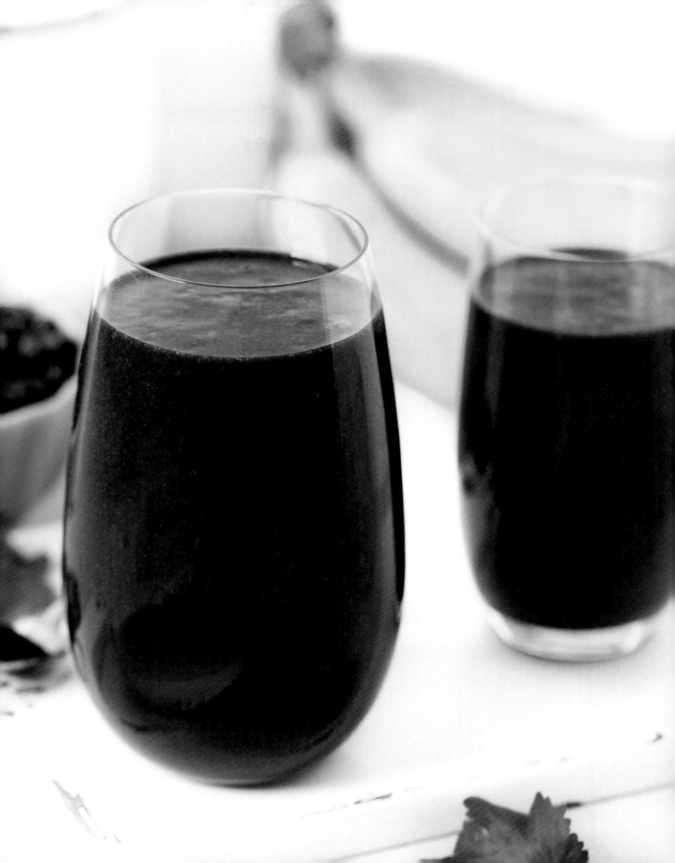

13. HEAVY METAL DETOX SMOOTHIE BOWL

Makes 1 serving

The Heavy Metal Detox Smoothie Bowl performs the same function as the Heavy Metal Detox Smoothie—it effectively removes toxic heavy metals from the brain and body. This delicious smoothie bowl gives you an alternative.

1½ cups fresh or frozen mango

2 cups frozen or fresh wild blueberries, or 2 ounces pure wild blueberry juice, or 2 tablespoons pure wild blueberry powder

½ cup fresh or frozen strawberries (optional)

1 cup tightly packed fresh cilantro

1 teaspoon barley grass juice powder

1 teaspoon spirulina

1 tablespoon Atlantic dulse or 2 dropperfuls Atlantic dulse liquid

1 tablespoon raw honey (optional)*

½ to 1 cup water, coconut water, or freshly squeezed orange juice (optional)

1 banana, sliced, for topping (optional)

¼ cup of fresh blueberries, raspberries, blackberries, and/or strawberries, for topping (optional)

Place the mango, blueberries, strawberries (if using), cilantro, barley grass juice powder, spirulina, Atlantic dulse, optional raw honey, and ½ cup water, coconut water, or orange juice (if using) in a high-speed blender and blend until smooth, at least 3 to 5 minutes. Add a bit more liquid if necessary to blend. Pour the smoothie into a bowl and top with banana slices and berries (if using). Serve immediately.

*If you're doing a Heavy Metal Detox Cleanse, you can use this recipe in place of the Heavy Metal Detox Smoothie if you leave out the raw honey. You can also use it in place of the Advanced Heavy Metal Detox Smoothie if you leave out the honey and increase the spirulina, barley grass juice powder, and cilantro to the amounts in the Advanced recipe in Chapter 10.

TIPS

- If the barley grass juice powder and spirulina taste is too strong for you, start with a smaller amount of each and work your way up.

- If you select fresh strawberries for this recipe, remove the greens before using.

- If you're in a part of the world where you can't access any form of wild blueberries, you can substitute blackberries, although blackberries do not uproot heavy metals. Read more in the previous recipe's tips.

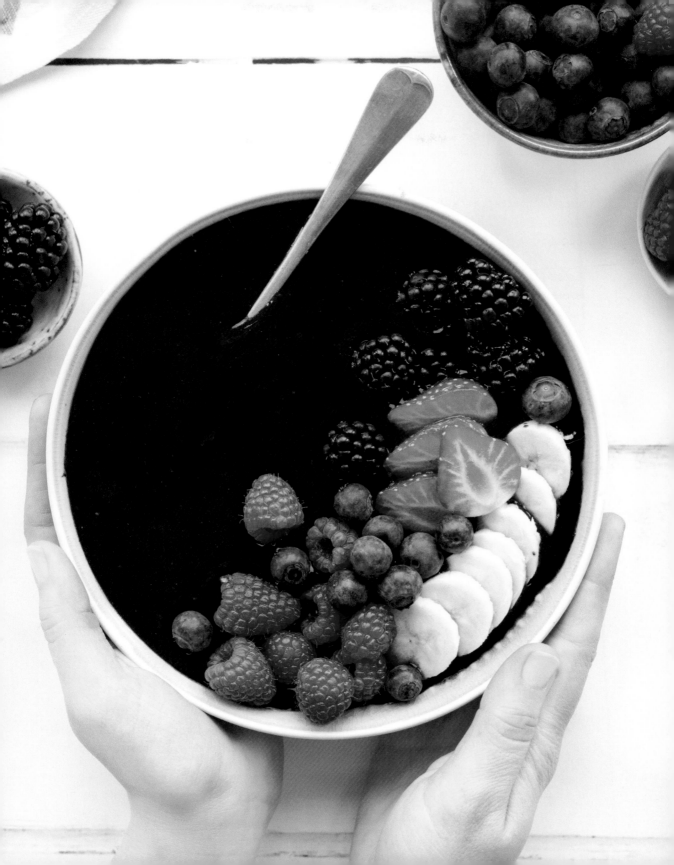

14. HEAVY METAL
DETOX SMOOTHIE POPS

Makes 8 pops

These fun pops give you an easy way to get the Medical Medium Heavy Metal Detox foods into your child's diet (or yours!). You might wish to double, triple, or quadruple this recipe so you have plenty of pops on hand ready to go.

1½ cups frozen or fresh wild blueberries or 8 ounces pure wild blueberry juice
½ cup diced mango (optional)
1 cup loosely packed fresh cilantro
1½ cups freshly squeezed orange juice
1 teaspoon barley grass juice powder
1 teaspoon spirulina
1 tablespoon Atlantic dulse or 2 dropperfuls Alantic dulse liquid
2 to 3 tablespoons raw honey or pure maple syrup (optional)

Combine all the ingredients in a blender and blend until smooth, 1 to 2 minutes. Taste and adjust sweetness if needed by adding more raw honey or maple syrup.

Pour the mixture into pop molds and freeze for at least 4 hours or until set.

Remove the pops from the molds and enjoy.

TIPS

- This recipe doesn't use the full amount of the five heavy metal detox foods that is best for removing heavy metals, so if you are using this recipe as an adult, it's important to include enough of the five heavy metal detox foods listed in Chapter 10, "Medical Medium Heavy Metal Detox," throughout your day in other ways.

- Because of wild blueberries' unique ability to set, you can try making these pops in the refrigerator instead of the freezer. In that case, allow the molds to set in the fridge for at least 3 hours, and keep in mind that the refrigerated pops won't be as solid as frozen pops when they're ready.

- These pops taste great with or without the mango. The mango gives the pops more creaminess, although the taste of the orange juice shines through more without the mango. Try this recipe both ways to discover which version is your family's favorite.

- If you're in a part of the world where you can't access any form of wild blueberries, you can substitute blackberries, although they do not uproot heavy metals.

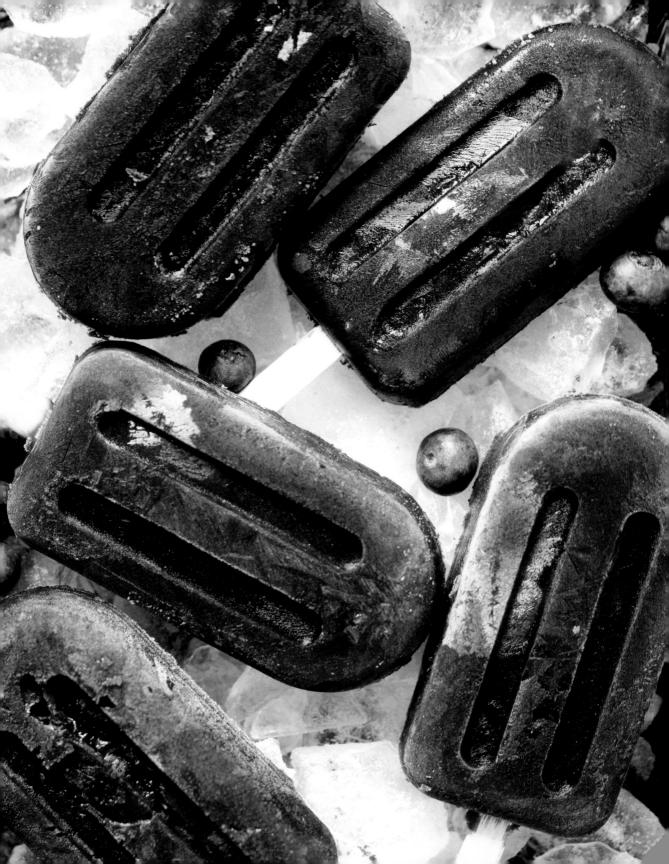

15. BRAIN DETOX TONIC

This two-part tonic helps remove ammonia gases that reach the brain from putrefied proteins and fats stuck on the walls of the intestinal tract lining and other foods that are fermenting in the intestinal tract. Following up the base recipe 15 minutes later with pure coconut water serves an important purpose: pushing the toxins out of the body.

2 cups (16 ounces) coconut water
1 teaspoon spirulina
1 teaspoon barley grass juice powder
2 teaspoons pure wild blueberry juice or 2 teaspoons pure wild blueberry powder
1 dropperful alcohol-free lemon balm tincture
1 cup (8 ounces) coconut water, for follow-up

Mix all the ingredients except the 1 cup of coconut water for follow-up.

Fifteen minutes after finishing your Brain Detox Tonic, drink the additional cup (8 ounces) of plain coconut water.

TIPS

- Avoid coconut water that is pink or red, which means it has gone off and is rancid. Also avoid coconut water with added flavors.

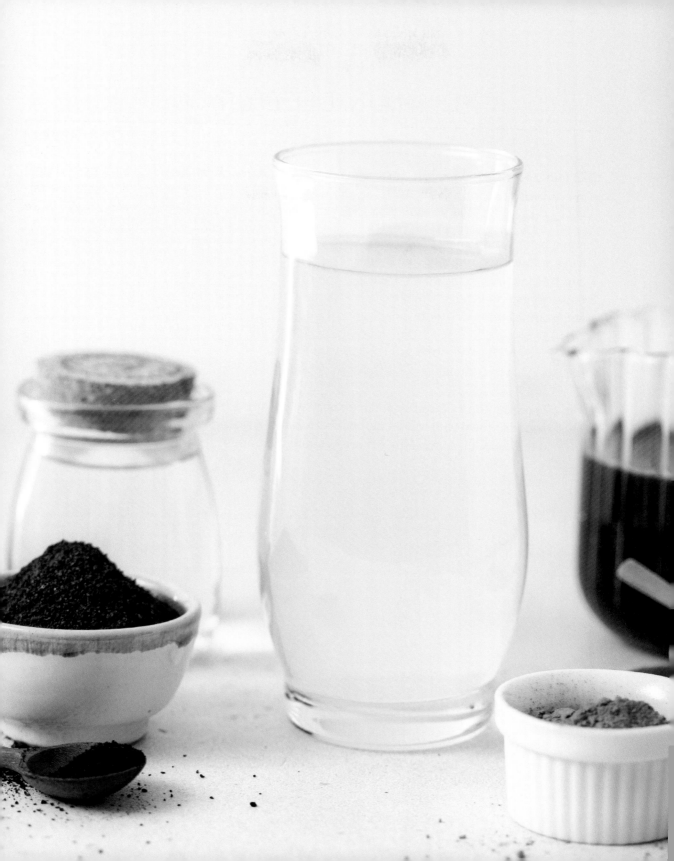

16. BRAIN FUELER SMOOTHIE

This fast and delicious recipe restores glucose and mineral salt reserves to easy-to-reach places inside the brain.

2 bananas or 2 cups mango or 2 cups freshly squeezed orange juice
1 cup fresh or frozen pitted cherries
2 cups spinach, mâche, or parsley
Juice from ½ lemon or 1 lime

Combine all the ingredients in a blender and blend until smooth.

Serve immediately.

TIPS

- Feel free to use additional bananas, mango, or fresh orange juice for a heartier snack or meal with more calories. For example, you may prefer to use 4 or 5 bananas in this recipe for a more satiating smoothie.

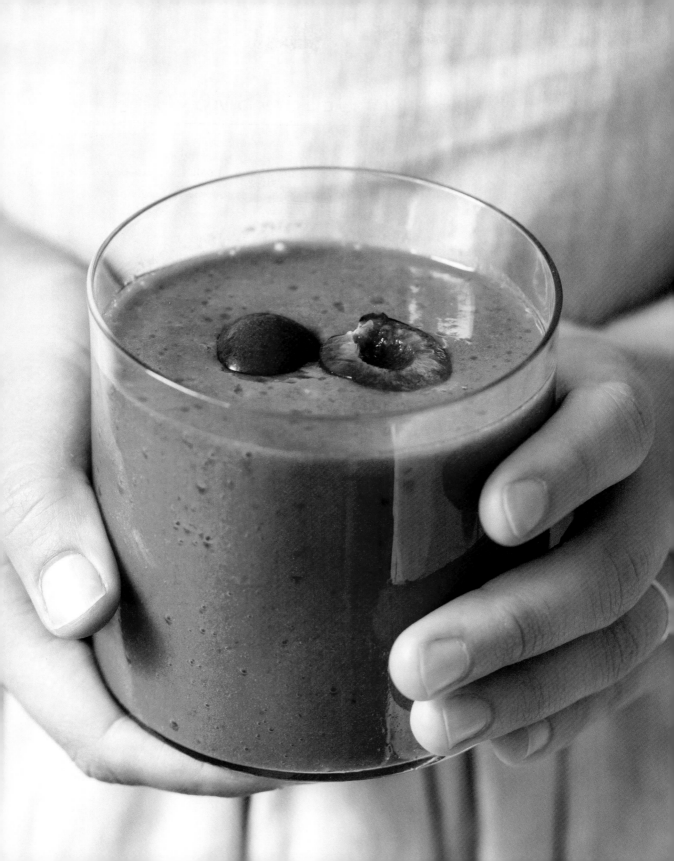

17. WILD BLUEBERRY "YOGURT"

Sweet with just a hint of tart from the lemon, this yogurt alternative is tasty and healing. Serve it in little glasses or jars for a more traditional yogurt experience. This is a great recipe to make a little extra of so you have a few days of snacks ready to go in your fridge for whenever you may want one.

2 bananas
1 cup frozen wild blueberries
1 teaspoon freshly squeezed lemon juice
½ teaspoon pure vanilla powder, cinnamon, or ground cardamom (optional)

Combine the bananas, wild blueberries, lemon juice, and the vanilla, cinnamon, or cardamom (if using) in a blender and blend until smooth, scraping down the sides as needed.

Pour into small glasses or jars. Refrigerate for at least 3 hours before serving, or ideally overnight.

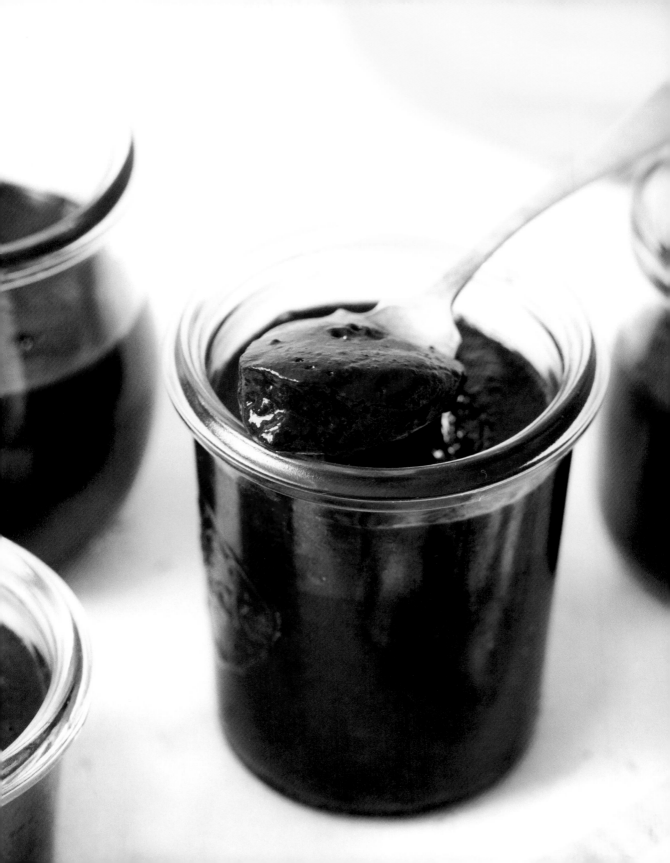

18. APPLESAUCE OR PEAR SAUCE

Makes 1 serving

Apples and pears are cleansing for the liver; they reduce friction from the liver overworking. Apples and pears are also hydrating for the bloodstream and reduce blood toxicity. Making fresh applesauce (or pear sauce) is a great way to assist in the body's healing process.

1 to 2 red apples or 3 ripe pears, diced
1 to 3 Medjool dates, pitted (optional)
1 stalk celery, chopped (optional)
¼ teaspoon cinnamon (optional)

Blend the diced red apple or diced pear and any other desired ingredients in a blender or food processor until a smooth, even applesauce or pear sauce forms.

Serve and enjoy immediately, or squeeze some fresh lemon juice over the top and seal tightly if you'd like to save it for later.

TIPS

- If you're making this recipe for a morning apple snack during a Heavy Metal Detox Cleanse (Simplified level or above), leave out the optional dates. As beneficial as dates are, you want to make sure you focus on the specified cleanse foods in the morning period of those cleanses.

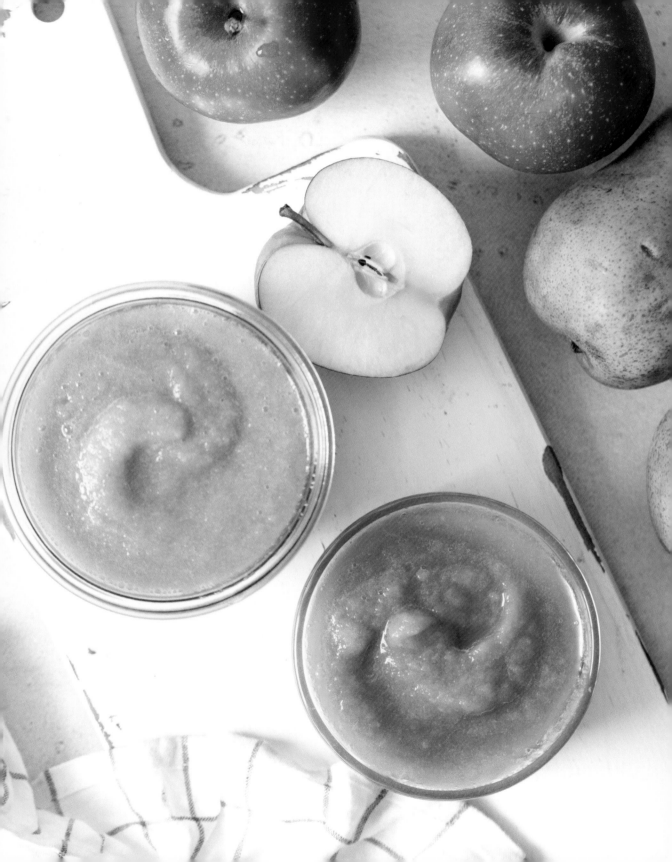

19. PEACHES AND CREAM

This healthy twist on peaches and cream is so delicious, especially if you use juicy, ripe fresh peaches. Enjoy this delicious recipe as a snack, or feel free to double the recipe to make it a more satisfying dish.

1 frozen banana
1 fresh banana
¼ to ½ cup cold water or coconut water
¼ teaspoon cinnamon or pure vanilla bean powder
2 to 3 ripe peaches, roughly chopped
1 to 2 teaspoons raw honey (optional)

Combine the frozen banana, fresh banana, ¼ cup water or coconut water, and cinnamon or vanilla in a food processor or blender. Blend until smooth, adding more water if needed to reach your desired consistency.

In a serving cup or glass, layer the banana cream and peaches. Drizzle with raw honey (if using) and serve immediately.

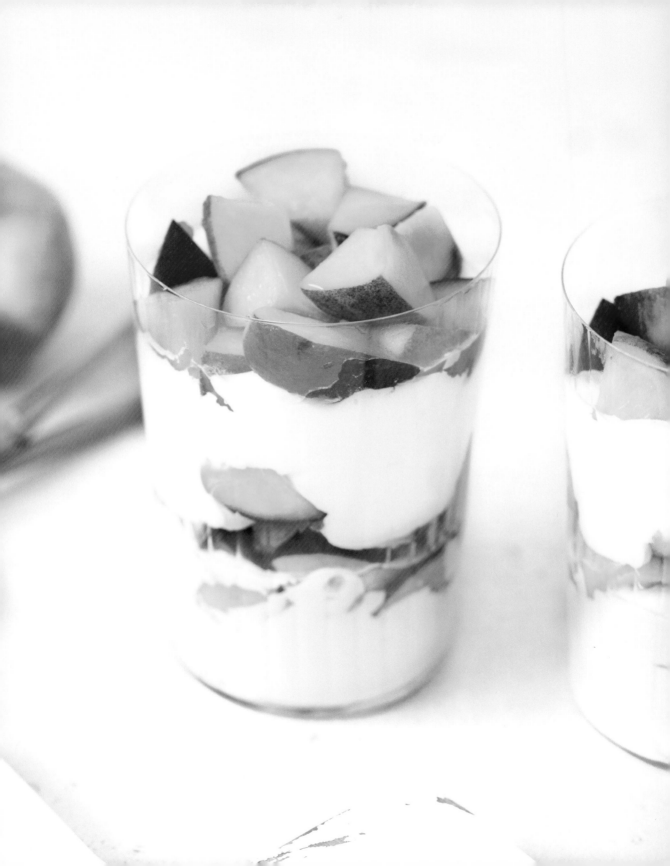

20. BANANA, MANGO, AND WILD BLUEBERRY TRIFLE

Makes 6 servings

Layers of sweet, heavenly fruits that will give your brain the fuel it needs. When you put this trifle in the fridge for a few hours or more, it firms up and becomes almost like a fruit cake with layers of banana "bread," sweet mango puree, and a wild blueberry–raw honey jam.

3 to 4 medium mangoes
5 cups thawed frozen wild blueberries
3 tablespoons raw honey
6 to 8 bananas
½ cup fresh blueberries or fresh or thawed frozen wild blueberries (optional)

Place the mango flesh in a blender and blend until smooth. Set aside.

Place the wild blueberries in a sieve over a jug or bowl to let all the liquid drain. Add the drained wild blueberries to the blender with the raw honey and blend until smooth. Use the leftover wild blueberry juice for another recipe or drink as a beverage.

If using a big trifle bowl, slice the bananas lengthwise into thick slices. If using small serving dishes, slice crosswise into rounds.

Add two layers of sliced banana to the bottom of your dish, overlapping slightly. Follow with a layer of mango puree; then spoon the wild blueberry jam evenly on top of the mango. Smooth out and repeat with the remaining ingredients.

Garnish with fresh blueberries or fresh or thawed frozen wild blueberries (if using). Refrigerate for a few hours or overnight.

TIPS

- You can eat this recipe immediately without refrigerating if you wish and it will still be delicious; however, time in the fridge allows it to firm up and taste even better.

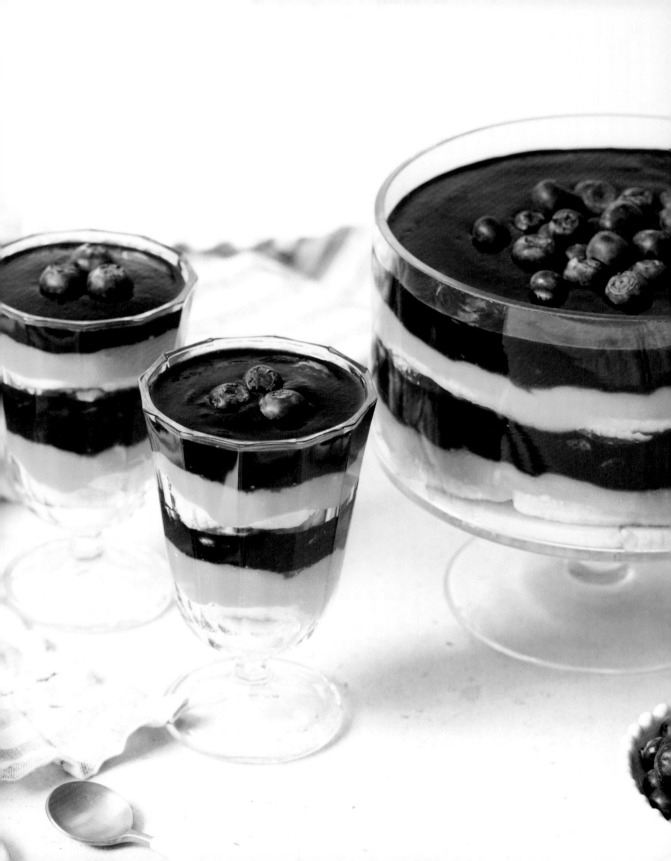

21. BRAIN SAVER SALAD

This healing salad helps minimize, reduce, and cleanse acids out of the brain and cerebro-spinal fluid. It also helps create alkalinity within all body systems.

1 cup loosely packed parsley leaves, roughly chopped

1 cup loosely packed cilantro leaves, roughly chopped

2 cups loosely packed spinach, roughly chopped

2 cups loosely packed kale leaves, finely chopped

2 cups loosely packed arugula, roughly chopped

4 to 6 cups loosely packed red leaf or green leaf lettuce, chopped

1½ cups fresh or steamed green peas

1½ cups thinly sliced cucumber

1 cup sprouts or microgreens

FOR THE DRESSING

1 cup freshly squeezed orange juice

2 tablespoons freshly squeezed lemon juice

2 tablespoons raw honey

1 sprig fresh rosemary, leaves only

¼ teaspoon cayenne, or more to taste

Combine all the salad ingredients in a bowl. Toss gently and set aside.

Combine the dressing ingredients in a blender and blend until smooth. Strain through a fine-mesh sieve into a small bowl or jug.

Pour the dressing on top of the salad. Toss gently and serve immediately.

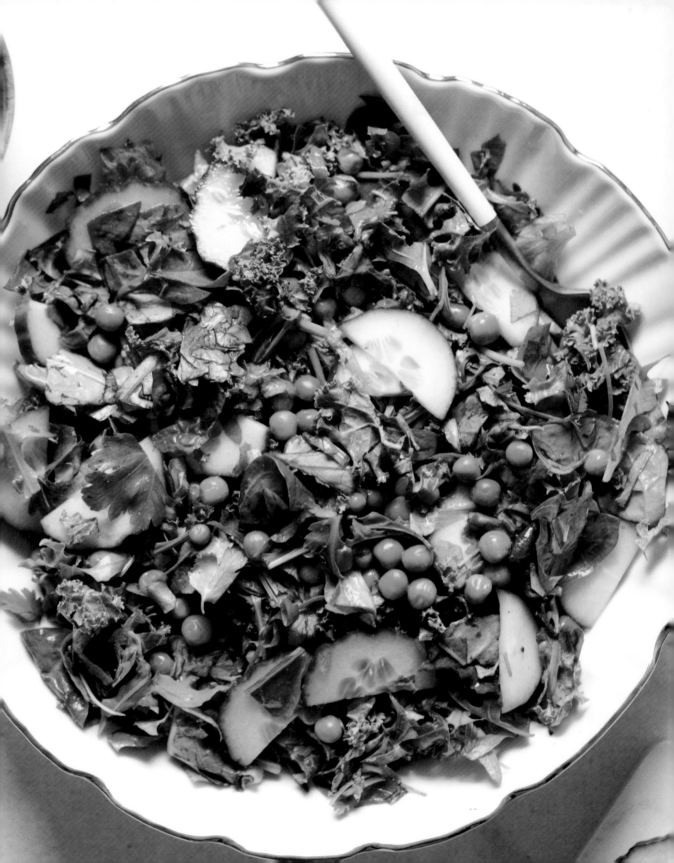

22. BRAIN ARMOR SALAD

Makes 2 servings

Rich in key antioxidants, this salad provides brain protection by helping to slow down and stop the oxidation process in glial cells. Interrupting the oxidation process allows brain cells to receive more nutrients and chemical compounds including neurotransmitter hormones, leading to clearer thinking.

1 cup chopped cucumber
1 cup chopped red bell pepper
⅓ cup finely chopped red onion
1 cup chopped apple
½ cup loosely packed fresh cilantro leaves, roughly chopped
6 to 8 cups loosely packed green leaf or butter leaf lettuce, chopped
1 cup berries of your choice, such as blackberries or wild blueberries

FOR THE DRESSING

1 cup diced mango or Maradol papaya
½ cup cherry tomatoes (about 4 to 5)
1 tablespoon freshly squeezed lime juice
2 teaspoons raw honey

Combine all the salad ingredients in a bowl. Toss gently and set aside.

Combine the dressing ingredients in a blender and blend until smooth.

Pour the dressing on top of the salad. Toss gently and serve immediately.

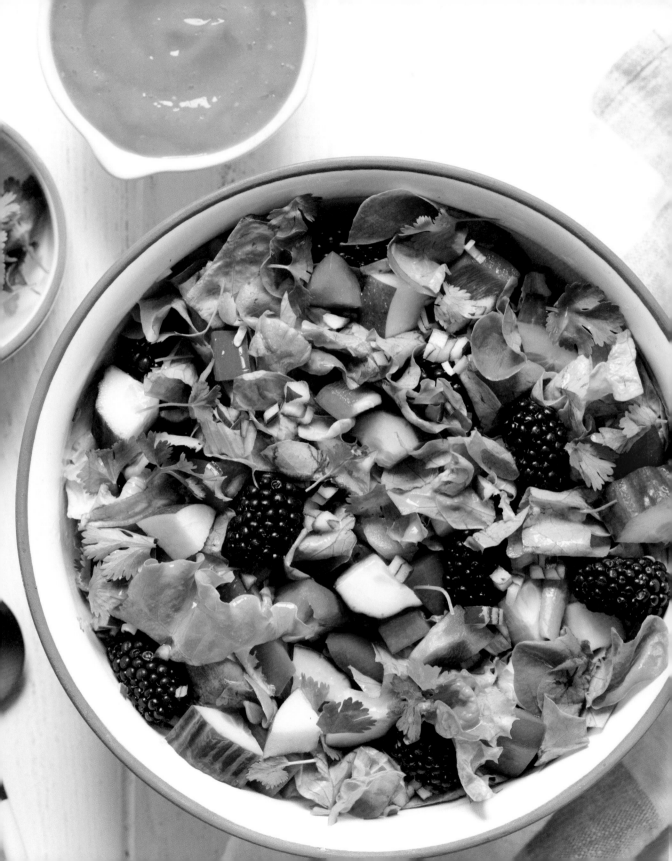

23. SPINACH SOUP

Makes 1 serving

This easy-to-make, richly flavored soup is a great way to incorporate more leafy greens into your day in an easily digestible form. Medical Medium Spinach Soup is a key healing tool for the brain and the rest of the body. Plus, with all of the minerals the spinach provides, it will also help curb any cravings for the foods you know don't serve your health right now.

1 pint grape tomatoes
1 stalk celery
1 garlic clove
1 orange, juiced
4 cups tightly packed baby spinach
2 basil leaves or a few sprigs of fresh cilantro
1 cucumber (optional)

Place the tomatoes, celery, garlic, and fresh orange juice in a high-speed blender and blend until smooth.

Add the spinach by the handful and blend until completely incorporated. Add the basil or cilantro and blend until smooth.

Serve alone as a soup, or if desired, serve the soup over cucumber noodles. You can use a spiralizer, julienne peeler, or vegetable peeler to create cucumber noodles. Place the noodles in a serving bowl. Pour the blended soup into the bowl and serve immediately.

TIPS

- If you can't use spinach, you can substitute butter leaf lettuce.

- If you can't use tomatoes, you can substitute ripe mango. If you can't get fresh, sweet mangoes, you can substitute thawed frozen mango.

- If neither tomato nor mango are options, you can blend up banana with greens instead. Be sure not to include both banana and tomato in the recipe, as they don't digest well together. Use banana only for this substitution.

- When using organic cucumber, you can leave the skin on or peel the cucumber first, depending on preference. With conventional cucumbers, peel the cucumber and discard the skin.

- English cucumbers are a fun option when making cucumber noodles because of their small seeds.

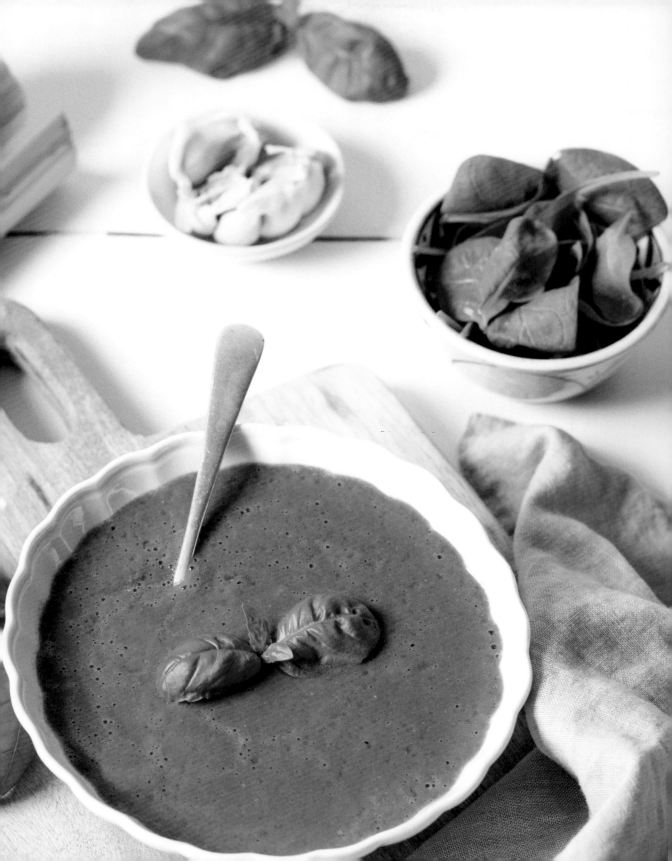

24. BRAIN SAVER WRAPS

Makes 1 serving

These wraps let the delicious natural flavors of the fruits and greens shine. They are simple and easy to throw together, but don't let this fool you—this snack or meal is packed with nutrients and feeds the brain with exactly what it needs. The hint of orange juice squeezed on top adds wonderful flavor while helping you to digest your meal at the best level of absorption possible.

6 large leafy lettuce leaves, such as green leaf, red leaf, butter leaf, or romaine
3 cups of toppings of your choice, such as cucumber slices, cucumber noodles, baby spinach, and/or sprouts or microgreens
3 cups sweet fruit of choice, such as banana slices, diced mango, and/or orange sections
2 cups berries of choice, such as raspberries, blackberries, and/or strawberries
Squeeze of orange juice (optional)

Arrange the lettuce leaves on a platter.

Top the lettuce leaves with cucumber slices, cucumber noodles, baby spinach, and/or sprouts.

Add your sweet fruit such as banana slices, diced mango, and/or orange sections. Then add your choice of berries.

Squeeze a little bit of orange juice on top, wrap, and serve.

TIPS

- While lettuce is preferred for this recipe, you can also use kale for the wraps.

- If you select fresh strawberries for this recipe, remove the greens before using. Read why on page 287.

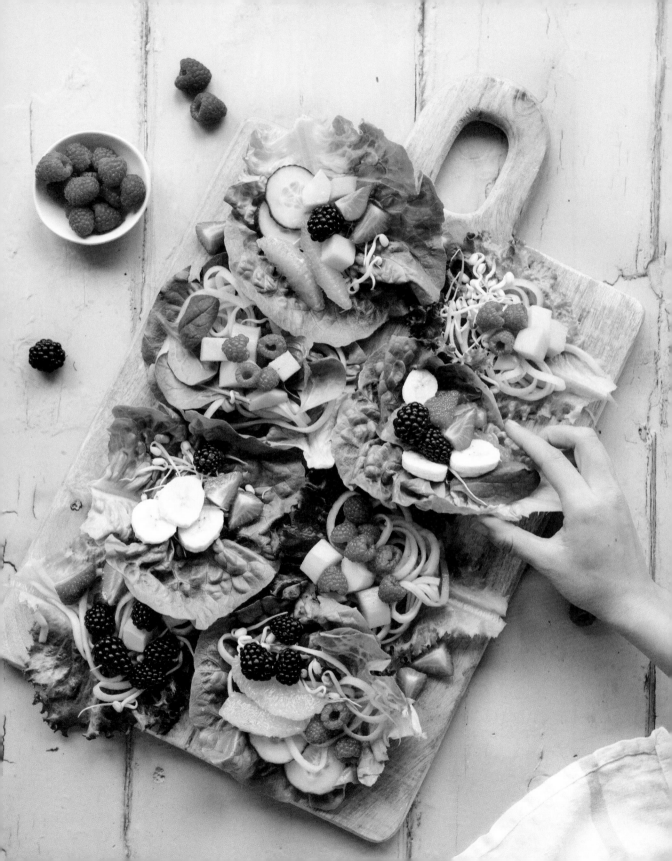

25. ASPARAGUS-SPINACH DIP

This wonderful, creamy dip is a fantastic way to get more essential leafy greens into your diet, along with healing herbs, asparagus, and more. This dip pairs beautifully with raw crudités, scooped into lettuce leaves, or served as a dip for steamed potatoes or sweet potatoes. It can also be enjoyed on its own as a healing raw soup.

1½ cups trimmed and roughly chopped
   raw asparagus
5 cups tightly packed spinach
½ cup cherry tomatoes
1 garlic clove, roughly chopped
2½ tablespoons freshly squeezed
   lemon juice
¼ cup loosely packed fresh cilantro leaves
¼ cup loosely packed fresh basil leaves
1 tablespoon raw honey or 2 pitted
   Medjool dates
¼ to ½ teaspoon cayenne or red
   pepper flakes

TO SERVE (OPTIONAL)

Bell pepper wedges (red, yellow, or orange)
Cucumber slices
Carrot sticks
Celery sticks
Lettuce leaves such as butter leaf, red
   leaf, green leaf, and romaine lettuce

Combine the asparagus, spinach, tomatoes, garlic, lemon juice, cilantro, basil, raw honey or dates, and cayenne or red pepper flakes in a food processor. Process until smooth and creamy but still with a little bit of texture, for 2 to 3 minutes, scraping down the sides as needed.

Serve immediately with the raw vegetables, fruits, and herbs or keep refrigerated until needed. The dip can also be served as soup or spooned into bell pepper halves or stuffed into scooped-out tomato halves or steamed for baked potatoes.

TIPS

- This recipe is best made in a food processor to produce a creamy dip that has a little bit of texture. If you don't have a food processor, you could also use a blender. The consistency will be different, but both are delicious.

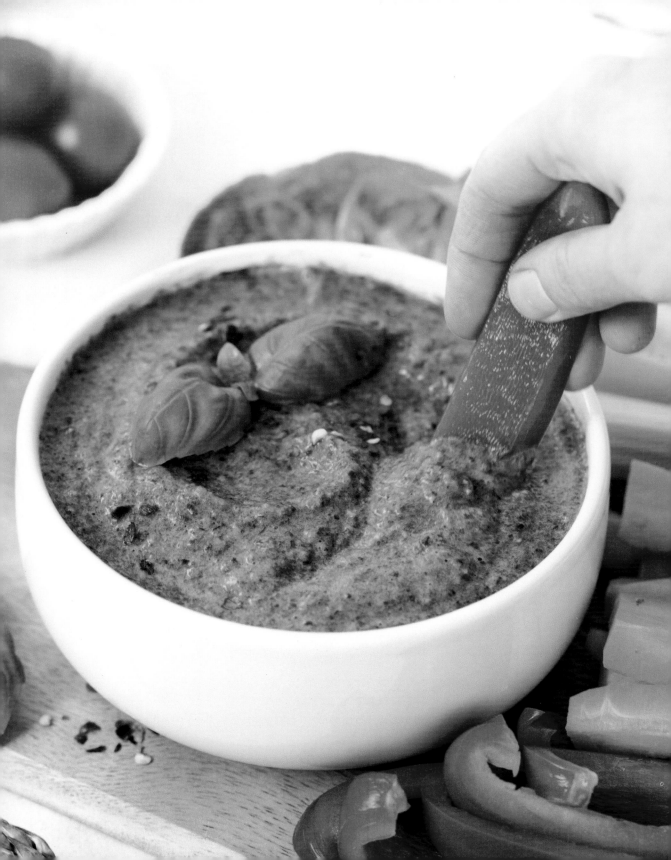

26. STUFFED TOMATOES WITH HERBED CAULIFLOWER RICE

Makes 2 servings

Tomatoes are often shunned or underrated when, really, they have so many healing properties to offer you. This recipe shines when you use the most flavorful tomatoes and produce you can find. Pick your favorite herb or combination of herbs, and enjoy the fragrance and simple flavors of this meal.

5 to 6 medium to large tomatoes
3 cups cauliflower florets
1 cup loosely packed fresh herb leaves, such as cilantro, parsley, and/or basil
1 tablespoon freshly squeezed lemon juice
½ tablespoon raw honey
½ to 1 teaspoon red pepper flakes
½ teaspoon garlic powder
½ teaspoon onion powder
1 teaspoon Atlantic dulse flakes (optional)

Prepare the tomatoes by cutting about ½ inch off the tops and scooping out the flesh. Set aside.

Make the cauliflower rice by combining the cauliflower florets, herbs, lemon juice, raw honey, red pepper flakes, garlic powder, onion powder, and Atlantic dulse flakes (if using) in a food processor. Pulse a few times until you get a rice-like texture.

Fill the tomatoes with the cauliflower herb rice, packing it in tightly. Serve immediately or keep refrigerated until needed. Enjoy!

TIPS

- Try to pick tomatoes that have the darkest red color. Heirloom tomatoes are very flavorful and work particularly well for this recipe, in which case, the tomatoes can be any color when ripe depending on their variety.

- You can keep the flesh of the tomatoes to blend into a salad dressing, soup, broth, or sauce, or chop it up and pour over the top of the stuffed tomatoes if you're not concerned with presentation and you're eating them right away.

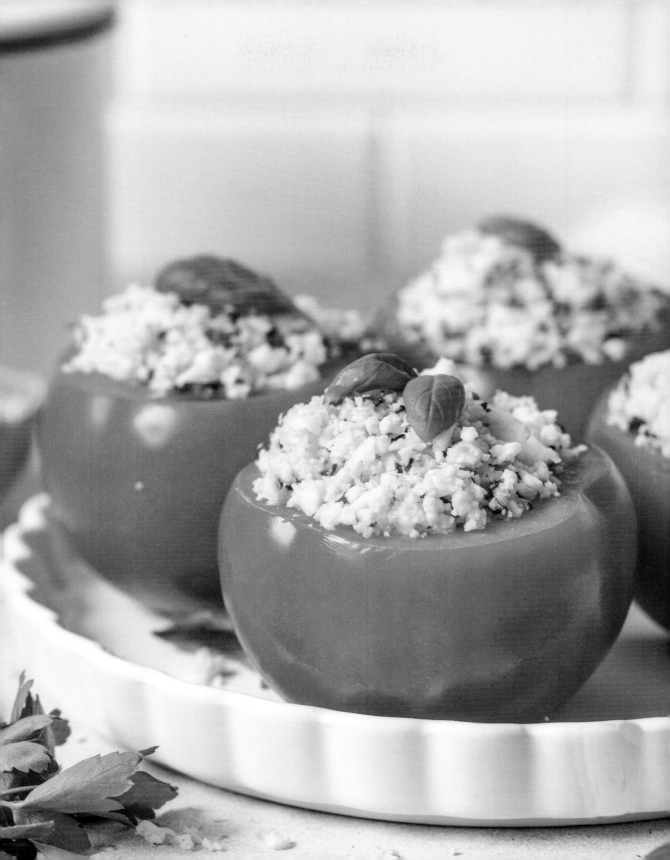

27. RAW "STIR-FRY"

Makes 2 servings

Sweet, savory, and full of flavor, this delicious Raw "Stir-Fry" is a wonderful way to get more raw fruits, herbs, and vegetables into your diet, which is the form in which they offer the greatest healing benefits.

¼ cup pineapple juice
¼ cup freshly squeezed lime juice
2 tablespoons raw honey
¼ cup diced mango
½-inch piece of fresh ginger
1 garlic clove
1 teaspoon Atlantic dulse flakes (optional)
¼ to ½ teaspoon cayenne or red pepper flakes
1 cup finely chopped broccoli
1 cup thinly sliced mushrooms*
1 cup finely shaved red cabbage
1 cup very thinly sliced red, orange, or yellow bell pepper
½ cup thinly sliced snap peas
½ cup very thinly sliced carrot
¼ cup loosely packed chopped green onions
2 tablespoons chopped fresh cilantro
2 tablespoons chopped fresh mint

To make the sauce, combine the pineapple juice, lime juice, raw honey, mango, ginger, garlic, Atlantic dulse flakes (if using), and cayenne or red pepper flakes in a blender. Blend until smooth and set aside.

Add the broccoli, mushrooms, red cabbage, bell pepper, snap peas, carrot, green onions, cilantro, and mint to a large bowl. Pour the sauce on top and toss gently until evenly mixed. Place in the fridge to marinate for at least 1 hour or up to 3 to 4 hours, stirring at the halfway mark.

Remove from fridge and divide between two bowls. Serve immediately.

*For the mushrooms, wash and rinse thoroughly with warm to hot water before slicing. Do not use slimy or decaying mushrooms. That's a sign of oxidizing and aging.

TIPS

- The key to this recipe is to chop the ingredients into very thin or small pieces and then let them marinate for at least an hour (or more) so the vegetables, herbs, and mushrooms become softer and easy to eat. It's important not to miss these steps.

- For the pineapple juice, you can either use freshly juiced pineapple or bottled pure, 100 percent pineapple juice with no additives, citric acid, or flavors.

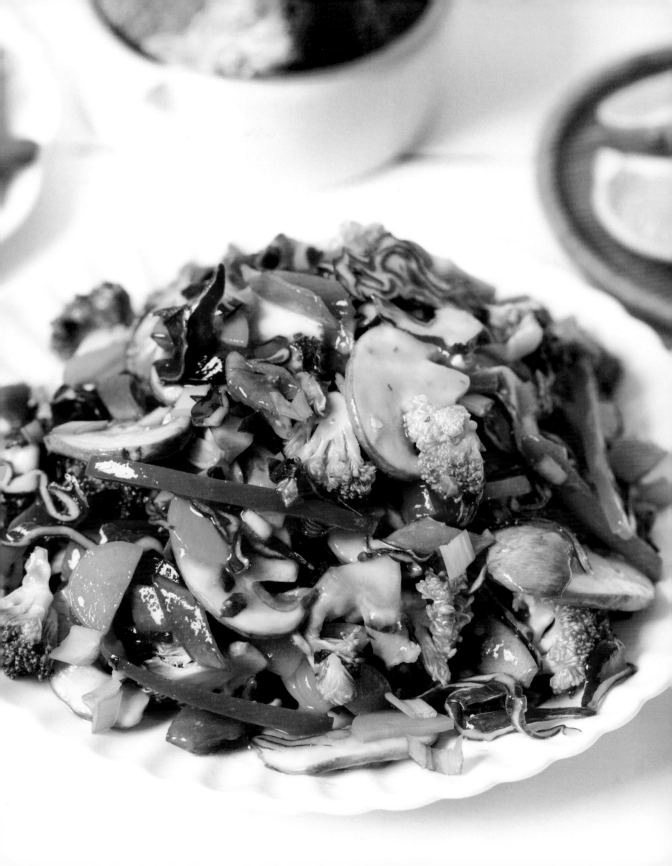

28. MANGO NORI WRAPS

Makes 1 to 2 servings

Sweet, juicy mango and fresh herbs make these nori wraps a standout. They are simple but full of flavor, especially when you can find high-quality mangoes and tomatoes. Roll your nori wraps and eat them right away, or pack them to go as a snack.

4 nori sheets
Squeeze of orange, lemon, or lime juice
1 mango, peeled and cut into thin strips
1 cucumber, julienned
2 tomatoes, cut into strips
4 spring onions
1 cup loosely packed microgreens or sprouts
1 cup loosely packed fresh cilantro leaves
1 cup loosely packed fresh mint leaves

Place a nori sheet shiny side down on a chopping board with the long edge close to you. Squeeze just a few drops of orange, lemon, or lime juice onto the nori sheet and use your fingers to roughly spread the juice over the nori sheet so that it's very lightly moistened.

Arrange ¼ of the mango slices, cucumber, tomatoes, spring onions, microgreens or sprouts, and herbs on one end of the sheet. Squeeze another drop or two of orange, lemon, or lime juice across the other end of the sheet; then roll up tightly. Cut the wrap in half.

Repeat with the remaining ingredients and serve.

TIPS

- If you can't find fresh mango, you can instead use papaya slices or use 4 dates, chopped. Divide the date pieces over the nori wraps.

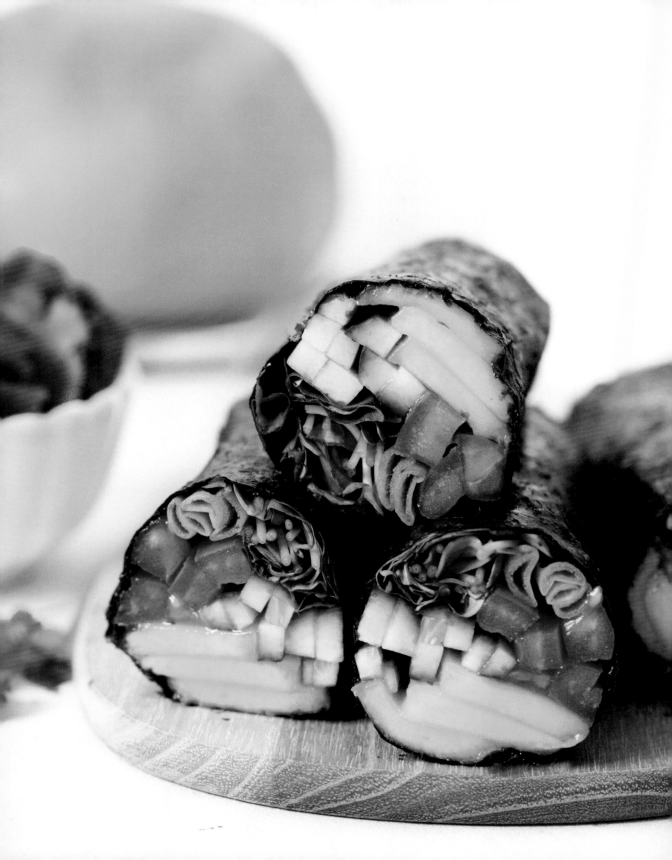

29. LEAFY GREEN AND BERRY SALAD

Fresh, light, and fruity, this vibrant salad is a fantastic choice for a meal or snack anytime of day. It offers you an explosion of nutrients from the leafy greens, mixed berries, wild blueberries, and well, every ingredient in this recipe!

6 cups loosely packed leafy greens, such as butter lettuce and spinach

2 cups mixed berries, such as strawberries, blueberries, mulberries, raspberries, and/or blackberries

1 mango, diced (about 1 cup) (optional)

1 large orange, peeled and cut into segments (about 1 cup) (optional)

1 banana, sliced (about 1 cup) (optional)

FOR THE WILD BLUEBERRY "VINAIGRETTE"

½ cup wild blueberries

¼ cup freshly squeezed orange juice

2 tablespoons freshly squeezed lemon juice

1 tablespoon raw honey

1 tablespoon roughly chopped shallots (optional)

½ teaspoon Atlantic dulse flakes (optional)

Combine the leafy greens, berries, mango (if using), orange segments (if using), and banana (if using) in a large bowl. Toss gently and divide between salad bowls. Set aside.

Combine the vinaigrette ingredients in a blender and blend until very smooth, 1 to 2 minutes. Drizzle onto salad and serve. Enjoy!

TIPS

- If you select fresh strawberries for this recipe, remove the greens before using. Read why on page 287.

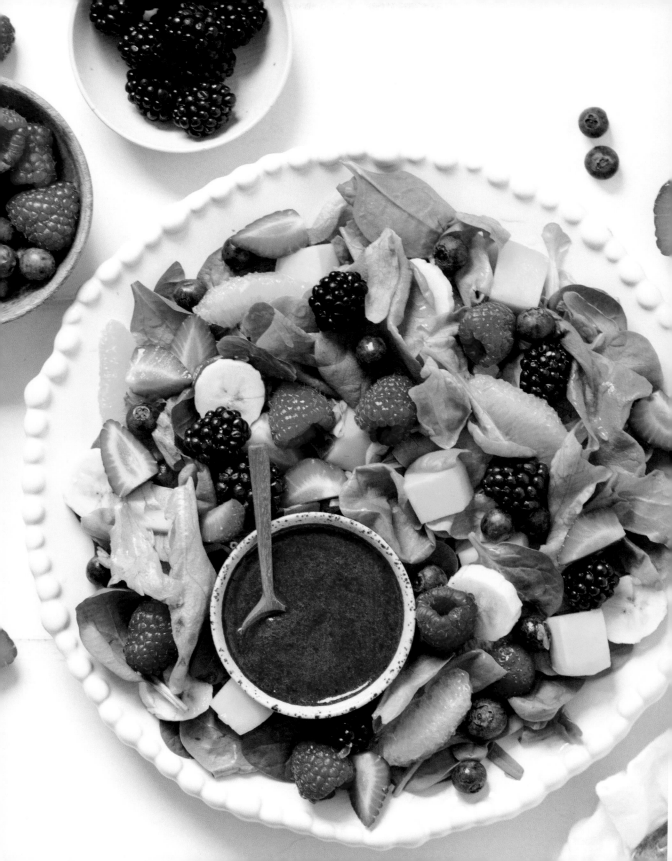

30. RAW CHILI

Makes 2 servings

If you're looking for a satisfying meal that's made only with raw ingredients, this Raw Chili might just do the trick! With a selection of spices and a kick of heat, this chili will bring some warmth to your belly without even having to heat your food!

FOR THE CHILI

½ cup tightly packed sun-dried tomatoes (oil-free and salt-free)
2½ cups roughly chopped cherry or plum tomatoes
1 Medjool date, pitted
1 teaspoon ground cumin
½ teaspoon ground coriander
½ teaspoon paprika
¼ to ½ teaspoon chili powder or cayenne
1 tablespoon fresh oregano or 1 teaspoon dried
1 garlic clove
½ tablespoon freshly squeezed lime juice
½ to 1 teaspoon Atlantic dulse flakes (optional)
1 to 2 tablespoons chopped ripe hot pepper (optional)
1 cup chopped zucchini
½ cup chopped red bell pepper
⅓ cup roughly chopped red onion
⅓ cup chopped celery
¼ cup loosely packed fresh cilantro leaves

FOR THE MUSHROOM MINCE

1½ cups roughly chopped mushrooms*
½ teaspoon ground cumin
½ teaspoon ground coriander
½ teaspoon paprika
½ teaspoon dried oregano
1 teaspoon freshly squeezed lime juice
1 teaspoon raw honey

TO SERVE

2 to 3 lime wedges
¼ cup loosely packed fresh cilantro
4 to 5 fresh ripe hot pepper slices (optional)

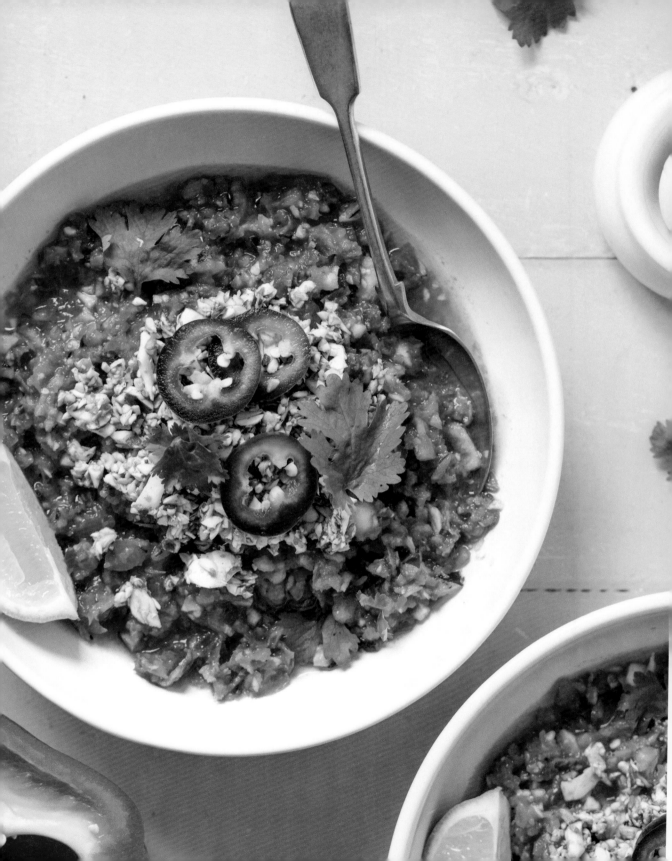

Place the sun-dried tomatoes in a heatproof bowl and cover with hot water. Let soak for 30 minutes.

Meanwhile, make the mushroom mince by combining the mushrooms, spices, oregano, lime juice, and raw honey in a food processor. Pulse a few times until roughly chopped. Remove from the food processor and set aside.

Drain the soaked sun-dried tomatoes and place in the food processor—you don't need to rinse them first. Add the cherry or plum tomatoes, date, ground cumin, ground coriander, paprika, chili powder or cayenne, oregano, garlic, lime juice, Atlantic dulse flakes (if using), and hot pepper (if using). Process for 2 to 3 minutes until very smooth, scraping down the sides as needed.

Add the zucchini, red bell pepper, red onion, celery, and cilantro leaves to the food processor. Pulse a couple of times until the sauce is combined but still chunky.

To serve, divide the chili between soup bowls and top with the mushroom mince, lime wedges, cilantro, and hot pepper slices (if using). Serve immediately.

*For the mushrooms, wash and rinse thoroughly with warm to hot water before chopping. Do not use slimy or decaying mushrooms. That's a sign of oxidizing and aging.

TIPS

- You can enjoy this Raw Chili as is, or if you want to make the meal even heartier, you could make the Stuffed Tomatoes with Herbed Cauliflower Rice recipe on page 342 and serve it with your chili.

31. RAW PORTOBELLO MUSHROOM BURGERS

Makes 1 to 2 servings

If you love to bite into a burger, this recipe gives you a fun and tasty way to have the burger experience with portobello mushrooms acting as the burger buns. Filled with flavor-packed sun-dried tomato spread, slices of fresh tomato, cucumber, onion, basil, and leafy greens, this burger offers you healing fuel with no drawbacks.

FOR THE SUN-DRIED TOMATO SPREAD

1 cup sun-dried tomatoes (oil-free and salt-free), soaked in warm water for at least 30 minutes
1 garlic clove
1 tablespoon fresh oregano or 1 teaspoon dried
1 tablespoon fresh thyme or 1 teaspoon dried
1½ tablespoons freshly squeezed lemon juice
1 tablespoon raw honey
2 to 3 tablespoons water, if needed to blend

FOR THE BURGERS

4 portobello mushrooms
2 to 3 tablespoons freshly squeezed lemon or orange juice
½ to 1 teaspoon Atlantic dulse flakes (optional)
½ cup loosely packed spinach and/or lettuce leaves
4 to 6 tomato slices
4 to 6 white or sweet onion slices
⅓ cup thinly sliced cucumber
4 basil leaves
½ teaspoon red pepper flakes (optional)

TIPS

- If your sun-dried tomatoes are very hard, try this method for soaking and softening: Place the tomatoes in a heatproof bowl and cover with boiling water. Soak for 30 minutes. You can also try this technique of soaking in boiled water if you have regular (less hard) sun-dried tomatoes that you'd like to soften more quickly than 30 minutes.

To make the sun-dried tomato spread, drain the soaked sun-dried tomatoes, then place in a blender or food processor. Add the garlic, oregano, thyme, lemon juice, and raw honey. Blend until well combined but still chunky, scraping down the sides and adding a spoonful of water as needed to blend. Keep refrigerated until needed.

Wash and rinse the portobello mushrooms thoroughly with warm to hot water. (Do not use slimy or decaying mushrooms. That's a sign of oxidizing and aging.) Pat dry, remove the stems, and place the caps on a cutting board. Drizzle the lemon or orange juice all over the underside of the mushrooms and sprinkle with the Atlantic dulse flakes (if using).

Add a few tablespoons of sun-dried tomato spread to the underside of two portobello mushrooms; then top both with the spinach and/or lettuce, tomato slices, onion slices, cucumber slices, fresh basil, and red pepper flakes (if using). Place a portobello mushroom cap on top of each burger so you have two burgers. If you like, you can add more sun-dried tomato spread to the underside of the two portobello mushroom tops before "capping" your burgers.

Serve immediately. Enjoy!

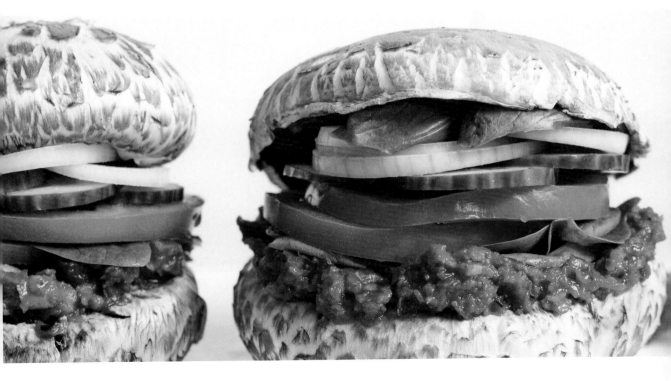

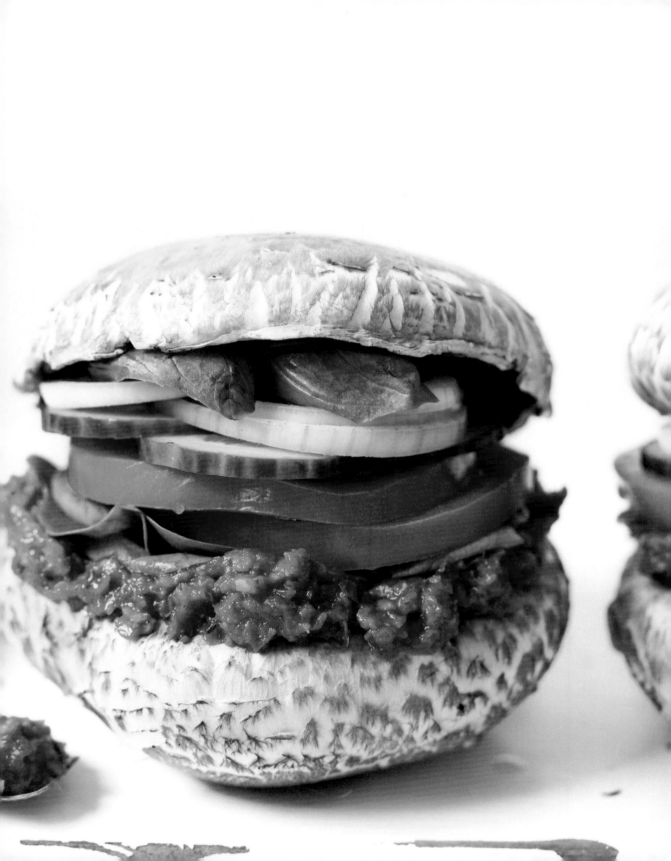

32. GREEN SALAD
WITH FRENCH DRESSING

Makes 2 servings

The stunning color of this dressing is reason enough to make it. Reminiscent of classic French dressing but without the vinegar, oil, and other problematic ingredients, this dressing tastes fantastic over a simple salad.

FOR THE DRESSING

1 cup diced mango
½ cup chopped red, yellow, or orange bell pepper
1 garlic clove
3 tablespoons freshly squeezed lemon juice
3 tablespoons tomato paste
2 tablespoons pure maple syrup
½ teaspoon mustard powder
1 teaspoon onion powder
½ teaspoon Atlantic dulse flakes

FOR THE SALAD

6 to 8 cups loosely packed leafy greens, such as mixed greens, spinach, arugula, butter lettuce, kale, and/or green leaf lettuce
½ cucumber, thinly sliced
3 to 4 medium tomatoes, thinly sliced
1 small onion, thinly sliced

Combine all the dressing ingredients in a blender and blend until smooth. Taste and adjust the flavor, adding more lemon juice or maple syrup as needed.

Add the leafy greens, cucumber, tomatoes, and onion to a salad or mixing bowl. Toss until evenly mixed.

Divide salad between salad plates and drizzle on the dressing. Serve immediately. Enjoy!

TIPS

- Look for a tomato paste that contains only tomato paste and no other ingredients, such as salt or citric acid.

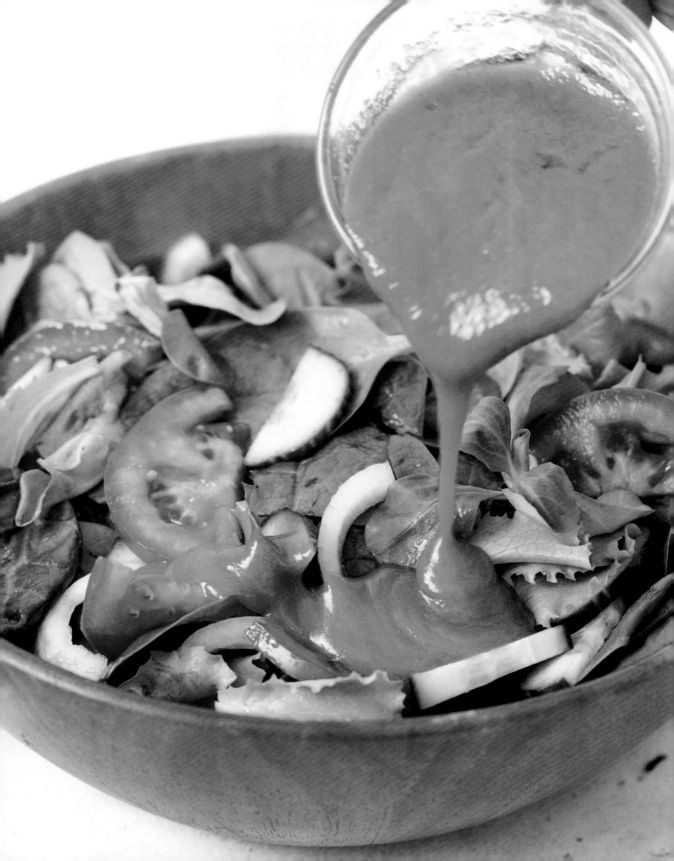

33. STRAWBERRY SALSA

This fun twist on regular salsa swaps out the tomato for strawberries! You can eat this wonderful salsa plain with a spoon, mix it into a salad, or scoop it into lettuce leaves, bell pepper halves, or onto cucumber slices. However you enjoy it, you'll find that this salsa is refreshing and a wonderful combination of sweet and savory.

2 cups finely chopped strawberries
¼ cup finely chopped red or white onions
2 tablespoons finely chopped jalapeño (preferably red)
¼ cup loosely packed cilantro leaves, finely chopped
2 tablespoons freshly squeezed lime juice
1 tablespoon raw honey (optional)
½ teaspoon garlic powder
Atlantic dulse flakes, to taste (optional)

Add the strawberries, onions, jalapeño, cilantro leaves, lime juice, raw honey (if using), garlic powder, and Atlantic dulse flakes (if using) to a large bowl.

Stir until the ingredients are evenly mixed. Cover and marinate for 20 to 25 minutes in the fridge.

Serve immediately or keep refrigerated until needed.

TIPS

- Remove the greens from the strawberries before using. Read why on page 287.

- Depending on how sweet your strawberries are, you may need to add some extra raw honey to the recipe.

- Marinating the salsa in the fridge intensifies the flavor, so don't skip this step.

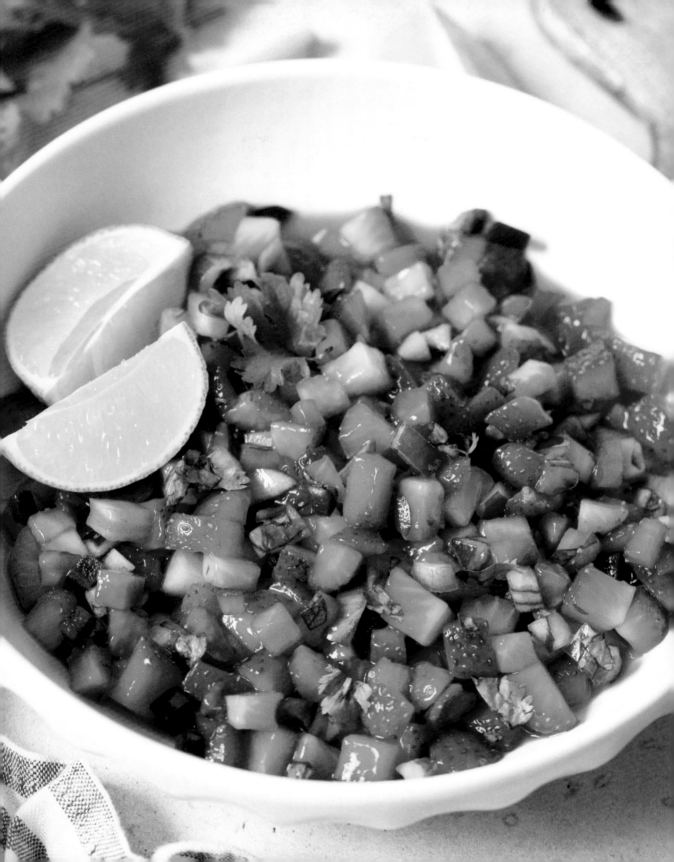

34. COBB SALAD

This Cobb Salad brings together crunchy romaine, refreshing cucumber, juicy cherry tomatoes, crispy eggplant-bacon bites, sprouts or microgreens, and optional chickpeas. You can choose from two dressings: a creamy ranch dressing made with cashews or a fat-free honey-mustard dressing for a light and bright option. You can omit the chickpeas to keep this recipe raw or add them for a heartier option.

6 cups tightly packed chopped romaine
   lettuce
1 cup chopped cucumber
1 cup cooked chickpeas (optional)
1 cup chopped cherry tomatoes
4 to 5 slices of eggplant bacon, chopped
   into bites (recipe on page 430)
½ cup sprouts or microgreens

FOR THE RANCH DRESSING

1½ cups raw, peeled, and diced zucchini
3 tablespoons raw cashews
1½ tablespoons freshly squeezed lemon juice
1 teaspoon garlic powder
½ teaspoon onion powder
½ teaspoon sea salt (optional)
1 tablespoon finely chopped dill
1 tablespoon finely chopped parsley

FOR THE HONEY-MUSTARD DRESSING

2 tablespoons freshly squeezed lemon juice
1½ tablespoons raw honey
1 teaspoon fresh thyme leaves or
   ½ teaspoon dried
¼ teaspoon mustard powder

Combine the romaine, cucumber, chickpeas (if using), cherry tomatoes, eggplant-bacon bites, and sprouts or microgreens in a large bowl. Stir until evenly mixed.

To make the ranch dressing, combine the zucchini, cashews, lemon juice, garlic powder, onion powder, and sea salt (if using) in a blender and blend until smooth. Stir in the dill and parsley.

To make the honey-mustard dressing, whisk the ingredients together in a bowl until smooth.

Divide the salad between the bowls and top with dressing. Serve immediately.

TIPS

- While high-quality sea salt or mountain rock salt is an optional inclusion in the ranch dressing, the recipe is more healing without salt. Over time, you may wish to reduce or exclude the salt.

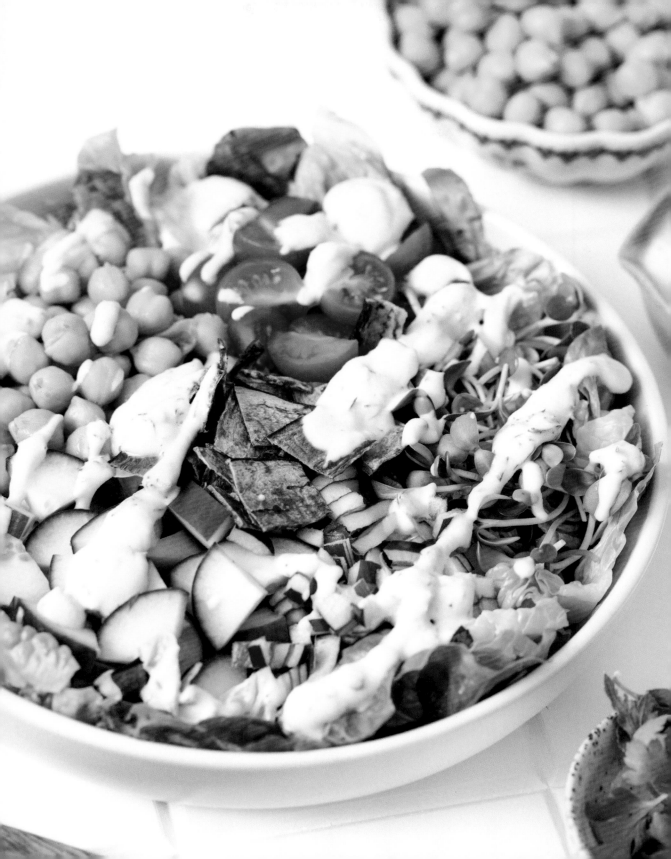

35. RAW CILANTRO CHUTNEY

This fresh and fragrant Raw Cilantro Chutney is an excellent way to get more of the healing and cleansing properties of cilantro into your diet. You can enjoy it as a dip, drizzled onto salads or crudités, as a condiment in any of the Medical Medium burger and sandwich recipes, or simply eat it straight off a spoon!

4 cups tightly packed cilantro leaves, roughly chopped
3 tablespoons freshly squeezed lime or lemon juice
2 tablespoons raw honey or 2 pitted Medjool dates
2-inch piece of ginger, roughly chopped
3 garlic cloves
1 teaspoon ground cumin
½ teaspoon sea salt (optional)
¼ to ½ teaspoon cayenne
1 to 2 tablespoons water, if needed to blend

Combine all the ingredients except the water in a food processor and process until smooth, scraping down the sides as needed. If needed, you can add the water to help the ingredients process smoothly; however, in most cases if you keep scraping down the sides of the food processor, you won't need the water. Serve immediately or refrigerate until needed.

TIPS

- While high-quality sea salt or mountain rock salt is an optional inclusion in this recipe, the recipe is more healing without salt. Over time, you may wish to reduce or exclude the salt.

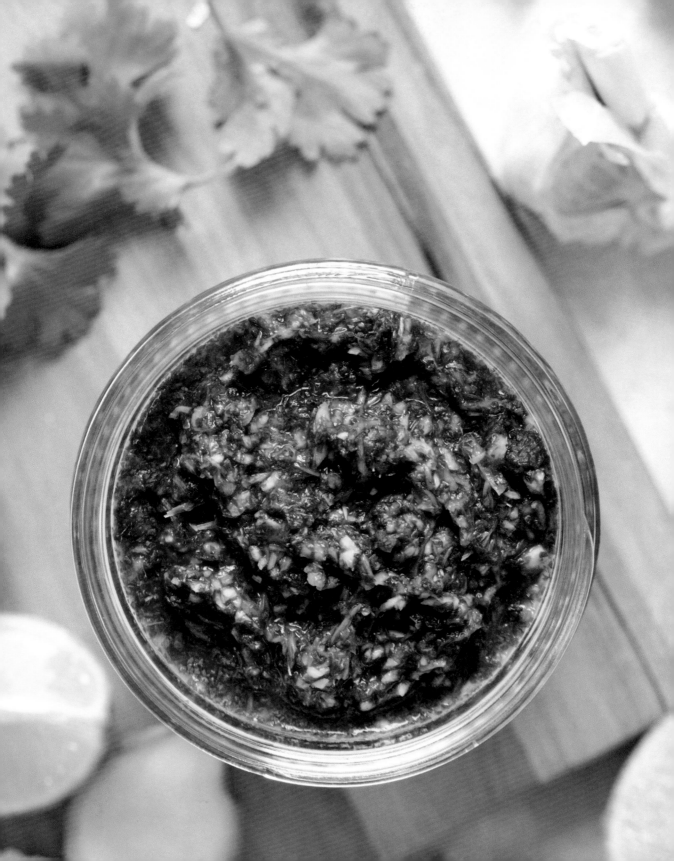

36. CAULIFLOWER CEVICHE

Makes 2 to 4 servings

Scoop this crunchy and juicy Cauliflower Ceviche into romaine lettuce leaves and enjoy every bite. A little bit spicy, a little bit salty, and with a hint of sweetness, this raw recipe has a balance of flavors and textures that is very satisfying.

1 small head cauliflower, finely diced (about 4 cups)
2 cups finely chopped tomatoes
½ cup finely chopped red onion
1 cup loosely packed cilantro leaves, finely chopped
½ red jalapeño, seeded and diced
½ cup freshly squeezed lime juice
2 teaspoons raw honey
1 teaspoon Atlantic dulse flakes
1 to 2 romaine lettuce heads, split into leaves

Combine the cauliflower, tomatoes, red onion, cilantro leaves, jalapeño, lime juice, raw honey, and Atlantic dulse flakes in a large bowl. Stir until evenly mixed; then cover and refrigerate for 1 to 2 hours.

Serve with romaine leaves.

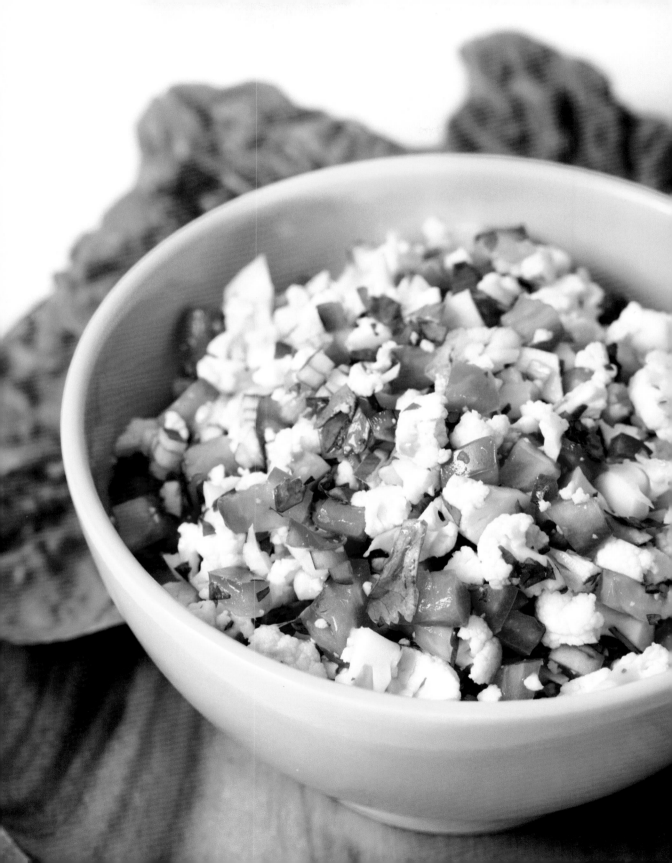

37. GREEK SALAD

This colorful salad is a sensory delight for the eyes and taste buds. It's beautiful, delicious, and aromatic. Enjoy it with the olives and avocado for a more filling option, or enjoy it without them for a fat-free meal that's also satisfying.

3 tablespoons freshly squeezed
  lemon juice
1 tablespoon raw honey
1 garlic clove, finely grated
1½ cups diced cucumber
1 cup orange cherry tomatoes, halved
1 cup red cherry tomatoes, halved
¾ cup diced avocado (optional)
½ cup diced red bell pepper
½ cup diced yellow bell pepper
½ cup thinly sliced red onion
½ cup raw pitted botija olives (optional)
2 tablespoons fresh oregano leaves or
  2 teaspoons dried
2 tablespoons fresh thyme leaves or
  2 teaspoons dried

Place the lemon juice, raw honey, and garlic in a large bowl. Whisk until well combined.

Place the cucumber, cherry tomatoes, avocado (if using), bell peppers, onion, botija olives (if using), oregano, and thyme in the bowl and toss to combine. Serve immediately.

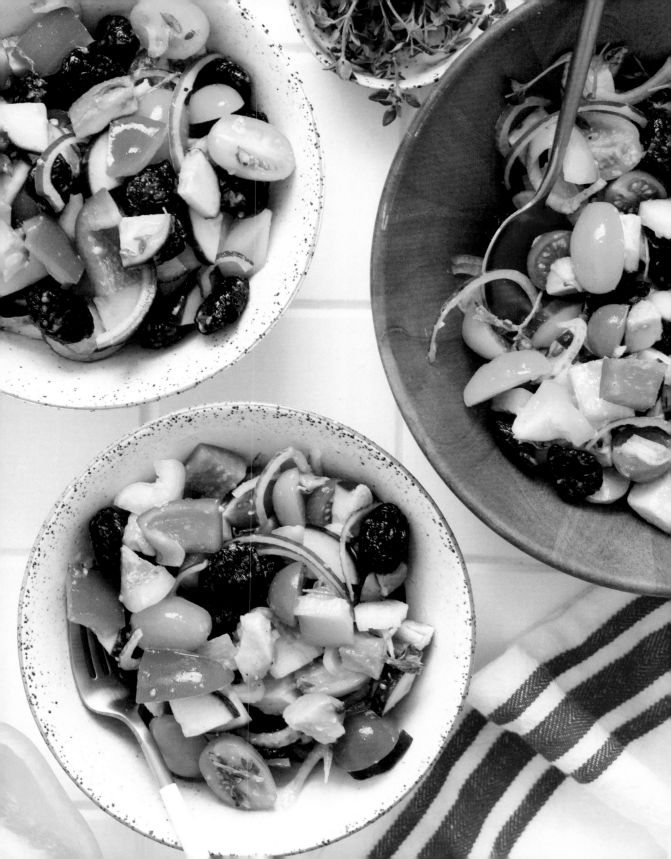

38. SESAME CUCUMBER NOODLES

Makes 2 servings

Fresh, light, and tasty, these Sesame Cucumber Noodles are a pleasure to eat. The cucumbers provide deep cellular hydration while the dressing and sesame seeds bring wonderful flavor and a hint of nuttiness to this simple recipe.

3 medium cucumbers, spiralized
2 medium carrots, julienned or spiralized
¼ cup loosely packed cilantro leaves, finely
  chopped

FOR THE DRESSING

1 tablespoon sesame seeds
3 tablespoons freshly squeezed lemon
  or lime juice
2 tablespoons raw honey
1 teaspoon finely grated fresh ginger
  or ½ teaspoon ginger powder
1 garlic clove, finely grated
¼ teaspoon cayenne or red pepper
  flakes (optional)

Add all the dressing ingredients to a large bowl and whisk together until smooth and combined.

Add the cucumbers, carrots, and cilantro to the bowl. Toss until evenly coated.

Divide between two bowls and serve immediately.

TIPS

- English cucumbers are the best cucumbers for spiralizing into noodles because of their small seeds, but any type of cucumber can be used.

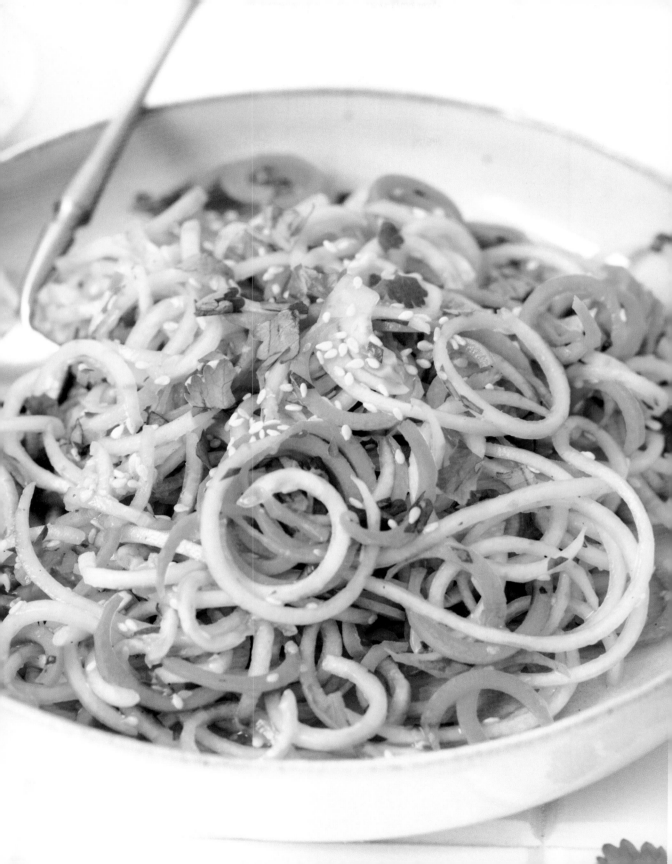

39. HEALING BROTH

Healing Broth is a powerful, mineral-rich liquid that carries the essence of vitally nutritious vegetables, herbs, and spices in a way that is easy for the body to digest, assimilate, and utilize. You will find this recipe as comforting as it is nourishing. The ingredients in this simple recipe provide tremendous healing benefits for both body and soul.

4 carrots, chopped, or 1 sweet potato, cubed

2 stalks celery, roughly chopped

2 onions, sliced

1 cup finely chopped parsley

1 cup shiitake mushrooms, fresh or dried (optional)*

2 tomatoes, chopped (optional)

1 medium bulb garlic (about 8 cloves), minced

1-inch piece of fresh ginger, finely sliced, minced, or grated

1-inch piece of fresh turmeric, finely sliced, minced, or grated

8 cups water

1 ripe hot pepper or ½ teaspoon red pepper flakes, or more to taste (optional)

Place all the ingredients in a large pot and bring to a gentle boil. Turn the heat down to low and allow to simmer for about 1 hour. Strain and sip for a mineral-rich, healing, and restorative broth.

*If using fresh mushrooms, wash and rinse thoroughly with warm to hot water. Do not use slimy or decaying mushrooms. That's a sign of oxidizing and aging.

TIPS

- As an alternative, you can blend the broth with the vegetables and herbs for a pureed soup. Or enjoy this recipe as a chunky vegetable and herb soup by leaving the ingredients whole within the broth.

- For convenience, make a batch of Healing Broth in advance and freeze it (consider pouring into ice cube trays for easy thawing) so you have it on hand.

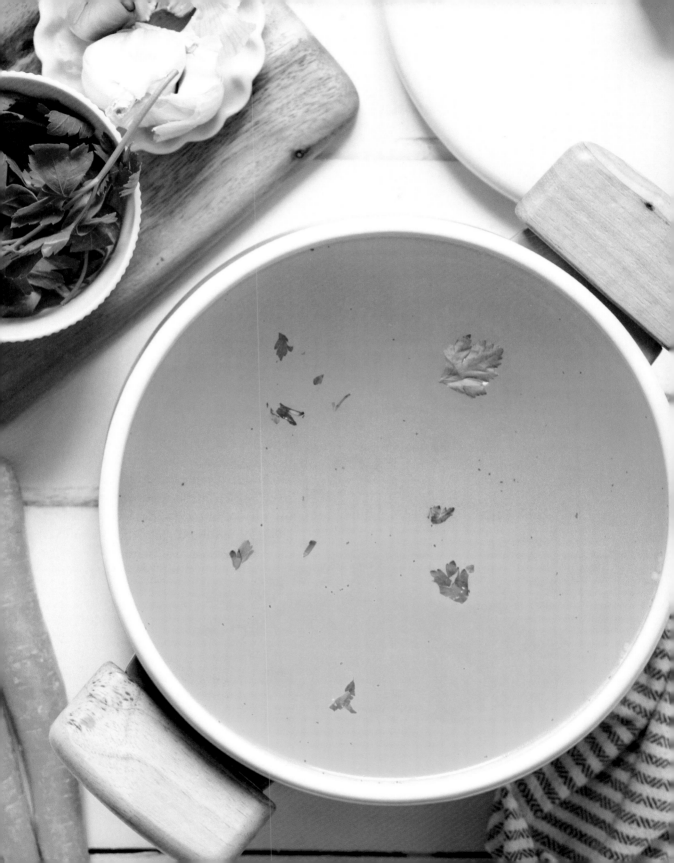

40. ROASTED TOMATO SOUP WITH POTATO CROUTONS

Makes 2 servings

Richly flavored roasted tomato soup topped with crispy potato croutons . . . what's not to love? Enjoy this soup alongside a big salad for a healing and satisfying lunch or dinner meal.

FOR THE SOUP

3 pounds plum or roma tomatoes, halved
8 garlic cloves, peeled
½ cup roughly chopped shallots
1 teaspoon dried oregano
1 teaspoon red pepper flakes
½ tablespoon raw honey
1½ cups Healing Broth (recipe on page 370) or water
1 cup loosely packed basil leaves, plus more to serve

FOR THE POTATO CROUTONS

3 to 4 medium potatoes, cut into 1-inch cubes
1 teaspoon onion powder
½ teaspoon garlic powder
½ teaspoon paprika

Preheat the oven to 400°F/200°C. Line a large baking sheet with parchment paper. Place halved tomatoes, garlic cloves, and shallots on the baking sheet. Roast for 40 to 50 minutes until browned on top.

To make the croutons, you can use either raw or steamed potatoes. Steamed potatoes that are then baked will produce crispier croutons, but both methods work well. Line another baking sheet with parchment paper. Combine the potato cubes (raw or steamed), onion powder, garlic powder, and paprika in a large bowl. Stir until evenly coated. Arrange the potato cubes in a single layer on the baking sheet and roast for 20 to 30 minutes (depending on your oven and whether you used raw or steamed potatoes) until browned and crispy. Set aside.

Once the tomatoes are done roasting, allow them to cool for 10 minutes, and then add them to a food processor or high-speed blender together with the dried oregano, red pepper flakes, raw honey, and Healing Broth or water. Blend until smooth. Add the basil leaves and blend again.

Divide soup between soup bowls and top with potato croutons. Serve immediately.

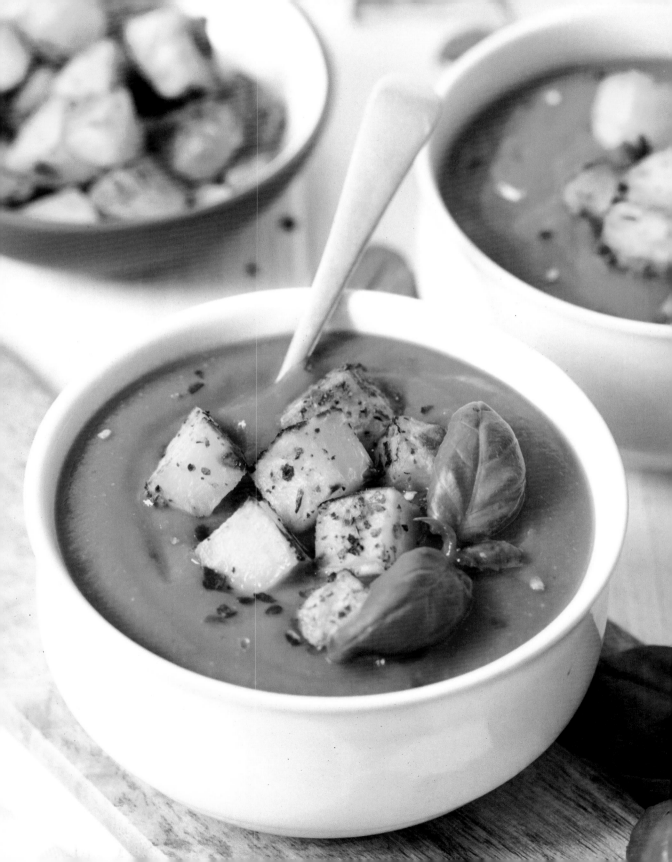

TIPS

- Look for a tomato paste that contains only tomatoes and no other ingredients, such as salt or citric acid.

- When you're choosing between Healing Broth and water for the ingredients, keep in mind that the broth will produce a richer flavor. Store-bought vegetable stock isn't called for because it's very difficult to find a variety that's free of oil, salt, natural flavors, and/or other additives. For convenience, make a batch of Healing Broth in advance and freeze it (consider pouring into ice cube trays for easy thawing) so you have it on hand for recipes like this.

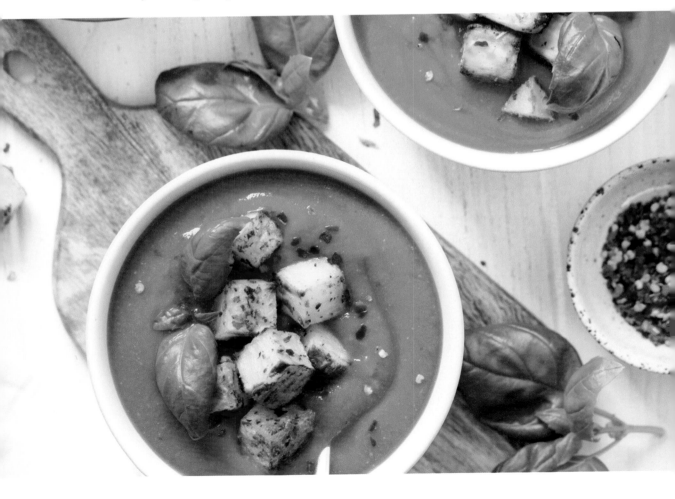

41. POT PIE SOUP

Makes 3 servings

This soup is the ultimate bowl of comfort! Creamy and warming, this Pot Pie Soup is a great choice when your soul needs a little soothing. There are two variations of this recipe: One is more decadent and richer with a coconut or almond milk base. The second is a fat-free version that gets its creaminess from a potato base.

FOR THE SOUP

1½ cups sliced carrots
1 cup finely chopped yellow onion
1 cup chopped celery
6 garlic cloves, roughly chopped
3 cups diced potatoes
1 tablespoon onion powder
1 teaspoon garlic powder
1 teaspoon paprika
1 teaspoon Atlantic dulse flakes
1½ tablespoons fresh thyme or 1½
   teaspoons dried
½ tablespoon chopped fresh rosemary or
   ½ teaspoon dried
1 bay leaf (optional)
4 to 6 cups Healing Broth (recipe on page
   370) or water
1 cup fresh or frozen peas
2 tablespoons freshly squeezed
   lemon juice
2 to 3 tablespoons finely chopped chives,
   to serve

FOR SLURRY OPTION #1

1½ cups unsweetened coconut or
   almond milk
¼ cup arrowroot powder or potato starch
½ teaspoon sea salt (optional)

FOR SLURRY OPTION #2

3 cups diced potatoes
½ teaspoon sea salt (optional)

Place a large ceramic nonstick pot on medium-high heat. Add the carrots, onion, and celery and cook for 5 to 7 minutes until the onion is soft. Add a bit of water if the ingredients start sticking to the pot.

Add the chopped garlic cloves and continue cooking for 1 to 2 minutes. Add in the potatoes, onion powder, garlic powder, paprika, Atlantic dulse flakes, thyme, rosemary, bay leaf (if using), and 6 cups of Healing Broth or water if making slurry #1 or 4 cups of Healing Broth or water if making slurry #2 (the fat-free potato option). Bring to a low simmer and cook for 15 to 20 minutes, uncovered, until the potatoes and onions are soft.

If you're making slurry #1, whisk together the coconut or almond milk and arrowroot powder. Add the peas to the soup, followed by the slurry. Stir until evenly mixed. Add the optional sea salt (if using). Bring to a simmer and cook for 1 to 2 minutes until thick. Stir in the lemon juice; then remove from the heat.

If you're making slurry #2 (the fat-free potato option), steam the diced potatoes until tender and place them in a blender. Remove as much liquid as possible from the soup and add the liquid to the blender. Blend until smooth; then pour back the mixture into the pot. Stir in the peas and lemon juice. Add the optional sea salt if using. Heat the soup until the peas are warmed through.

Divide the soup between three bowls and top with chives.

TIPS

- When you're choosing between Healing Broth and water for the ingredients, keep in mind that the broth will produce a richer flavor. Store-bought vegetable stock isn't called for because it's very difficult to find a variety that's free of oil, salt, natural flavors, and/or other additives. For convenience, make a batch of Healing Broth in advance and freeze it (consider pouring into ice cube trays for easy thawing) so you have it on hand for recipes like this.

- While high-quality sea salt or mountain rock salt is an optional inclusion in this recipe, the recipe is more healing without salt. Over time, you may wish to reduce or exclude the salt.

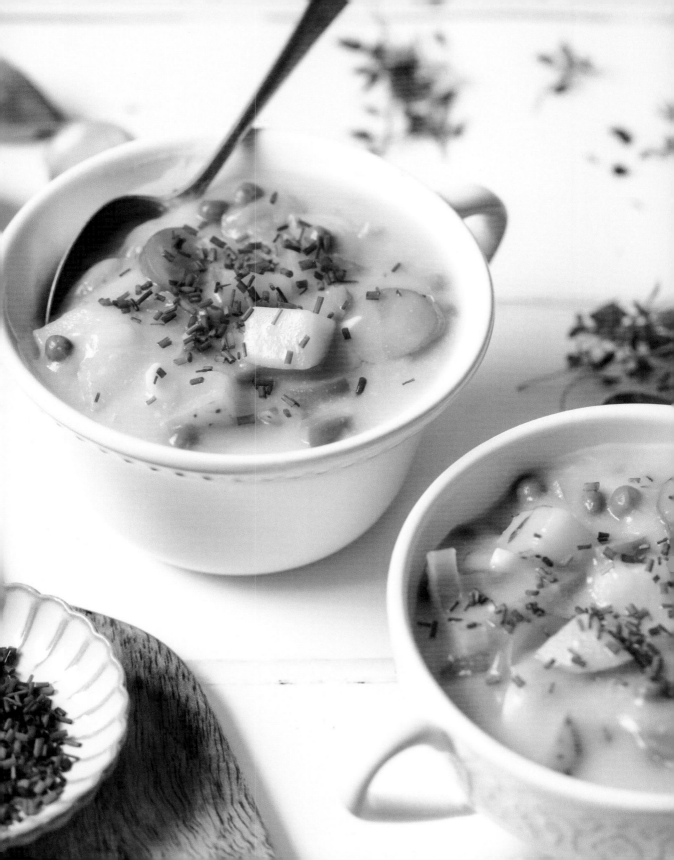

42. CHICKPEA DUMPLING SOUP

Makes 2 servings

Chickpea dumplings and tender vegetables and herbs are nestled in a savory broth that's packed full of vital minerals and vitamins. If you've grown up eating dumpling soup of any variety, this recipe might be a new alternative for you to enjoy.

FOR THE SOUP

1 cup diced onion
1 cup diced carrot
1 cup diced celery
8 cups Healing Broth
    (recipe on page 370) or water
½ tablespoon onion powder
1 teaspoon garlic powder
½ teaspoon ground turmeric
1 teaspoon dried oregano
¼ to ½ teaspoon sea salt (optional)
¼ cup chopped fresh parsley, to serve

FOR THE DUMPLINGS

1 cup chickpea flour
¼ teaspoon aluminum-free baking powder
½ teaspoon paprika
2 tablespoons finely chopped parsley
⅓ cup water

Place a large ceramic nonstick pot on medium-high heat. Add the onion, carrot, and celery and cook for 5 to 7 minutes until the onion is soft. Add a bit of water if the ingredients start sticking to the pot.

Add the Healing Broth or water, onion powder, garlic powder, turmeric, and dried oregano; add the optional sea salt if using. Bring the soup base to a simmer and cook for 13 to 18 minutes.

While the soup simmers, make the dumpling batter. Whisk all the ingredients together, stirring in the water a little at a time until you get a thick dough. Make the batter into small balls (they will puff up in the soup). After the soup base has simmered for 13 to 18 minutes, gently drop the dumpling balls into the soup. Cook for another 8 to 12 minutes, until a toothpick inserted into the middle of a dumpling comes out clean.

Ladle the soup into bowls, sprinkle the fresh parsley on top, and serve. This soup is best eaten on the day it is made.

TIPS

- While high-quality sea salt or mountain rock salt is an optional inclusion in this recipe, the recipe is more healing without salt. Over time, you may wish to reduce or exclude the salt.

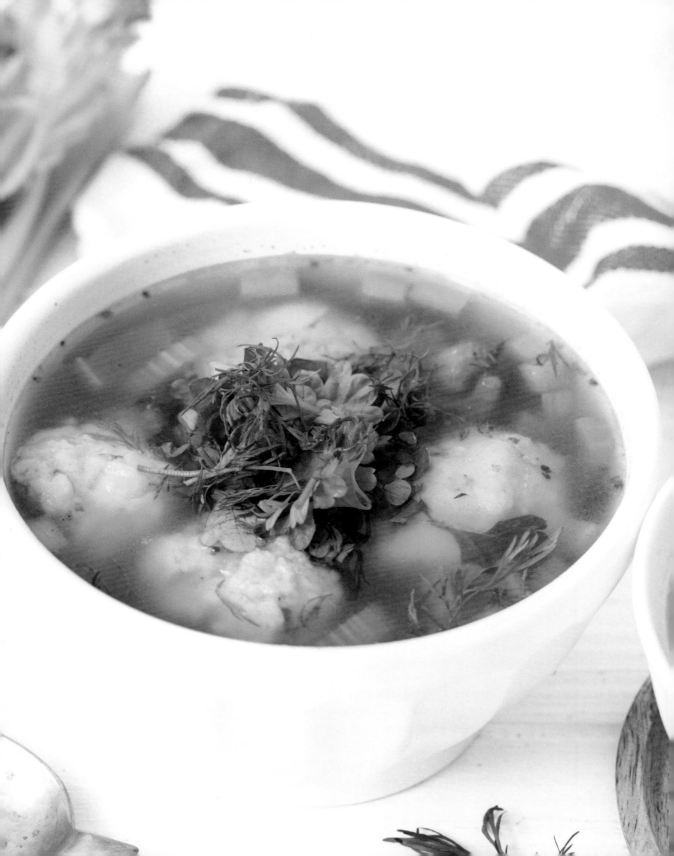

43. SWEET POTATO NACHO CHEESE SOUP

Makes 2 servings

This creamy and flavorful soup offers a fantastic combination of flavors in each mouthful. Enjoy it alongside a salad for a satisfying and healing meal.

6 to 7 cups peeled and diced sweet potatoes (about 2 pounds)
2¼ cups heated Healing Broth (recipe on page 370) or water
1 tablespoon chopped fresh ripe hot pepper
2 garlic cloves
1½ tablespoons onion powder
1 teaspoon paprika
¼ to ½ teaspoon cayenne
½ teaspoon dried oregano
2 tablespoons freshly squeezed lime juice
1 tablespoon tomato paste
¼ cup loosely packed chopped cilantro leaves, to serve
¼ cup loosely packed chopped green onion, to serve

Place the sweet potato in a steamer basket set over a pot of boiling water, cover, and steam for 15 to 18 minutes, until tender. Remove and cool for 5 minutes.

Add the steamed sweet potato into a high-speed blender together with the hot Healing Broth or water, fresh hot pepper, garlic, onion powder, paprika, cayenne, oregano, lime juice, and tomato paste. Blend until very smooth, 2 to 3 minutes on high speed.

Divide between soup bowls and garnish with the cilantro and green onion. Serve immediately.

TIPS

- Look for a tomato paste that contains only tomatoes and no other ingredients, such as salt or citric acid.

- When you're choosing between Healing Broth and water for the ingredients, keep in mind that the broth will produce a richer flavor. Store-bought vegetable stock isn't called for because it's very difficult to find a variety that's free of oil, salt, natural flavors, and/or other additives. For convenience, make a batch of Healing Broth in advance and freeze it (consider pouring into ice cube trays for easy thawing) so you have it on hand for recipes like this.

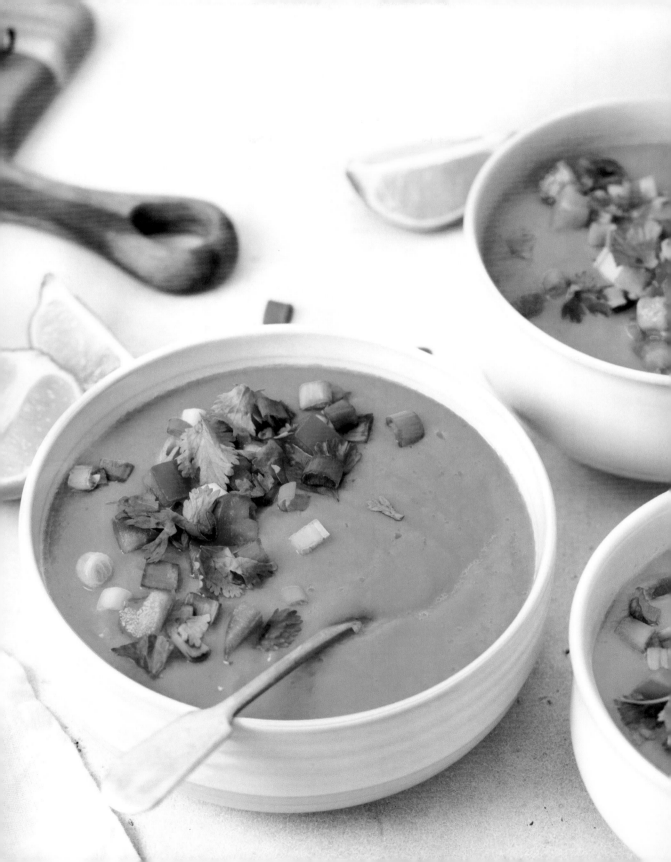

44. ZUCCHINI LASAGNA SOUP

Makes 2 servings

A delicious tomato and herb broth with zucchini ribbons, dollops of potato cheese, and topped with mushroom "mince," this recipe brings you the flavors of lasagna in a fragrant soup. Enjoy a big bowl for lunch or dinner, or pair it with one of the salad recipes and/or the Rosemary Potato Flatbread (recipe on page 414) for a heartier meal.

FOR THE SOUP

1 cup diced onion
6 garlic cloves, finely chopped
2 tablespoons tomato paste
5 cups Healing Broth (recipe on page 370) or water
3 cups jarred crushed tomatoes or 4 cups diced fresh tomatoes
½ cup sun-dried tomatoes (oil-free and salt-free)
1 tablespoon dried oregano
2 teaspoons dried basil
½ teaspoon red pepper flakes
1 medium zucchini, cut into ribbons with a vegetable peeler
½ cup loosely packed fresh basil leaves, to serve

FOR THE POTATO CHEESE

2 cups finely diced potatoes
2 tablespoons onion powder
2 teaspoons garlic powder

FOR THE MUSHROOM MINCE

4 cups finely diced mushrooms*
½ teaspoon garlic powder
½ teaspoon onion powder
½ teaspoon paprika
2 tablespoons tomato paste
1 tablespoon freshly squeezed lemon juice

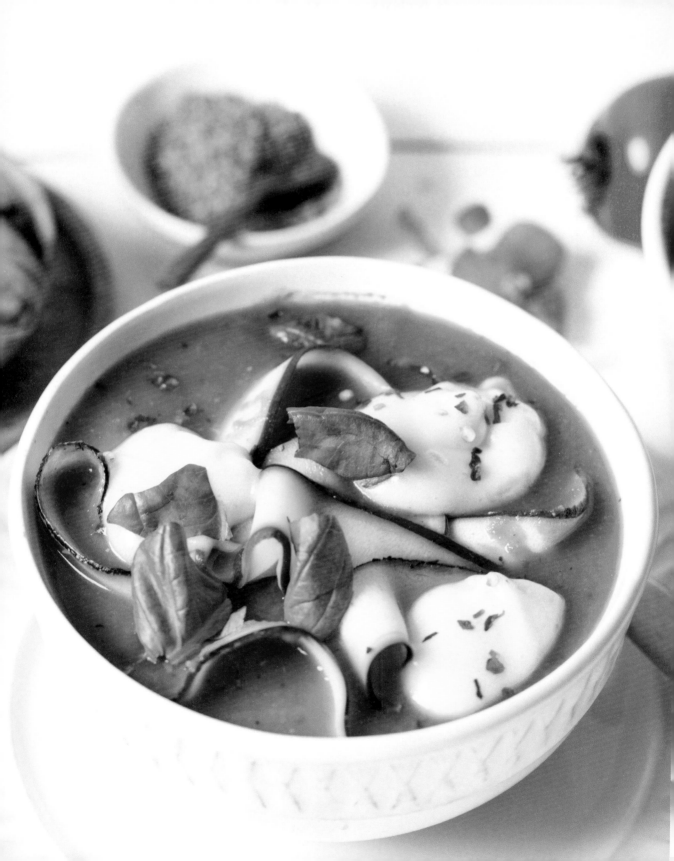

Place a ceramic nonstick soup pot on medium-high heat. Add a small splash of water, then add the onion and cook for 3 to 5 minutes until softened. Add the garlic and tomato paste and cook for a further 2 to 3 minutes until the tomato paste starts to caramelize and turns a darker color.

Add the Healing Broth or water, crushed and sun-dried tomatoes, dried oregano, dried basil, and red pepper flakes. Bring to a simmer and cook, uncovered, for 20 to 30 minutes.

While the soup is cooking, add 3 inches of water to a medium pot, insert a steaming basket, add the potatoes, and cover. Steam the potatoes for 15 to 20 minutes until soft. Remove the potatoes and place them in a blender or food processor together with the onion powder and garlic powder. Blend until smooth, scraping down the sides as needed. Set aside.

To make the mushroom mince, place a ceramic nonstick skillet on medium-high heat. Add the diced mushrooms and cook for 5 to 8 minutes until soft. Add the garlic powder, onion powder, paprika, tomato paste, and lemon juice and cook for a further 1 to 2 minutes until all the liquid has evaporated and the mushrooms are browned.

Add the zucchini ribbons to the soup and continue cooking for 3 to 5 minutes until soft.

Divide soup between two bowls and top with the potato cheese, mushroom mince, and fresh basil. Serve immediately.

*For the mushrooms, wash and rinse thoroughly with warm to hot water before dicing. Do not use slimy or decaying mushrooms. That's a sign of oxidizing and aging.

TIPS

- Look for a tomato paste that contains only tomatoes and no other ingredients, such as salt or citric acid.

- When you're choosing between Healing Broth and water for the ingredients, keep in mind that the broth will produce a richer flavor. Store-bought vegetable stock isn't called for because it's very difficult to find a variety that's free of oil, salt, natural flavors, and/or other additives. For convenience, make a batch of Healing Broth in advance and freeze it (consider pouring into ice cube trays for easy thawing) so you have it on hand for recipes like this.

45. CURRY POTATO SAMOSAS

Makes 8 to 10 samosas

These oil-free and grain-free samosas are made with the ever-versatile potato. Filled with a curried pea and potato or cauliflower filling, these samosas are a fantastic snack or finger food, or pair them with a soup or salad for a main meal.

1 pound potatoes, peeled and roughly chopped
¾ to 1 cup potato starch

FOR THE FILLING

¼ cup finely chopped onion
1 teaspoon finely chopped fresh ginger
½ teaspoon curry powder
½ teaspoon garlic powder
¼ teaspoon red pepper flakes or cayenne
¾ cup finely chopped potato or cauliflower
1 cup Healing Broth (recipe on page 370) or water
¼ cup fresh or frozen peas
1 tablespoon roughly chopped fresh cilantro
1 teaspoon freshly squeezed lemon juice

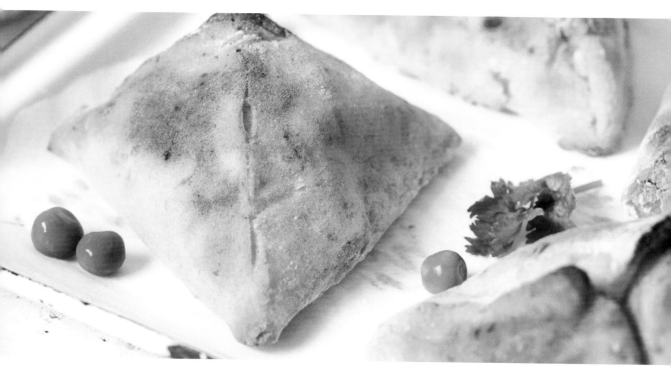

Add 3 inches of water to a medium pot, insert a steaming basket, add the potatoes, and cover. Steam the potatoes for 20 to 25 minutes until soft. Place in a large bowl and mash until smooth. Add the potato starch and knead until you get a soft dough that's not sticky. Add more starch if necessary.

While the potatoes are steaming, make the filling by placing a ceramic nonstick skillet on medium-high heat. Add the onions and cook for 3 to 5 minutes until softened. Add the ginger, curry powder, garlic powder, red pepper flakes, potato or cauliflower, and Healing Broth or water. Stir well; then cover and simmer for 10 to 15 minutes until the potatoes or cauliflower are tender. Stir in the peas, cilantro, and lemon juice and cook for a further 2 to 3 minutes until the peas are bright green and the Healing Broth or water has completely evaporated. Remove from heat and set aside.

Preheat the oven to 400°F/200°C. Line a large baking sheet with parchment paper.

Sprinkle potato starch generously onto a work surface. Divide the dough in half. Working with one piece of dough at a time, roll the dough into a ¼-inch-thick circle that's about 8 inches in diameter.

Cut each circle of dough into quarters, making 8 wedges in total. Place a tablespoon of filling in the center of each wedge. Bring the two bottom corners together over the filling and press to form a seam. Bring the third corner to join the other two, and then gently pinch to close. Transfer the samosa to the baking sheet and repeat with the remaining dough.

Bake samosas for 25 to 30 minutes until browned on top. Cool for 5 minutes before serving.

TIPS

- All types of potatoes are options for this recipe. One great variety of potato to try here is Yukon gold.

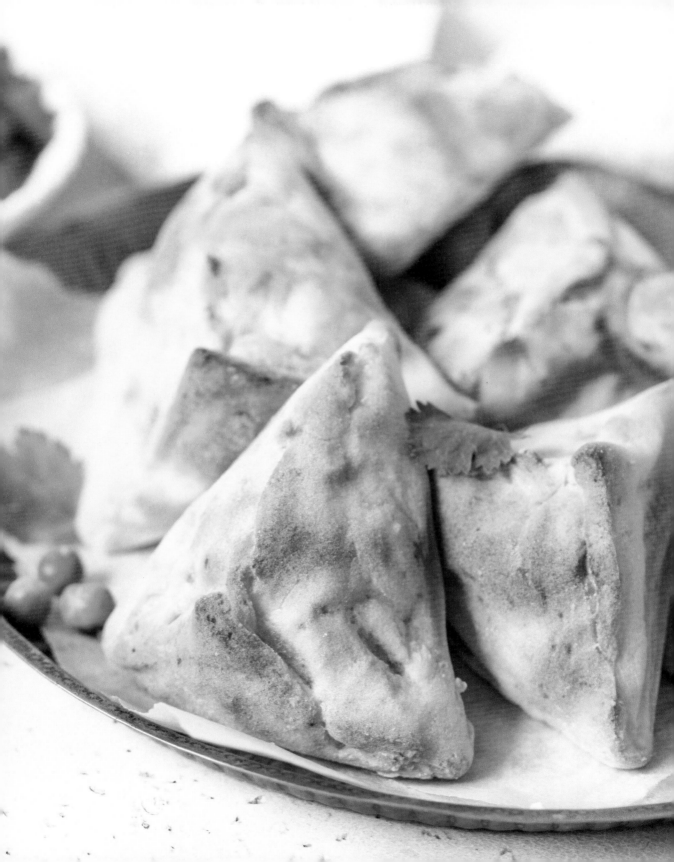

46. SPICED SQUASH SOUP

Makes 2 to 3 servings

A creamy butternut squash soup made with warming spices, a kick of heat, and finished with fresh herbs and a squeeze of lime juice. This soup is an easy dinner option for cool nights or simply when you want a cozy, comforting, and nourishing bowl of soup. Make extra to feed the whole family or to have plenty left over for lunch or dinner the next day.

½ cup diced onion

4 garlic cloves

1½ tablespoons roughly chopped fresh ginger

1 tablespoon roughly chopped long red hot pepper

1 teaspoon ground cumin

1 teaspoon ground coriander

¼ to ½ teaspoon cayenne pepper

6 cups peeled and seeded butternut squash

2 cups Healing Broth (recipe on page 370) or water

1 tablespoon freshly squeezed lime juice

¼ cup loosely packed parsley or cilantro leaves, to serve

Place a ceramic nonstick soup pot on medium-high heat. Add the onion, garlic, fresh ginger, and hot pepper and cook for 3 to 5 minutes, or until the onion is soft. Add a bit of water if needed to prevent sticking.

Add the spices and squash and cook for another 1 to 2 minutes until the spices are fragrant.

Add in the Healing Broth, cover, and simmer for 20 to 30 minutes until the butternut squash is very soft. Add in the lime juice and blend with an immersion blender until smooth. Alternatively, you can do this in a jug blender (in batches if needed).

Divide the soup between two or three bowls and top with parsley or cilantro. Serve immediately.

TIPS

- When you're choosing between Healing Broth and water for the ingredients, keep in mind that the broth will produce a richer flavor. Store-bought vegetable stock isn't called for because it's very difficult to find a variety that's free of oil, salt, natural flavors, and/or other additives. For convenience, make a batch of Healing Broth in advance and freeze it (consider pouring into ice cube trays for easy thawing) so you have it on hand for recipes like this.

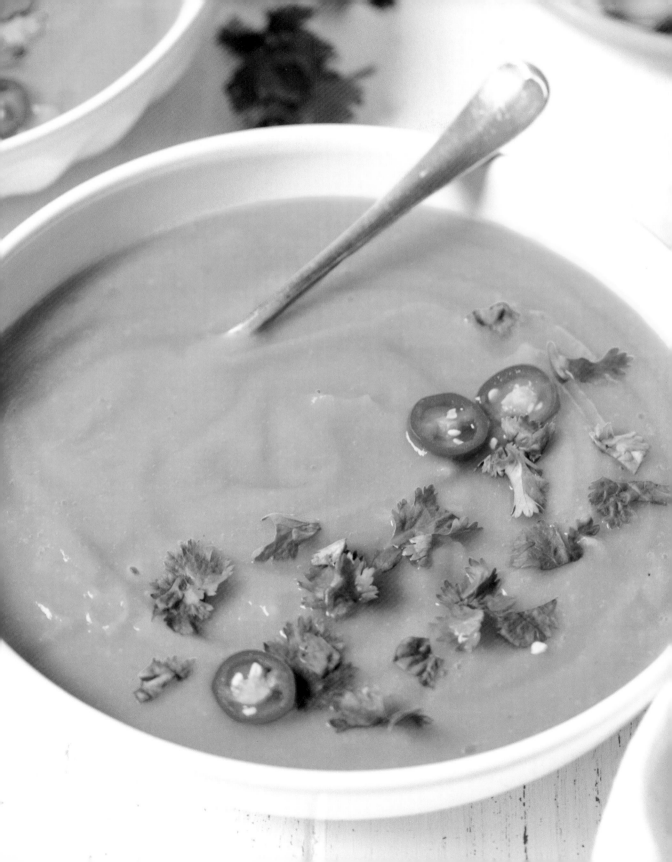

47. BABA GANOUSH

This creamy dip made with roasted eggplants is a Middle Eastern favorite. This recipe omits the oil and heavy amounts of tahini normally used in baba ganoush in order to bring you a truly healing dip option. Enjoy this dip with your favorite crudités, such as celery sticks, carrot sticks, cucumber slices, lettuce leaves, or asparagus spears, or enjoy it with the Rosemary Potato Flatbread (recipe on page 414).

2 medium eggplants, cut in half
2 garlic cloves, roughly chopped
1 tablespoon tahini (optional)
Zest of 1 lemon
¼ cup freshly squeezed lemon juice
½ pitted Medjool date
¼ teaspoon sea salt (optional)
¼ cup fresh parsley leaves, finely chopped
¼ cup fresh mint leaves, finely chopped,
   plus more to serve
¼ cup pomegranate seeds, to serve

Preheat the oven to 400°F/200°C. Line a baking sheet with parchment paper.

Arrange the eggplant halves on the baking sheet, flesh-side facing down; then bake for 40 to 45 minutes, or until soft. Remove the eggplant from the oven; then put aside to cool.

Once the eggplant is cool, peel it and place in a food processor. Add the garlic, tahini (if using), lemon zest, lemon juice, and date. Add the optional sea salt if using. Process until smooth but still with a bit of texture. Add the parsley and mint and pulse briefly until incorporated.

Place the dip in a serving bowl and top with pomegranate seeds and a bit more finely chopped mint. Serve immediately or keep refrigerated until needed.

TIPS

- The tahini makes the Baba Ganoush creamier and richer; however, if you are trying to lower your fats, you can keep it out and you'll still get a great result.

- While high-quality sea salt or mountain rock salt is an optional inclusion in this recipe, the recipe is more healing without salt. Over time, you may wish to reduce or exclude the salt.

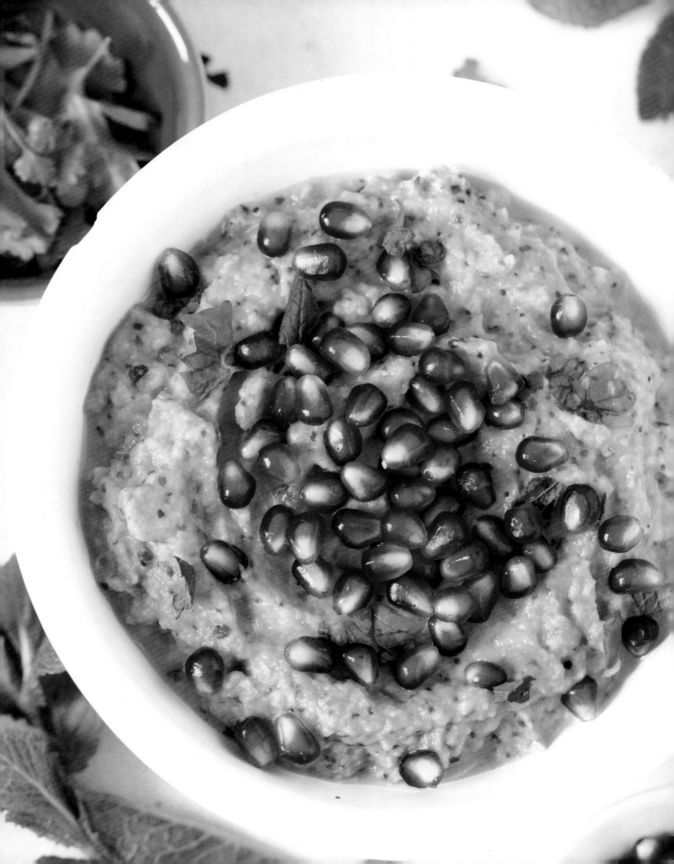

48. CAULIFLOWER AND SQUASH BOWL

This Buddha bowl–style recipe gives you a variety of flavors and ingredients to enjoy together in one bowl. While there are a few different parts to this recipe, each component is quite quick to prepare, and the result is a very tasty meal. This bowl pairs beautifully with a simple leafy green salad.

FOR THE CAULIFLOWER RICE

½ medium cauliflower, cut into florets

FOR THE SQUASH

3 cups peeled or unpeeled diced kabocha, acorn, sweet dumpling, butternut, or delicata squash
½ teaspoon ground cumin
½ teaspoon ground coriander
½ teaspoon cinnamon
2 tablespoons finely chopped fresh cilantro
1 teaspoon freshly squeezed lemon or lime juice
½ teaspoon raw honey

FOR THE ZUCCHINI

3 cups diced zucchini
1 tablespoon finely chopped fresh parsley
1 tablespoon finely chopped fresh basil
½ teaspoon garlic powder
½ teaspoon onion powder
1 teaspoon freshly squeezed lemon or lime juice

FOR THE CAULIFLOWER

3 cups cauliflower florets
½ teaspoon paprika
½ teaspoon garlic powder
¼ teaspoon ground turmeric
2 tablespoons finely chopped fresh cilantro
1 teaspoon freshly squeezed lemon or lime juice

FOR THE ONIONS AND GARLIC

1 cup diced onion
4 garlic cloves, minced
1 teaspoon ground cumin
½ teaspoon ground turmeric
½ teaspoon red pepper flakes
1 tablespoon freshly squeezed lemon or lime juice

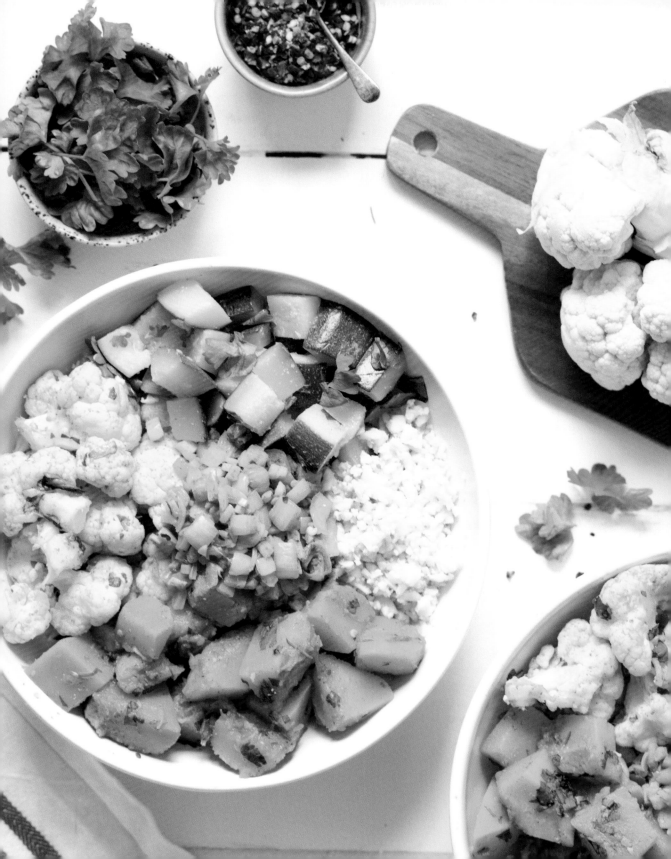

To make the cauliflower rice, place the florets in a food processor. Pulse a few times until you get a rice-like texture. Place a large ceramic nonstick frying pan on medium-high heat and add the cauliflower rice. Cook, stirring frequently, for 5 to 7 minutes, or until tender. Remove from the heat and set aside.

To make the squash, add 3 inches of water to a medium pot, insert a steaming basket, add the squash, and cover. Steam the diced squash for 10 to 15 minutes, or until soft. Place in a bowl and add the cumin, coriander, cinnamon, cilantro, lemon or lime juice, and raw honey. Stir gently until evenly coated. Set aside.

To make the zucchini, add 3 inches of water to a medium pot, insert a steaming basket, add the zucchini, and cover. Steam the diced zucchini for 3 to 5 minutes, or until soft. Place in a bowl and add the parsley, basil, garlic powder, onion powder, and lemon or lime juice. Stir gently until evenly coated. Set aside.

To make the cauliflower, add 3 inches of water to a medium pot, insert a steaming basket, add the cauliflower, and cover. Steam the cauliflower florets for 4 to 6 minutes, or until soft. Place in a bowl and add the paprika, garlic powder, turmeric, cilantro, and lemon or lime juice. Stir gently until evenly coated. Set aside.

To make the onions and garlic, place a medium ceramic nonstick skillet on medium-high heat. Add the onion and cook for 3 to 5 minutes, or until soft. Add the garlic, cumin, turmeric, red pepper flakes, and lemon or lime juice. Cook for another 1 to 2 minutes until the garlic is soft and the spices are fragrant. Remove from heat.

To serve, divide the cauliflower rice between two bowls and top with the squash, zucchini, cauliflower, and the onions and garlic. Serve immediately.

TIPS

- If you would like to enjoy this recipe for multiple meals or days, you may wish to double, triple, or quadruple the recipe so you have extra of each of the vegetable components. You can simply reheat them on the stove to put together another bowl the next time you'd like to enjoy it.

49. POTATO LETTUCE SANDWICHES

These lettuce sandwiches really hit the spot when you're looking for a fresh and simple option. Load up your layered lettuce leaves with potato slices, fresh tomato, onion, cucumber, and radish, all topped off with mustard and/or ketchup.

FOR THE POTATO SLICES

2 to 3 medium potatoes
2 teaspoons garlic powder
2 teaspoons onion powder
2 teaspoons paprika
2 teaspoons dried oregano or basil
½ teaspoon chili powder

TO SERVE

8 to 12 green or red leaf lettuce leaves
2 to 3 tablespoons Potato Mustard (optional)
2 to 3 tablespoons Ketchup (optional)
½ cup thinly sliced tomato
⅓ cup thinly sliced onion
½ cup thinly sliced cucumber (optional)
½ cup thinly sliced radish (optional)
½ cup sprouts or microgreens (optional)

FOR THE POTATO MUSTARD (OPTIONAL)

½ cup peeled and diced steamed potato
2 teaspoons mustard powder
½ garlic clove, roughly chopped
⅛ teaspoon ground turmeric
3 tablespoons lemon juice
2½ tablespoons raw honey
1 tablespoon water

FOR THE KETCHUP (OPTIONAL)

3 ounces tomato paste
¼ teaspoon onion powder
¼ teaspoon garlic powder
¼ teaspoon dried oregano
¼ teaspoon cayenne (optional)
3 tablespoons apple juice
1 tablespoon freshly squeezed lemon juice
1 teaspoon raw honey

Add 3 inches of water to a medium pot, insert a steaming basket, add the potatoes, and cover. Steam the whole potatoes 40 to 50 minutes until soft. Remove and cool completely.

Slice the potatoes into thin slices lengthwise and place on a cutting board or platter in a single layer. Sprinkle spices and herbs generously on top.

To make the optional Potato Mustard, combine the mustard ingredients in a blender and blend until smooth. Serve immediately, or keep refrigerated until needed.

To make the optional Ketchup, combine the ketchup ingredients in a small bowl and whisk until evenly mixed and smooth. Serve immediately, or keep refrigerated until needed.

To assemble the sandwiches, layer 2 to 3 lettuce leaves on top of each other to create a sturdy base. Add a few potato slices, ketchup and/or mustard (if using), tomato, onion, and the cucumber, radish, and/or sprouts or microgreens (if using). Place another 2 to 3 lettuce leaves on top. Repeat with the remaining ingredients and serve immediately.

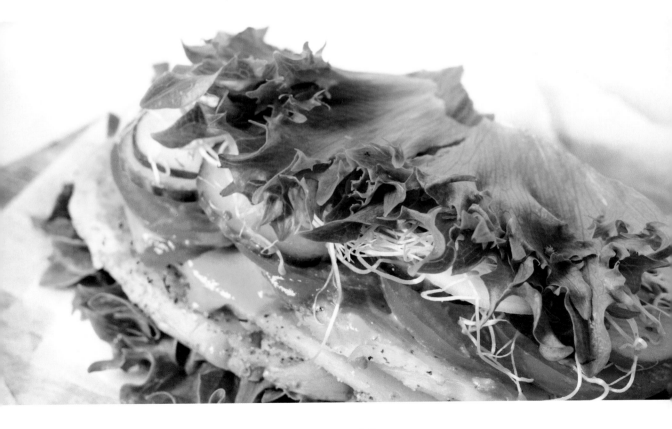

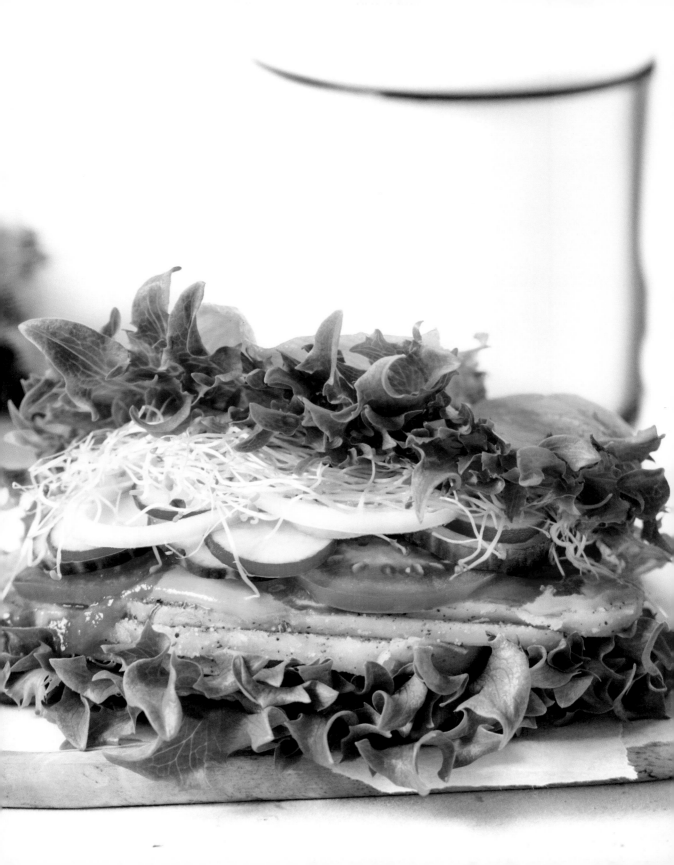

50. SWEET POTATO NORI WRAPS

Makes 1 to 2 servings

These Sweet Potato Nori Wraps taste fantastic on their own, or if you like, you can dip them into any of the sauces or dips in this book, such as the Potato Mustard (recipe on page 395), Baba Ganoush (recipe on page 390), Raw Cilantro Chutney (recipe on page 362), or Asparagus-Spinach Dip (recipe on page 340).

1 pound sweet potatoes (any color) or winter squash (any variety other than spaghetti squash), peeled and cut into thick sticks

4 nori sheets

2 to 3 tablespoons freshly squeezed lemon, lime, or orange juice

4 cups tightly packed leafy greens

1 cup julienned red, yellow, or orange bell pepper

1 cup julienned cucumber

1 cup sprouts

1 cup loosely packed cilantro leaves

Add 3 inches of water to a medium pot, insert a steaming basket, add the sweet potatoes or winter squash sticks, and cover. Steam the potatoes or squash 13 to 16 minutes until soft. Remove and cool completely.

Place a nori sheet shiny side down on a chopping board with the long edge facing you. Squeeze just a few drops of lemon, lime, or orange juice onto the nori sheet and use your fingers to roughly spread the juice over the nori sheet so that it's very lightly moistened.

Arrange the sweet potato or winter squash sticks, leafy greens, prepared bell pepper and cucumber, sprouts, and cilantro leaves on one end of the sheet. Squeeze a few more drops of lemon, lime, or orange juice across the end of the sheet; then roll up tightly and cut in half. Repeat with the remaining ingredients and serve immediately.

TIPS

- While steamed sweet potatoes offer the most healing benefits, you can also bake your sweet potatoes to include in these nori wraps if you like.

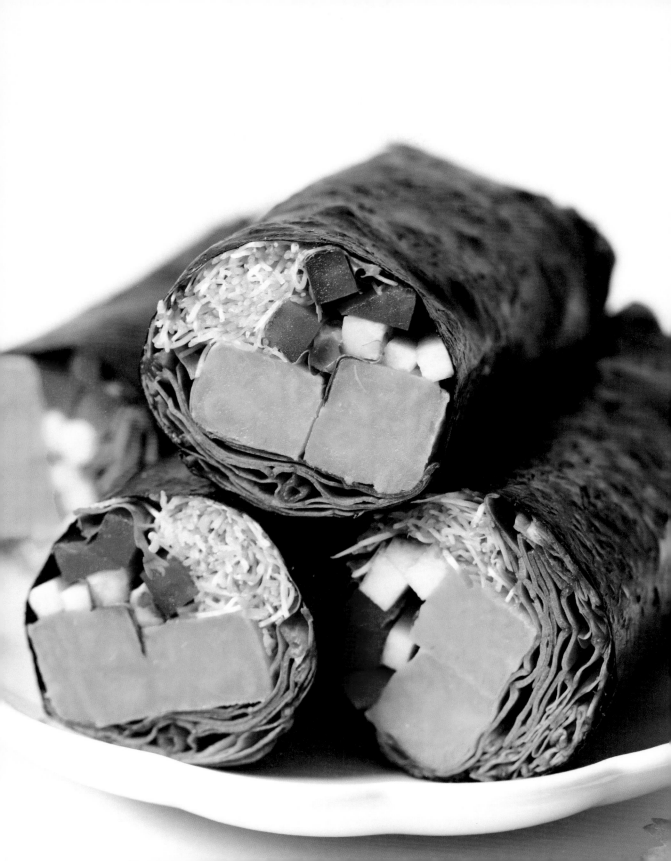

51. ZUCCHINI NOODLES WITH MARINARA SAUCE

Makes 2 servings

Satisfy a craving for pasta with marinara sauce with this far more healing option. It's rich in both flavor and nutrients, and you won't feel heavy after eating it!

¼ cup finely chopped yellow onion or shallot
4 garlic cloves, thinly sliced
2 tablespoons tomato paste
2 pounds fresh plum or cherry tomatoes, roughly chopped, or 2 cups jarred crushed or diced tomatoes
2 teaspoons dried oregano
½ teaspoon red pepper flakes
¼ cup loosely packed basil leaves
2 zucchinis, spiralized

Place a ceramic nonstick pot on medium-high heat. Add the onion or shallot and cook, stirring occasionally, until very soft, 8 to 10 minutes. Add a bit of water if needed to prevent sticking.

Add the garlic and cook, stirring occasionally, until very soft, about 5 minutes. Add the tomato paste and cook for 1 to 2 minutes until the paste begins to caramelize.

Add the tomatoes, dried oregano, and red pepper flakes. Stir until evenly mixed. Reduce the heat, cover, and simmer gently, stirring occasionally, until the tomatoes are soft, 30 to 40 minutes. Remove the lid and cook for a further 10 minutes until the sauce is thick. If using jarred tomatoes, then you can reduce the overall cooking time by half.

Transfer the sauce to a blender or food processor, add the basil leaves, and pulse a few times until you get a chunky sauce. Set aside.

Place a ceramic nonstick frying pan on medium-high heat and add the spiralized zucchini. Sauté while tossing the noodles with tongs until al dente, 2 to 3 minutes.

Divide noodles between two bowls and top with the sauce. Garnish with a bit of basil and serve immediately.

TIPS

- Look for a tomato paste that contains only tomatoes and no other ingredients, such as salt or citric acid.

- A good quality jarred fat-free marinara sauce without citric acid, oil, preservatives, natural flavors, or other problematic ingredients can be used when you don't have time to make your own.

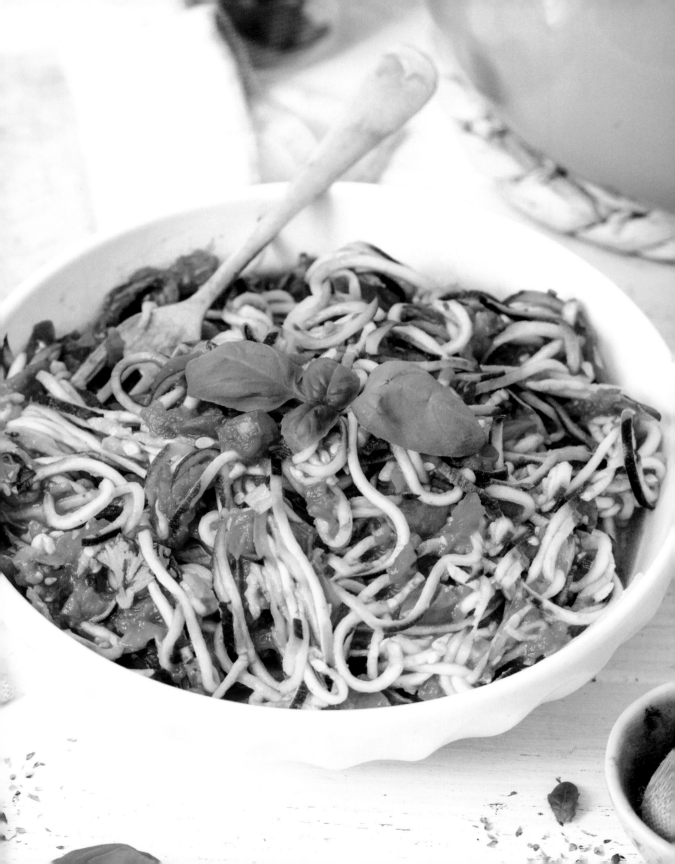

52. ASIAN-INSPIRED POTATO SKILLET

Asian flavors bring this potato skillet recipe to life. Savory, a little bit spicy, and with a hint of sweetness, this is a great lunch or dinner choice, and it can even be enjoyed as a savory cooked breakfast.

½ cup finely chopped spring or
   yellow onion
2 garlic cloves, finely sliced
½ teaspoon finely chopped ripe
   hot pepper
1½ cups thinly sliced shiitake or
   button mushrooms*
2 pounds potatoes or sweet potatoes
   of any variety, thinly sliced
1 cup Healing Broth (recipe on page
   370) or water
½ teaspoon Atlantic dulse flakes
1 cup chopped sugar snap peas or
   green beans
¼ cup roughly chopped cilantro leaves,
   to serve
5 to 6 fresh ripe hot pepper slices,
   to serve

FOR THE SAUCE

2 tablespoons freshly squeezed lime juice
2 tablespoons pure maple syrup
2 tablespoons tomato paste
½ tablespoon finely grated fresh ginger
¼ teaspoon red pepper flakes
2 tablespoons water

TIPS

- When you're choosing between Healing Broth and water for the ingredients, keep in mind that the broth will produce a richer flavor. Store-bought vegetable stock isn't called for because it's very difficult to find a variety that's free of oil, salt, natural flavors, and/or other additives. For convenience, make a batch of Healing Broth in advance and freeze it (consider pouring into ice cube trays for easy thawing) so you have it on hand for recipes like this.

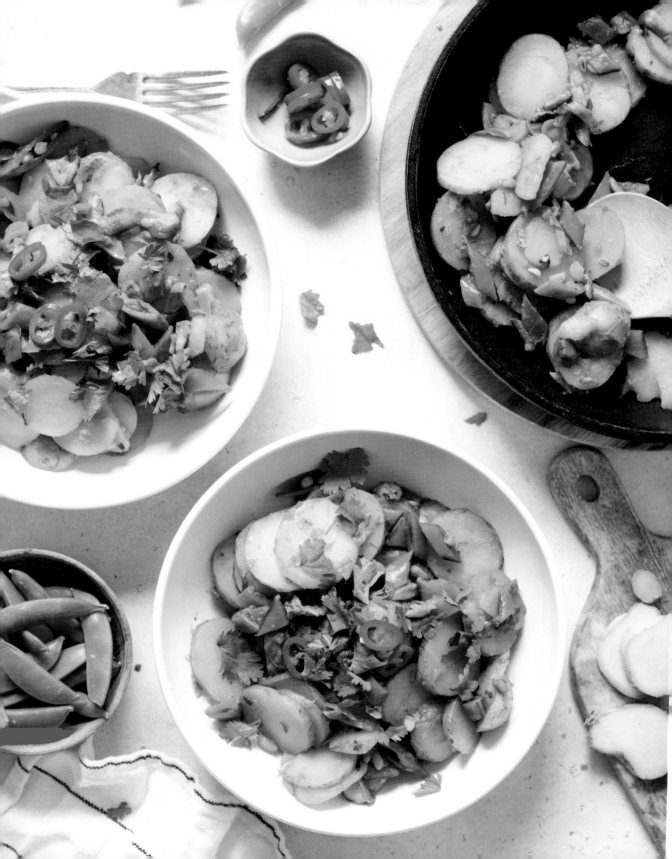

Asian-Inspired Potato Skillet continued

Place a ceramic nonstick skillet on medium-high heat. Add the spring onion or yellow onion, garlic, hot pepper, and mushrooms, and cook for 5 to 8 minutes until the mushrooms are soft, adding a bit of water if needed to prevent sticking. Add the potatoes, Healing Broth or water, and Atlantic dulse flakes to the pan. Stir until evenly mixed, then cover, turn the heat to low, and simmer for 10 to 15 minutes until the potatoes are almost tender.

Combine the sauce ingredients in a small bowl and whisk until smooth.

When the potatoes are almost ready, stir in the sauce and sugar snap peas or green beans. Cook for 2 to 3 minutes until the liquid has evaporated.

Divide between two or three bowls and top with the fresh cilantro and hot pepper slices. Serve immediately.

*For the mushrooms, wash and rinse thoroughly with warm to hot water before slicing. Do not use slimy or decaying mushrooms. That's a sign of oxidizing and aging.

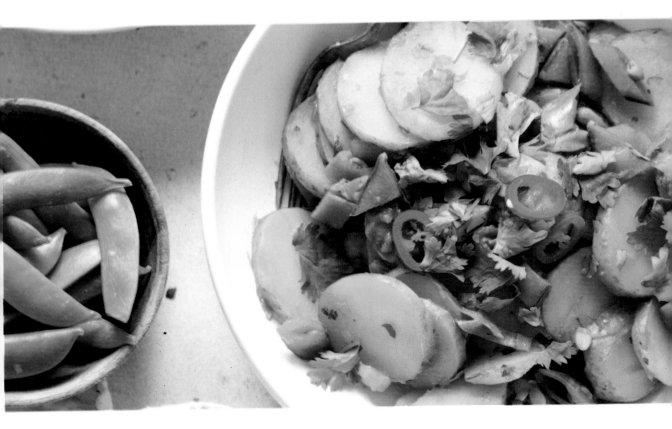

53. STEAMED CABBAGE ROLLS

Makes 2 servings

These cabbage rolls are tasty and beautiful, especially if you use savoy cabbage with its gorgeous aesthetic. It's a great way to get more vegetables into your diet in a unique way.

1 large savoy or green cabbage, broken
   into leaves
⅔ cup finely chopped shiitake or button
   mushrooms*
½ cup chopped spring onions
4 garlic cloves, finely chopped
1 tablespoon finely chopped fresh ginger
½ to 1 teaspoon red pepper flakes
1 cup finely chopped potato
½ cup finely chopped cauliflower
⅔ cup finely chopped red, yellow, or
   orange bell pepper
½ teaspoon sea salt (optional)
1 cup water
½ cup finely chopped sugar snap peas

FOR THE SAUCE

3½ tablespoons raw honey
3 tablespoons freshly squeezed lime juice
½ to 1 teaspoon red pepper flakes
½ teaspoon garlic powder
½ teaspoon paprika
1 teaspoon finely grated fresh ginger

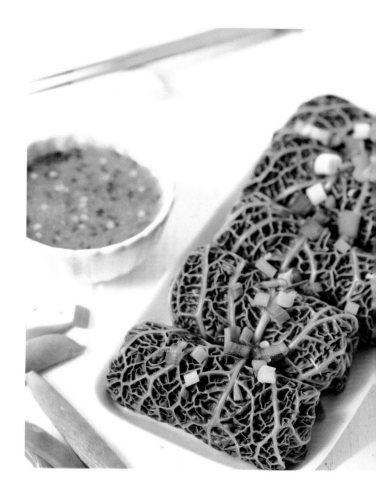

Add 3 inches of water to a medium pot, insert a steaming basket, add the cabbage leaves, and cover. Steam the cabbage leaves for 2 to 3 minutes, or until just pliable. Remove and rinse under cold water. Set aside.

Make the filling by placing a ceramic nonstick skillet on medium-high heat. Add the mushrooms, spring onions, garlic, ginger, and red pepper flakes and cook for 3 to 5 minutes until the mushrooms are softened. Add the potato, cauliflower, and bell pepper. Add the optional sea salt if using. Cook for another 1 to 2 minutes, stirring frequently; then add the water, cover, and cook for 10 to 12 minutes, or until the potatoes are tender. Stir in the sugar snap peas. Remove from the heat and place the filling in a bowl.

Mash the mixture a few times with a potato masher to get a filling that holds together when shaped.

Working with 1 cabbage leaf at a time, place about ¼ cup of filling toward the stem end, fold the sides over the mixture, and roll up tightly. Place the roll end-down in a steamer. Repeat with the remaining leaves and filling.

Steam the cabbage rolls for 10 to 12 minutes until completely tender.

While the rolls are steaming, whisk together all the sauce ingredients until smooth.

Serve the cabbage rolls immediately with the sauce.

*For the mushrooms, wash and rinse thoroughly with warm to hot water before chopping. Do not use slimy or decaying mushrooms. That's a sign of oxidizing and aging.

TIPS

- While high-quality sea salt or mountain rock salt is an optional inclusion in this recipe, the recipe is more healing without salt. Over time, you may wish to reduce or exclude the salt.

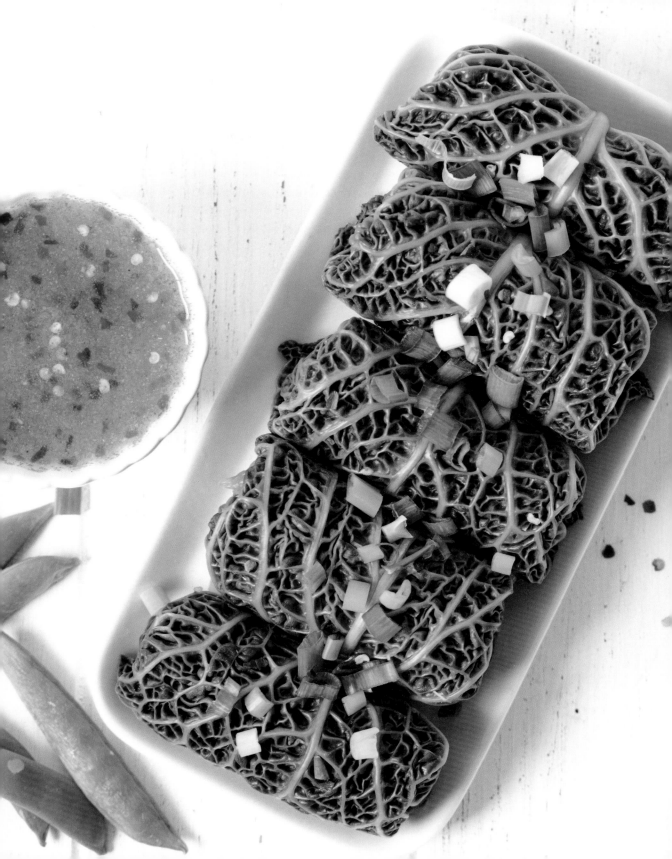

54. BAKED MAC AND CHEESE

Makes 4 to 6 servings

This Baked Mac and Cheese is a perfect choice for children or adults who want a hearty and fun meal, and yet it doesn't include any cheese, cream, milk, gluten, oil, or refined sugar. It's fat-free, and can even be grain-free if you choose a pasta made without grains, such as cassava, pea, lentil, or chickpea pasta. You may wish to pair this dish with a leafy green salad for a meal.

4 cups roughly chopped potatoes

2 cups diced carrots

12 ounces gluten-free, corn-free elbow pasta

3 tablespoons onion powder

1 tablespoon garlic powder

1 tablespoon paprika

¼ teaspoon cayenne (optional)

1½ tablespoons freshly squeezed lemon juice

¾ to 1 teaspoon sea salt (optional)

Preheat the oven to 400°F/200°C.

Add 3 inches of water to a medium pot, insert a steaming basket, add the chopped potatoes and carrots, and cover. Steam for 15 to 20 minutes until tender. Cook the pasta according to package instructions, drain, and place back in the pot.

Once the potatoes and carrots are tender, remove them from the heat and place in a food processor along with the onion powder, garlic powder, paprika, cayenne (if using), lemon juice, and sea salt (if using). Process until smooth. Pour the sauce onto the pasta in the pot and stir until evenly coated.

Transfer the sauced pasta to a medium baking dish and smooth the top. Bake for 25 to 30 minutes until browned on top. Cool for 5 minutes before serving.

TIPS

- While high-quality sea salt or mountain rock salt is an optional inclusion in this recipe, the recipe is more healing without salt. Over time, you may wish to reduce or exclude the salt.

- A gluten-free pasta made with grains such as millet, quinoa, or brown rice is an option for this recipe. Be sure that your pasta does not contain corn or egg.

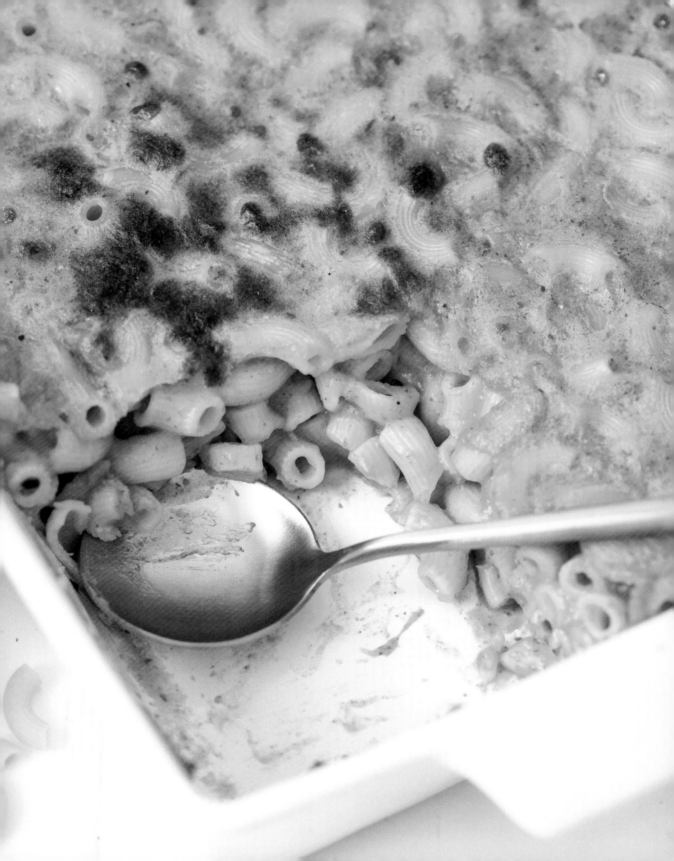

55. MINI FRITTATAS

Makes 12

These Mini Frittatas are free of eggs and dairy—two foods that feed the pathogens behind so many chronic illnesses. Made with chickpea flour and colorful veggies, fruits, and herbs, these tasty bites are great to serve with a big salad for a meal or to include in lunch boxes as a snack.

2 cups chickpea flour
1 teaspoon aluminum-free baking powder
2 teaspoons onion powder
1 teaspoon garlic powder
1 teaspoon paprika
¼ to ½ teaspoon red pepper flakes
   or cayenne
1 teaspoon dried basil or oregano
1¾ cups water
½ tablespoon freshly squeezed
   lemon juice
½ cup finely chopped red bell pepper
½ cup finely chopped red or yellow onion
½ cup finely chopped zucchini
⅓ cup finely chopped carrot

Preheat the oven to 350°F/180°C.

In a large bowl, combine the chickpea flour, baking powder, onion powder, garlic powder, paprika, red pepper flakes, and dried basil or oregano. Mix well.

Whisk in the water and lemon juice. Add the bell pepper, onion, zucchini, and carrot, stirring to combine.

Using a ¼-cup measuring cup, scoop the batter into a nonstick muffin pan, filling all 12 cups.

Place the frittatas in the oven and bake for 30 to 35 minutes until a toothpick inserted in the frittatas comes out clean.

Remove the frittatas from the oven and cool in the muffin pan for at least 10 minutes. Remove the frittatas from the pan and place on a cooling rack until cool enough to eat.

Serve immediately, or keep in an airtight container at room temperature until needed.

TIPS

- If you have produce that needs to be used, this is a good recipe in which to do so. For example, if you have broccoli, cauliflower, or mushrooms on hand, you could replace the zucchini with them in this recipe.

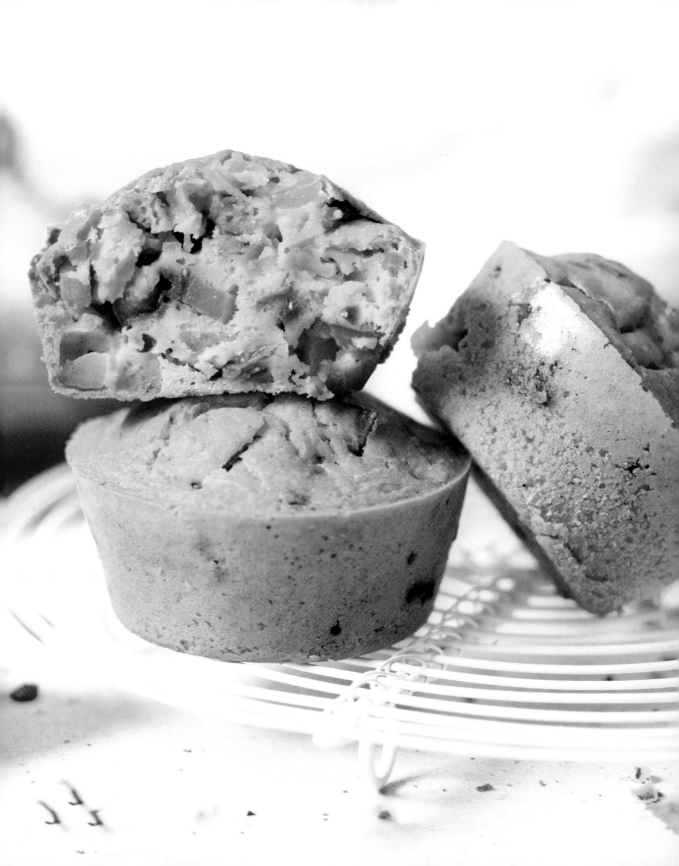

56. PEA HUMMUS

Makes 2 to 3 servings

Peas, lemon juice, herbs, and spices combine together to make a creamy and pretty dip in this recipe. It is satisfying and flavorful without needing any oil or fat.

3 cups frozen green peas

4 to 5 tablespoons freshly squeezed lemon juice, to taste

⅓ cup loosely packed cilantro leaves

1 teaspoon onion powder

1 garlic clove, roughly chopped, or ½ teaspoon garlic powder

½ teaspoon paprika

½ teaspoon ground cumin

¼ to ½ teaspoon cayenne

¼ to ½ teaspoon sea salt (optional)

1 to 2 tablespoons cold water, to desired consistency (optional)

4 cups vegetable crudités, to serve (optional)

Place a dry skillet on medium-high heat and add the peas. Cook for 3 to 5 minutes, stirring often, until the peas are bright green and hot. If you overcook the peas, the dip will lose its pretty bright green color.

Place the peas in a food processor and add the lemon juice, cilantro leaves, onion powder, garlic or garlic powder, paprika, cumin, cayenne, and sea salt (if using). Process on high speed until the dip is as smooth as possible. If you need to add a tablespoon or two of cold water to get the consistency you want, go ahead and do that. Taste and adjust the spices as desired.

Serve immediately with crudités, or keep refrigerated until needed.

TIPS

- Whenever possible, it's best to look for organic frozen green peas.

- While high-quality sea salt or mountain rock salt is an optional inclusion in this recipe, the recipe is more healing without salt. Over time, you may wish to reduce or exclude the salt.

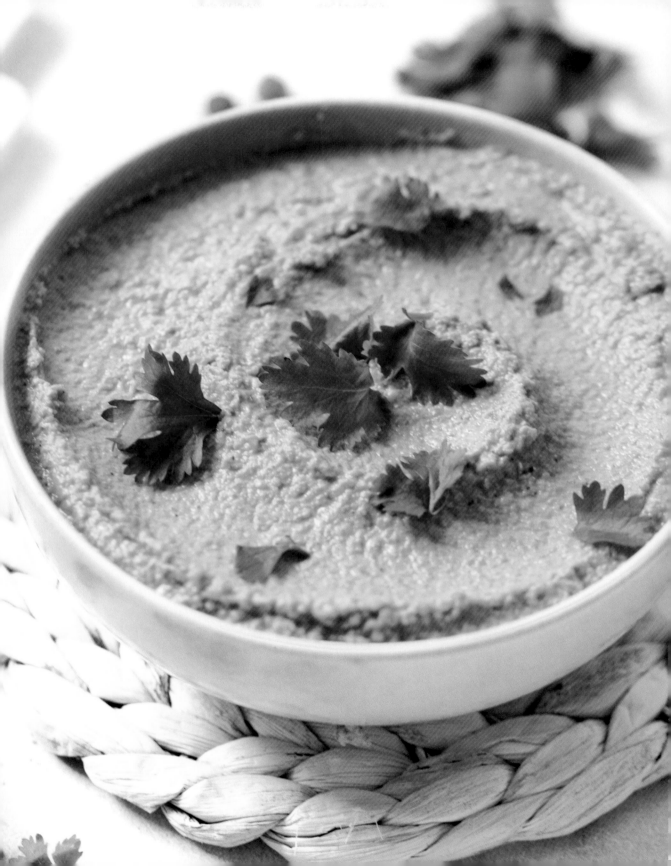

57. ROSEMARY POTATO FLATBREAD

Makes 2 to 3 servings

This flatbread tastes amazing and is incredibly versatile. Enjoy it on its own, with a dip such as the Sun-Dried Tomato Spread (recipe on page 353), Baba Ganoush (recipe on page 390), Raw Cilantro Chutney (recipe on page 362), or Asparagus-Spinach Dip (recipe on page 340). It's also perfect to cut into large squares and use as a bread for a sandwich with fillings like lettuce, tomato, onion, and Potato Mustard (recipe on page 395). It's also a great side to soup or salad.

2 pounds potatoes, roughly chopped
½ teaspoon onion powder
½ teaspoon garlic powder
½ teaspoon paprika
½ cup cassava flour
⅓ cup potato starch, more if needed
2 to 3 tablespoons chopped rosemary

Add 3 inches of water to a medium pot, insert a steaming basket, add the potatoes, and cover. Steam the potatoes for 20 to 25 minutes until soft. Remove the potatoes and place them in a bowl or pot together with the onion powder, garlic powder, and paprika. Mash until smooth. Set aside for 10 minutes to cool.

Preheat the oven to 400°F/200°C. Line a baking sheet with parchment paper. Add the cassava flour and potato starch to the mashed potatoes, and knead until you get a soft dough that isn't sticky, adding more potato starch as needed.

Place the dough on the prepared baking sheet and spread out evenly to about ½ inch thick. Sprinkle the rosemary on top and press it in slightly. Bake for 25 to 35 minutes until browned on top. Cool for 15 minutes before slicing.

TIPS

- Feel free to swap out the rosemary for a different herb if you'd like, such as thyme, parsley, oregano, or sage.

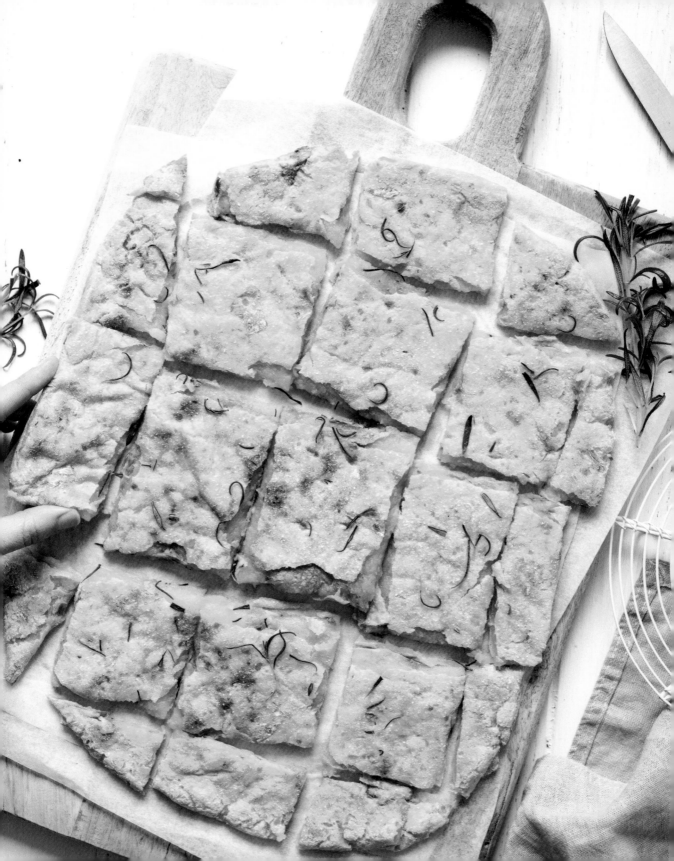

58. MILLET SUSHI

Makes 2 to 3 servings

These simple and tasty sushi rolls are made with millet and fresh fillings, their flavor elevated by marinated ginger and wasabi. Enjoy these sushi rolls as part of a meal or for a snack.

FOR THE SUSHI

1 cup millet
2 cups water
2 to 3 nori sheets
1 cup julienned cucumber
1 cup julienned carrots
1 cup thinly sliced red cabbage

FOR THE MARINATED GINGER

2 tablespoons freshly squeezed orange or lemon juice
1 teaspoon raw honey
1-inch piece of ginger, peeled and very thinly sliced

FOR THE WASABI

1 teaspoon wasabi powder
1 to 2 tablespoons water

TIPS

- You can make extra marinated ginger to add to meals if you wish, such as salads, steamed vegetables, or stir-fries. You can store the marinated ginger in an airtight container in the fridge for up to a week.

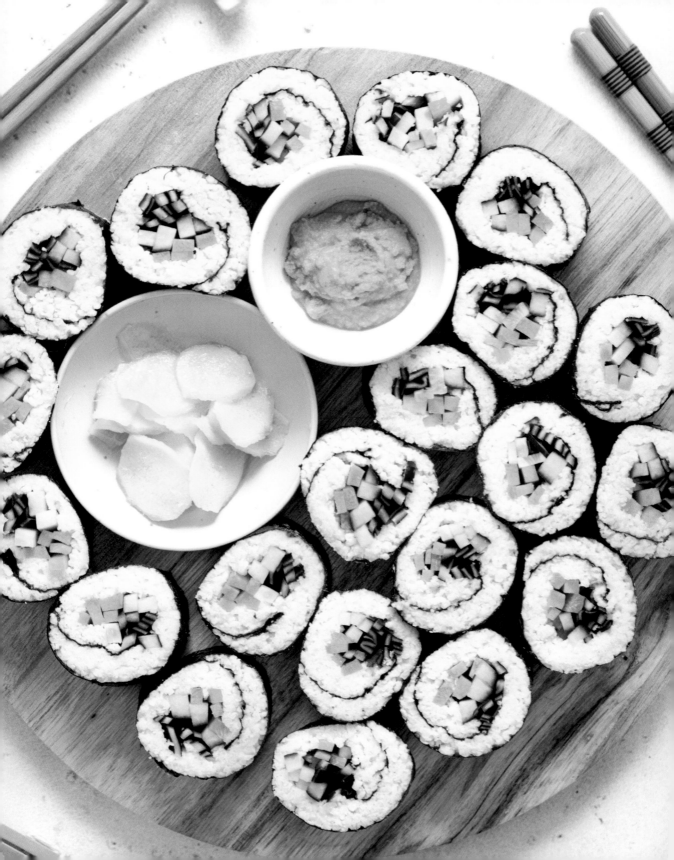

To make the marinated ginger, combine the orange or lemon juice and raw honey in a small bowl and whisk until well combined. Add the thinly sliced ginger and submerge in the liquid. Set aside for at least 1 hour to marinate.

Combine the millet and water in a small saucepan. Cover and simmer for 10 to 15 minutes until the millet is cooked. Remove from the heat and cool completely.

Place one sheet of nori on a cutting board, long edge facing you. Scoop about ¾ cup of millet onto the end of the nori sheet closest to you and spread it over the sheet in an even layer, leaving about a 1-inch border at the top of the sheet. Arrange the fillings on the middle section of the millet layer.

Carefully lift the nori from the bottom edge close to you and begin rolling it tightly toward the top. Just before finishing the roll, dip your finger in the ginger marinade and run it along the top edge of the sheet. Using a sharp knife, slice each sushi roll into even pieces. Repeat with the remaining ingredients.

Mix the wasabi powder and water until you get a smooth paste.

Serve the millet sushi immediately with the wasabi and marinated ginger.

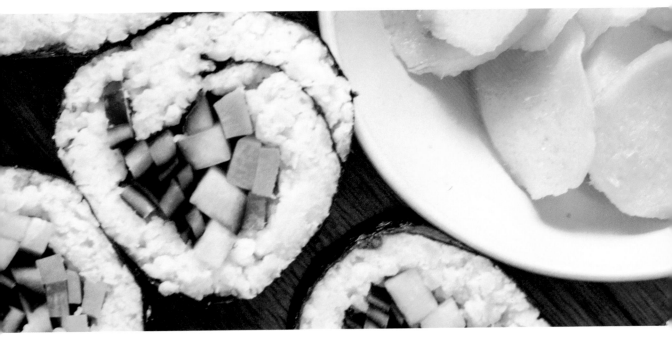

59. POTATO MOUSSAKA

Makes 4 to 6 servings

This Potato Moussaka is hearty, comforting, and so satisfying. It's the perfect meal when you feel like you need some comfort food that will fill your belly but not hold you back from healing. For an even more nourishing meal, try pairing it with a leafy green salad.

2 medium eggplants, cut into ½-inch discs
1 large zucchini, cut into ½-inch discs
3 medium tomatoes, cut into ½-inch slices

FOR THE POTATO LAYER

3 pounds potatoes, roughly chopped
1 tablespoon onion powder
1 teaspoon garlic powder

FOR THE TOMATO SAUCE

3½ cups finely chopped mushrooms*
½ cup diced onion
½ cup finely chopped sun-dried tomatoes (oil-free and salt-free)
⅓ cup finely chopped celery
3 garlic cloves, finely chopped
1½ cups jarred diced or crushed tomatoes or 2 cups fresh tomatoes, diced
1 teaspoon fresh thyme or ½ teaspoon dried
1 teaspoon fresh oregano or ½ teaspoon dried
¼ teaspoon red pepper flakes
¼ to ½ teaspoon sea salt (optional)

TIPS

- While high-quality sea salt or mountain rock salt is an optional inclusion in this recipe, the recipe is more healing without salt. Over time, you may wish to reduce or exclude the salt.

Preheat the oven to 400°F/200°C. Line two baking sheets with parchment paper.

Layer half the eggplant slices and all the zucchini slices in a single layer on the prepared baking sheets. Bake for 15 to 20 minutes until tender. Remove and set aside.

While the eggplant and zucchini are baking, add 3 inches of water to a medium pot and insert a steaming basket. Add the potatoes, cover, and steam for 20 to 25 minutes until soft. Remove and place the potatoes in a large bowl together with the onion powder and garlic powder. Mash until smooth. Set aside.

To make the sauce, place a large ceramic nonstick skillet on medium-high heat. Add the mushrooms, onion, sun-dried tomatoes, celery, and garlic. Cook for 5 to 8 minutes until the mushrooms are soft and browned. Add the tomatoes, thyme, oregano, and red pepper flakes. Add the optional sea salt if using. Lower the heat and cook for 10 to 12 minutes, stirring occasionally, until the sauce is thick.

Add a layer of cooked zucchini and eggplant to the bottom of a medium lasagna dish, overlapping slightly. Top with half of the potato mash, spreading it out evenly, followed by half the tomato sauce. Repeat with another layer of eggplant and zucchini slices, followed by the tomato sauce, and finish with the mashed potatoes on top. Arrange the remaining raw tomato and leftover raw eggplant slices on top. Bake for 30 to 35 minutes until lightly browned on top. Cool for 10 to 15 minutes before slicing.

*For the mushrooms, wash and rinse thoroughly with warm to hot water before slicing. Do not use slimy or decaying mushrooms. That's a sign of oxidizing and aging.

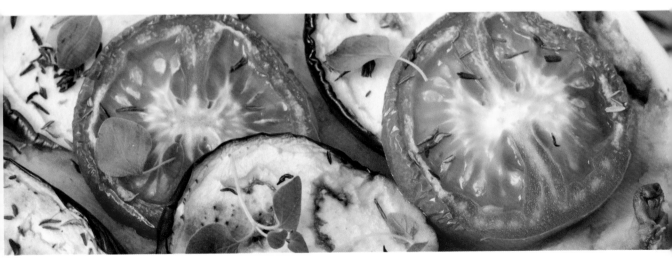

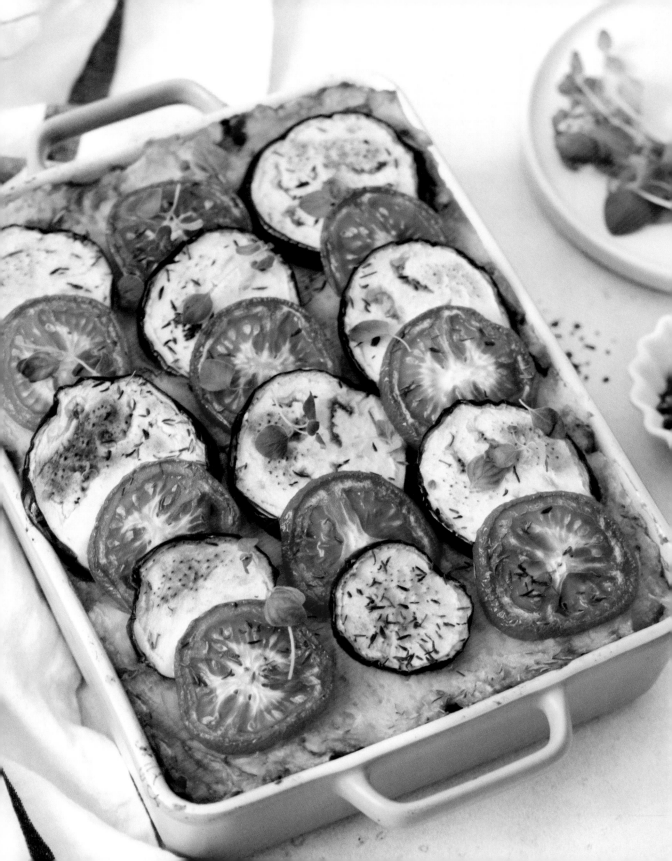

60. EMPANADAS

These gluten-free and grain-free Empanadas are made with a potato dough that's baked until golden. With a savory tomato filling with optional black beans, you may find these empanadas keep you coming back for more!

1 pound potatoes (any variety; e.g. Yukon gold), peeled and roughly chopped
¾ to 1 cup potato starch, more if needed

FOR THE FILLING

½ cup finely chopped onions
½ cup finely chopped red, yellow, or orange bell pepper
¼ cup finely chopped tomato
¼ cup black beans (optional)
½ teaspoon ground cumin
½ teaspoon paprika
½ teaspoon garlic powder
¼ teaspoon chipotle powder
1 tablespoon finely chopped fresh cilantro
1 teaspoon freshly squeezed lime juice

Add 3 inches of water to a medium pot, insert a steaming basket, add the potatoes, and cover. Steam the potatoes for 20 to 25 minutes until soft. Place in a bowl and mash until smooth. Add the potato starch and knead until you get a soft dough that's not sticky. Add more starch if necessary.

While the potatoes are steaming, make the filling by placing a ceramic nonstick skillet on medium-high heat. Add the onions and cook for 3 to 5 minutes until softened. Add the bell peppers, tomato, black beans (if using), cumin, paprika, garlic powder, and chipotle powder. Cook for a further 5 to 8 minutes until the peppers and beans are soft. Stir in the cilantro and lime juice. Remove from the heat and set aside.

Preheat the oven to 400°F/200°C. Line a large baking sheet with parchment paper.

To make the empanadas, sprinkle potato starch generously onto a work surface and roll out the dough to about ¼ inch thick. Cut circles about 4 inches in diameter. One at a time, place each circle on the prepared baking sheet and place 1 to 2 tablespoons of filling onto the dough. Gently fold one side of the dough over the filling and seal the empanada by gently pressing the edges together with a fork. Pinch the dough together if there are any cracks. Repeat with the remaining dough and filling.

Bake the empanadas for 25 to 30 minutes until browned on top. Cool for 5 minutes before serving.

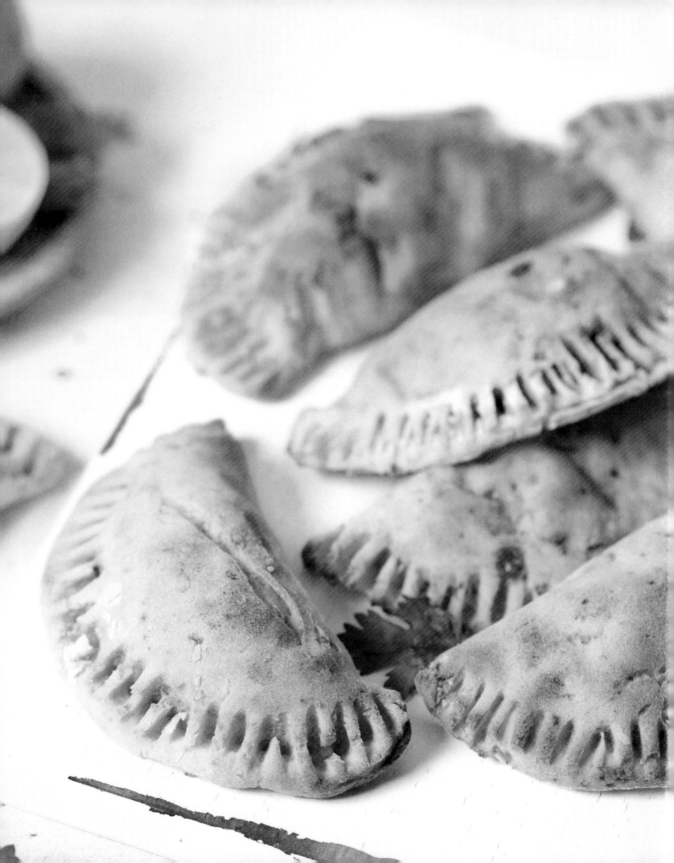

61. FALAFEL WAFFLES

Makes 2 to 3 servings

These savory waffles are cooked until golden and topped with a naturally creamy pureed cauliflower sauce. Cherry tomatoes and cucumber add freshness and juiciness.

1 pound potatoes, diced
¾ cup cooked chickpeas
3 tablespoons chickpea flour
¼ cup loosely packed fresh parsley and/or cilantro leaves, roughly chopped, plus more to serve
1 teaspoon ground cumin
1 teaspoon ground coriander
1 teaspoon garlic powder
1 teaspoon freshly squeezed lemon juice
1 teaspoon pure maple syrup
1 cup roughly chopped cherry tomatoes and/or sliced cucumber, to serve
½ teaspoon red pepper flakes (optional), to serve

FOR THE CAULIFLOWER SAUCE

2 cups cauliflower florets
1 teaspoon garlic powder
1 teaspoon onion powder
¼ teaspoon paprika
1 tablespoon freshly squeezed lemon juice
1 tablespoon water or 3 tablespoons unsweetened almond or coconut milk, more if needed

Add 3 inches of water to a medium pot, insert a steaming basket, add the potatoes, and cover. Steam for 15 to 20 minutes until the potatoes are tender when pierced with a fork. Remove and cool completely.

Add the potatoes to a large bowl together with the chickpeas, chickpea flour, parsley or cilantro, cumin, coriander, garlic powder, lemon juice, and maple syrup. Mash with a potato masher until combined and lump-free.

Heat a ceramic nonstick waffle machine to high heat. Place the mash onto the base of the waffle machine, making sure the base is evenly covered; then close the machine and cook until the waffle is crispy, 10 to 15 minutes. Repeat with the remaining mash.

To make the sauce, steam the cauliflower florets for 4 to 8 minutes until tender. Place in a blender or food processor together with the garlic powder, onion powder, paprika, lemon juice, and water or almond or coconut milk. Blend until smooth. Serve the waffles immediately with the sauce, cherry tomatoes, cucumber, red pepper flakes (if using), and fresh cilantro.

TIPS

- For a creamier and more indulgent recipe, make the cauliflower sauce with the almond or coconut milk option. For a fat-free recipe, use water only in the sauce.

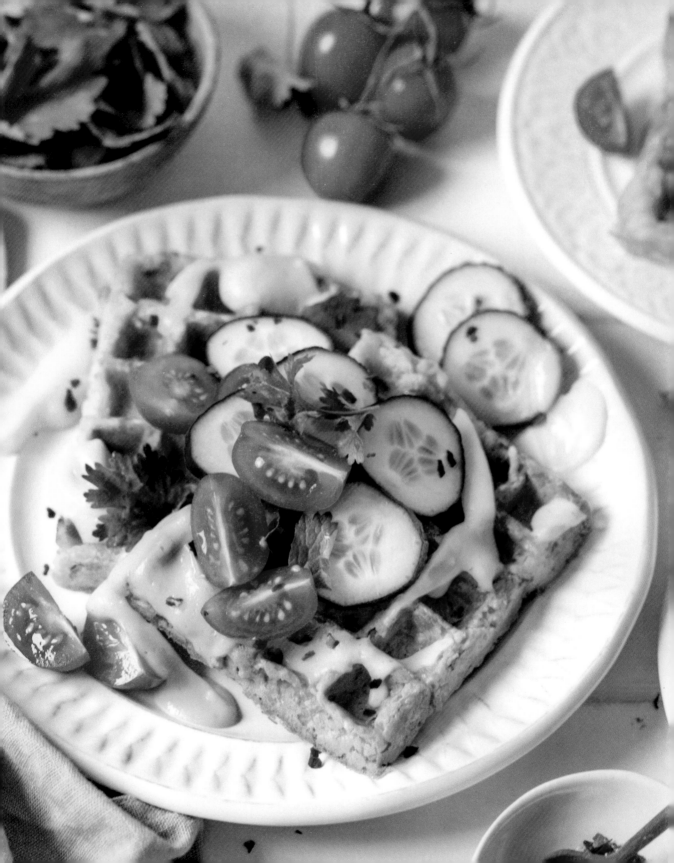

62. ZUCCHINI PIZZA BOATS

Makes 2 servings

Roasted zucchini is the base for pizza sauce and roasted toppings in this delicious recipe. You'll find this recipe helps satisfy a pizza craving while keeping you moving forward with your healing.

4 medium zucchini

FOR THE PIZZA SAUCE

½ cup tomato paste
1 teaspoon dried oregano
½ teaspoon dried thyme
1 teaspoon raw honey
⅓ cup water

FOR THE TOPPINGS

¼ cup thinly sliced onion
½ cup cherry tomatoes, halved
¼ cup olives (oil-free and citric acid–free), pitted and sliced in half lengthwise (optional)
4 to 5 sun-dried tomatoes, roughly chopped
¼ cup diced red bell pepper
4 button mushrooms, thinly sliced*
1 teaspoon red pepper flakes (optional)
¼ cup thinly sliced fresh basil, to serve

Preheat the oven to 400°F/200°C. Line a baking sheet with parchment paper.

Trim the ends off each zucchini; then cut in half lengthwise. Carefully scoop out the flesh from the center of each half to form a cavity. Place each half, cut side up, on the baking sheet. Discard the flesh or set aside to use in other dishes.

Make the pizza sauce by mixing together the tomato paste, oregano, thyme, raw honey, and water. Divide the pizza sauce between the zucchini halves and add different topping combinations to each.

Bake for 20 to 25 minutes until the zucchini is tender but not mushy. Sprinkle zucchini boats with fresh basil and serve.

*For the mushrooms, wash and rinse thoroughly with warm to hot water before slicing. Do not use slimy or decaying mushrooms. That's a sign of oxidizing and aging.

TIPS

- For a fat-free recipe, omit the olives. If you do choose to include olives, look for sun-dried botija olives or another variety that doesn't contain oil, citric acid, or table salt.

- Look for a tomato paste that contains only tomatoes and no other ingredients, such as salt or citric acid.

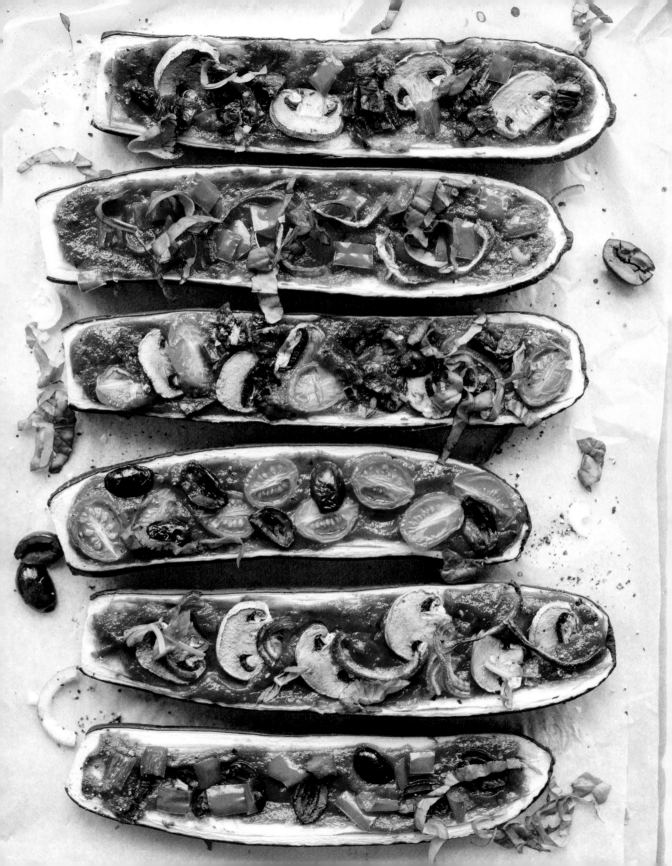

63. BUTTERNUT POTATO HASH

Makes 2 to 3 servings

Fresh herbs complement the potatoes and naturally sweet butternut squash in this hash. This recipe is simple, easy to make, and flavorful. Enjoy it for any meal of the day, for a snack, or as a side along with any other recipe of your choosing.

½ cup diced onion
3 cups diced potato
3 cups peeled and diced butternut squash
2 tablespoons fresh thyme or 2 teaspoons dried
2 tablespoons chopped fresh rosemary or 1 teaspoon dried
2 teaspoons garlic powder
2 teaspoons paprika
½ cup Healing Broth (recipe on page 370) or water
1 tablespoon freshly squeezed lemon juice
1 tablespoon chopped fresh parsley leaves

Place a ceramic nonstick skillet on medium-high heat. Add the onion and cook for 3 to 5 minutes until soft, adding a bit of water if needed to prevent sticking.

Add the potatoes, butternut squash, thyme, rosemary, garlic powder, paprika, and Healing Broth or water to the pan. Stir until evenly mixed, then cover, turn the heat to low, and simmer for 10 to 15 minutes until the potatoes and butternut squash are tender. Uncover and cook until all the liquid has evaporated and the potatoes and squash are slightly browned.

Stir in the lemon juice and parsley. Remove from the heat and divide between two or three bowls. Serve immediately.

TIPS

- When you're choosing between Healing Broth and water for the ingredients, keep in mind that the broth will produce a richer flavor. Store-bought vegetable stock isn't called for because it's very difficult to find a variety that's free of oil, salt, natural flavors, and/or other additives. For convenience, make a batch of Healing Broth in advance and freeze it (consider pouring into ice cube trays for easy thawing) so you have it on hand for recipes like this.

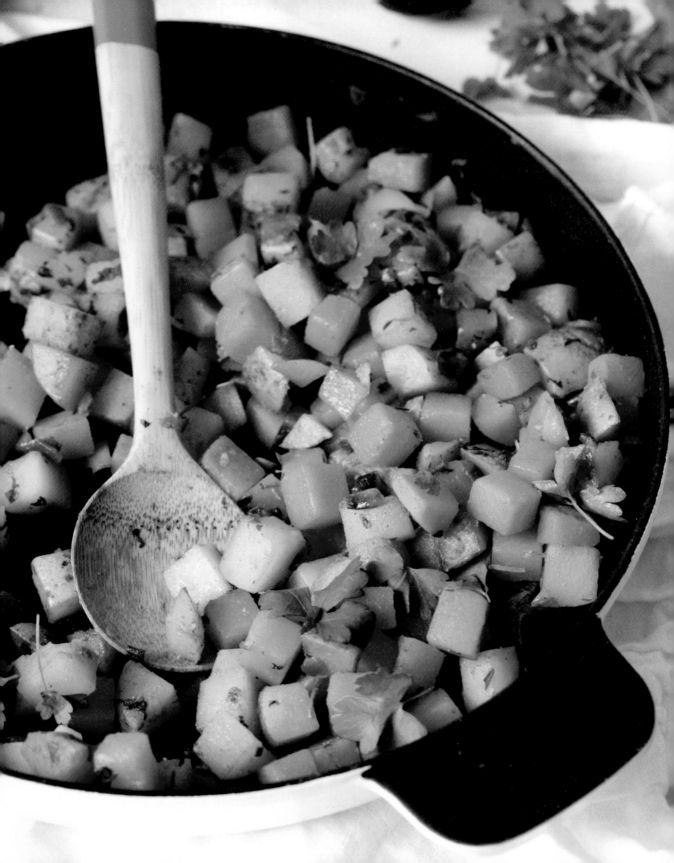

64. EGGPLANT BACON

Makes 2 servings, about 20 bacon strips

Marinated in spices, maple syrup, lemon juice, and tomato paste, these crispy strips of eggplant can be enjoyed alone or used in your favorite recipes for some exra flavor, texture, and depth.

1 tablespoon pure maple syrup
1 tablespoon freshly squeezed
   lemon juice
1 teaspoon tomato paste
½ teaspoon garlic powder
½ teaspoon paprika
½ teaspoon onion powder
⅛ teaspoon chipotle powder,
   or more to taste
1 medium eggplant

Preheat the oven to 250°F/120°C. Line a large baking sheet with parchment paper.

Whisk together the maple syrup, lemon juice, tomato paste, garlic powder, paprika, onion powder, and chipotle powder in a small bowl. Set aside.

Cut off the ends of the eggplant, then slice lengthways into quarters. Lay each quarter down flat on a sturdy surface and use a sharp knife to cut the eggplant quarter into slices as thin as possible. You can also use a mandolin.

Arrange the eggplant slices on the prepared baking sheet and brush the marinade on top. Flip and brush the other side as well.

Bake for 40 to 60 minutes, flipping the slices halfway, until crispy. Keep an eye on them for the last 10 minutes to make sure they don't burn. Alternatively, you can dehydrate them at 285°F/140°C for 4 to 6 hours, or until crispy.

Cool the strips completely on a wire rack after baking. Store in an airtight container at room temperature for 3 to 4 days.

TIPS

- You can enjoy the eggplant bacon in long strips or break them up into pieces that you can use in other recipes, such as the Cobb Salad (recipe on page 360) and Spaghetti Carbonara (recipe on page 443), or in any other recipe you wish.

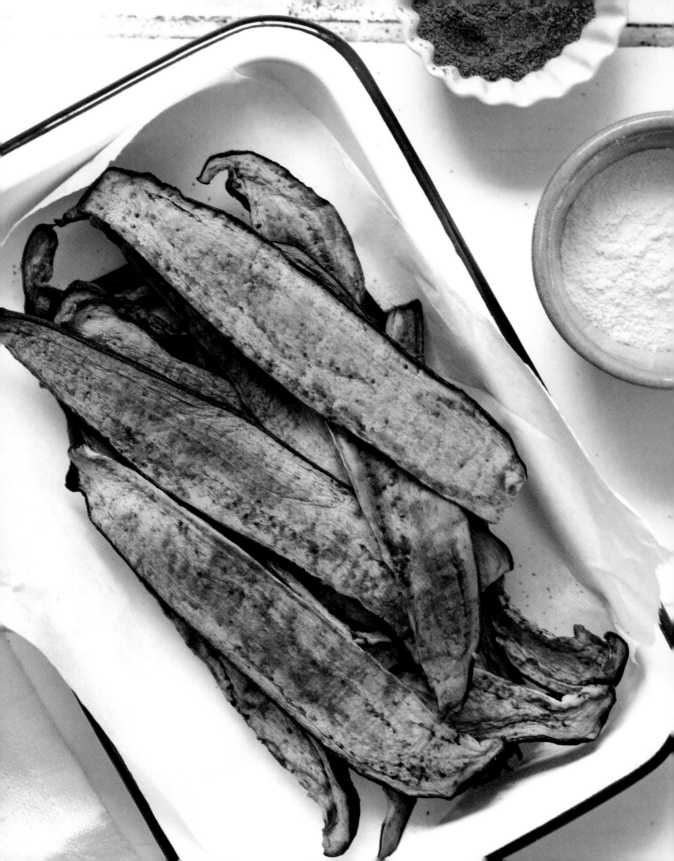

65. LOADED CRINKLE-CUT FRIES

Makes 2 servings

These fun crinkle-cut fries are loaded with all the goodies: creamy potato-based nacho cheese sauce, crispy eggplant-bacon bites, optional black beans, juicy tomato, spicy jalapeño, and fresh green onions. Every bite offers texture and flavor to enjoy! Serve these fries already fully loaded or put each ingredient in its own bowl and let everyone build their own loaded fries. They'll be a hit either way!

2 pounds potatoes (4 to 5 potatoes)
1 teaspoon paprika
1 teaspoon garlic powder
1 teaspoon onion powder
1 teaspoon dried oregano
4 to 5 eggplant-bacon slices, chopped into bites, to serve (recipe on page 430)
1 cup diced tomato, to serve
1 to 2 tablespoons red jalapeño slices, to serve
½ cup cooked black beans, to serve (optional)
¼ cup chopped green onions, to serve

FOR THE NACHO CHEESE SAUCE

1½ cups diced potato
1 cup diced carrot
½ teaspoon garlic powder
½ teaspoon onion powder
½ teaspoon cayenne
¼ teaspoon ground turmeric
1 tablespoon freshly squeezed lemon or lime juice
1 to 2 tablespoons water, to desired thickness

Preheat the oven to 400°F/200°C. Line a large baking sheet with parchment paper. Using a crinkle cutter, cut the potatoes into slices; then cut them into individual fries.

Place the fries in a large bowl and add the seasonings and oregano. Toss until evenly coated.

Spread the fries on the prepared baking sheet and bake for 20 to 30 minutes, flipping halfway, until crispy. Alternatively, you can make these in an air fryer at 400°F/200°C for 20 to 25 minutes, tossing the potatoes every 5 minutes until crispy.

While the potatoes are baking, make the sauce. Add 3 inches of water to a medium pot and insert a steaming basket. Add the diced potato and carrot, cover, and steam for 15 to 20 minutes until soft. Transfer to a blender or food processor together with the garlic powder, onion powder, cayenne, turmeric, and lemon or lime juice. Blend until very smooth, adding a tiny bit of water if needed.

Arrange the fries on a platter or individual plates and top with the nacho cheese sauce, eggplant-bacon bites, diced tomato, red jalapeño slices, black beans (if using), and green onions. Serve immediately.

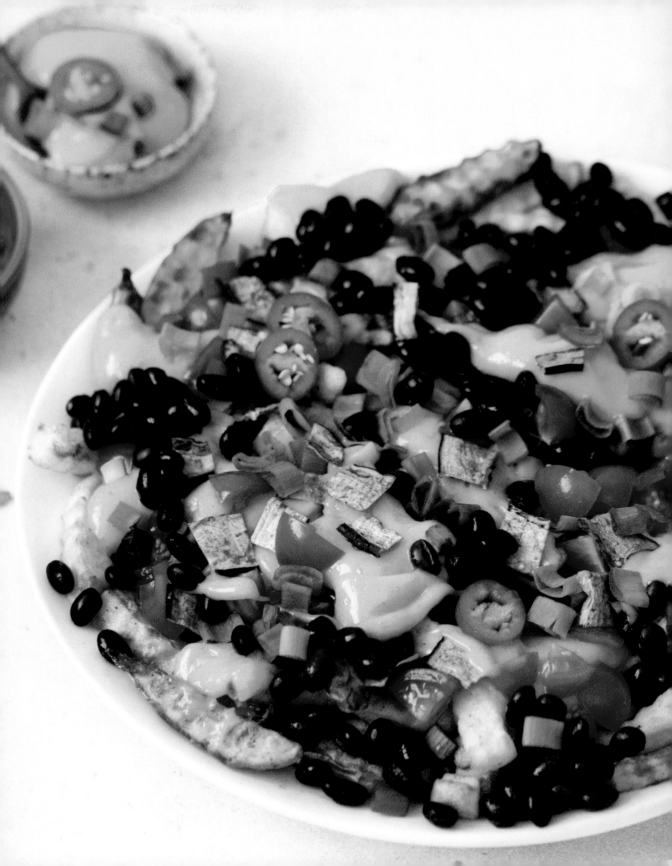

66. SWEET CHILI BROCCOLI

Makes 2 servings

This Sweet Chili Broccoli makes a perfect side dish. Coated in a spicy-sweet sauce, it's a great way to get some extra produce into your diet, and it works not only for broccoli but also for other vegetables of your choice, such as cauliflower, asparagus, or brussels sprouts.

1 large head of broccoli, cut into florets

FOR THE SAUCE

2 tablespoons tomato paste
½ cup orange juice
¼ cup raw honey
¼ cup freshly squeezed lime juice
1 tablespoon chopped ripe hot peppers of choice
1 tablespoon onion powder
2 teaspoons finely grated fresh ginger
2 garlic cloves, finely grated
½ teaspoon cayenne
½ teaspoon Atlantic dulse flakes
2 teaspoons arrowroot powder or potato starch

Add 3 inches of water to a medium pot and insert a steaming basket. Add the broccoli, cover, and steam until bright green and tender, 5 to 8 minutes. Remove from the heat and set aside.

Whisk together all the sauce ingredients in a small saucepan. Place on medium-high heat and cook, stirring often, until thick. Stir in the broccoli and remove from the heat. Serve immediately.

TIPS

- Look for a tomato paste that contains only tomatoes and no other ingredients, such as salt or citric acid.

- Depending on which variety of hot pepper you choose, you will need to adjust how much you use according to your tastes.

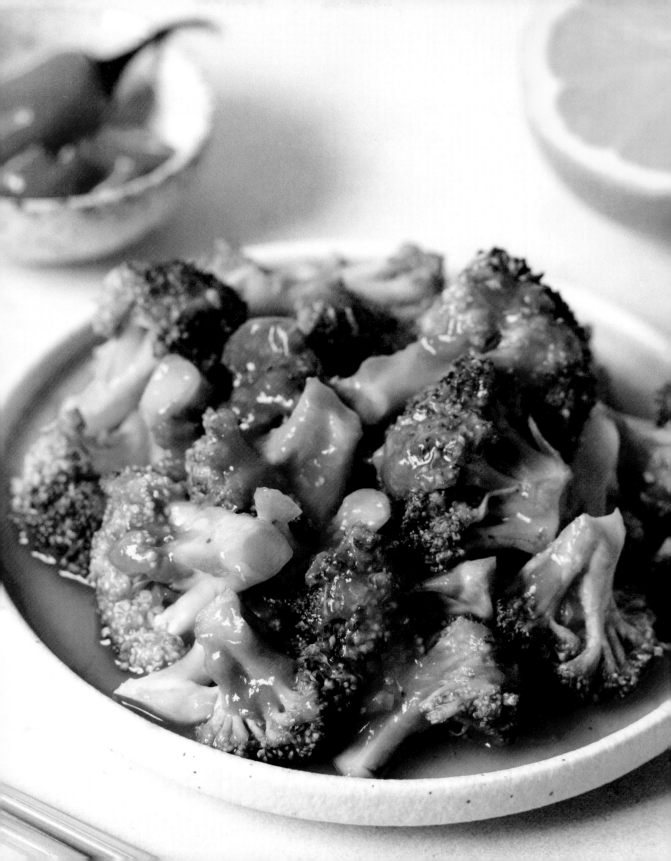

67. NIÇOISE SALAD

Fresh and bright, this attractive salad offers a bit of everything: tender greens, crunchy radishes, juicy tomatoes, creamy potatoes, succulent green beans, savory olives, and fragrant fresh herbs—all covered in a slightly sweet, slightly tangy dressing.

1 pound baby potatoes, halved
1 cup green beans, trimmed
4 cups tightly packed leafy greens, such as mâche, arugula, or butter lettuce
1½ cups cherry tomatoes, halved
½ cup thinly sliced radish
¼ cup pitted olives (oil-free and citric acid–free; optional)
¼ cup loosely packed basil leaves, roughly chopped
2 tablespoons loosely packed fresh thyme leaves

FOR THE DRESSING

2 tablespoons freshly squeezed lemon juice
1½ tablespoons raw honey
1 teaspoon fresh thyme leaves or ½ teaspoon dried
¼ teaspoon mustard powder
½ tablespoon finely chopped shallots (optional)

Add 3 inches of water to a medium pot, insert a steaming basket, add the potatoes, and cover. Steam for 15 to 18 minutes until tender. Remove the potatoes and cool.

Add 3 inches of water to a medium pot, insert a steaming basket, add the green beans, and cover. Steam for 4 to 5 minutes until bright green and tender. Remove and cool.

Whisk together all the ingredients for the dressing.

Arrange the leafy greens, potatoes, green beans, cherry tomatoes, radishes, olives (if using), basil, and thyme on plates. Drizzle the dressing over the salad and serve.

TIPS

- For a fat-free recipe, omit the olives. If you do choose to include the olives, look for sun-dried botija olives or another variety that doesn't contain any oil, citric acid, or table salt.

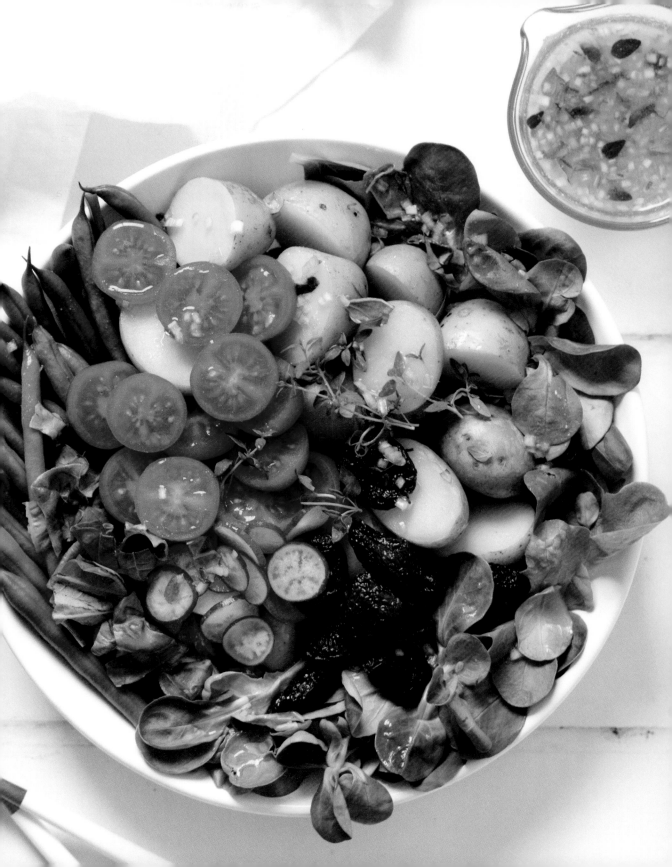

68. POTATO AND CHERRY TOMATO BAKE

Makes 4 servings

This simple bake is both pretty and tasty. It is a wonderful side dish when you want an alternative to mashed potatoes, whether it's for a holiday meal, lunch or dinner with family or friends, or a simple but yummy meal for yourself.

2½ pounds potatoes, roughly chopped
1 tablespoon onion powder
2 teaspoons garlic powder
½ tablespoon freshly squeezed lemon juice
1 teaspoon fresh thyme or 1 teaspoon dried
1 teaspoon fresh oregano or 1 teaspoon dried
1 teaspoon raw honey
2 cups cherry tomatoes, halved

Preheat the oven to 350°F/180°C.

Add 3 inches of water to a medium pot, insert a steaming basket, add the potatoes, and cover. Steam for 15 to 18 minutes until tender. Cool for 10 minutes.

Place the potatoes in a large bowl together with the onion powder, garlic powder, lemon juice, thyme, oregano, and raw honey. Mash until almost smooth (some bigger chunks are okay).

Place the mashed potatoes in a 10-inch quiche pan or baking dish of a similar size. Press the tomato halves evenly on top.

Bake for 50 to 55 minutes until browned on top. Cool for 10 minutes before serving.

TIPS

- This bake is not meant to be sliced; it won't hold its shape. The best way to serve this dish is to scoop out spoonfuls of the bake.

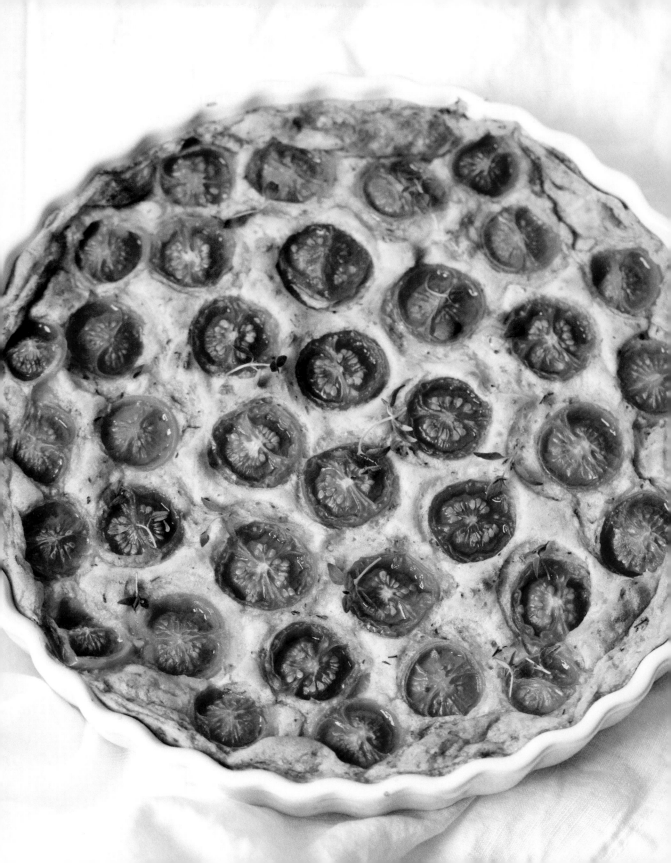

69. MUSHROOM AND HERB MILLET RISOTTO

If you're a fan of risotto, try this upgraded version made with millet, which is a superior grain to rice for someone who is working on healing. It's also a tasty grain with a slightly nutty flavor. Mushrooms, onions, garlic, and herbs add healing nutrients and flavor to this meal that is best enjoyed for dinner alongside a leafy green salad.

1 medium onion, finely chopped

1½ cups thinly sliced mushrooms*

2 garlic cloves, finely chopped

1 cup millet

1 teaspoon paprika

1 tablespoon fresh thyme or
  1 teaspoon dried

1 tablespoon fresh oregano
  or 1 teaspoon dried

3 to 4 cups Healing Broth (recipe on
  page 370) or water

1 cup loosely packed fresh parsley
  and/or basil, finely chopped

¼ teaspoon sea salt (optional)

Place a large ceramic nonstick pot on medium-high heat. Add the onion and mushrooms and cook for 3 to 5 minutes until softened.

Add the garlic and cook for another 2 to 3 minutes. Reduce the heat to medium-low.

Add the millet, paprika, thyme, oregano, and 1 cup of Healing Broth or water. Stir until evenly mixed. Cook for 17 to 20 minutes, stirring every few minutes and adding more Healing Broth or water as needed.

When the millet is cooked, stir in the fresh parsley or basil. Add the sea salt if using and stir.

Serve immediately.

*For the mushrooms, wash and rinse thoroughly with warm to hot water before slicing. Do not use slimy or decaying mushrooms. That's a sign of oxidizing and aging.

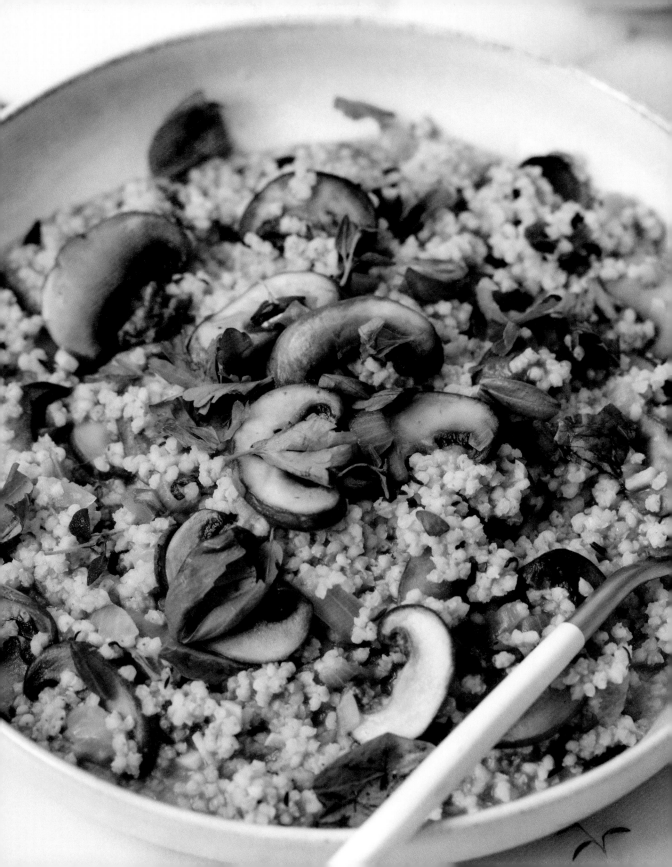

TIPS

- When you're choosing between Healing Broth and water for the ingredients, keep in mind that the broth will produce a richer flavor. Store-bought vegetable stock isn't called for because it's very difficult to find a variety that's free of oil, salt, natural flavors, and/or other additives. For convenience, make a batch of Healing Broth in advance and freeze it (consider pouring into ice cube trays for easy thawing) so you have it on hand for recipes like this.

- While high-quality sea salt or mountain rock salt is an optional inclusion in this recipe, the recipe is more healing without salt. Over time, you may wish to reduce or exclude the salt.

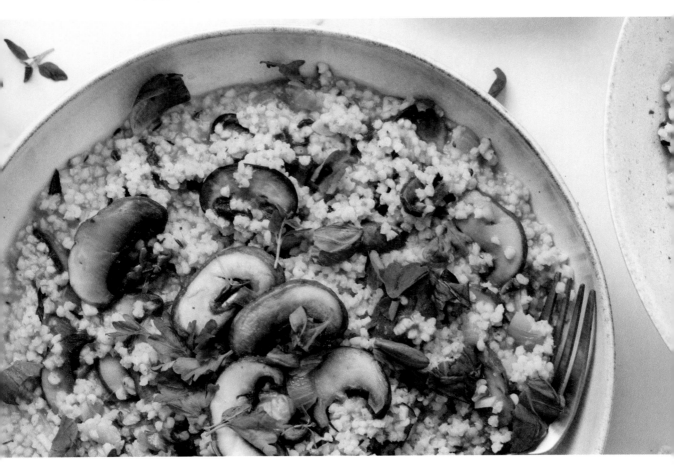

70. SPAGHETTI CARBONARA

Makes 2 to 4 servings

This creamy pasta dish is so satisfying and delicious! There are so many cleaner pasta options now that you can pair with a fantastic sauce made only with healthy ingredients, such as this carbonara sauce. If you love your pasta, you don't have to go without!

4 cups roughly chopped potatoes
4 cups cauliflower florets
12 ounces gluten-free, corn-free spaghetti
2 tablespoons onion powder
2 teaspoons garlic powder
½ teaspoon paprika
½ teaspoon grated lemon zest
2 tablespoons freshly squeezed
  lemon juice
¼ to ½ teaspoon sea salt (optional)
1 cup fresh or frozen green peas (optional)
8 to 10 pieces of eggplant bacon, finely
  chopped (recipe on page 430)
3 tablespoons finely chopped fresh parsley

Add 3 inches of water to a medium pot, insert a steaming basket, add the potatoes, and cover. Steam for 10 minutes. Add the cauliflower to the steaming basket and continue steaming for a further 8 to 10 minutes until both the potatoes and cauliflower are tender.

While the vegetables are steaming, cook the pasta according to package instructions. Drain and place back in pot.

Once the vegetables are tender, remove them from the heat and place in a food processor along with the onion powder, garlic powder, paprika, lemon zest, and lemon juice. Add the sea salt if using. Process until smooth.

If using peas, steam them separately for 3 to 5 minutes until bright green and tender.

Pour the sauce onto the pasta and stir until evenly coated. Add the peas (if using) to the pasta, together with the eggplant bacon and chopped parsley. Stir until evenly mixed.

Divide between two to four bowls and serve immediately.

TIPS

- Look for pasta that is grain-free, such as cassava, pea, lentil, or chickpea pasta. Alternatively, a gluten-free pasta that is made with grains such as millet, quinoa, or brown rice is also an option. Be sure to check that your pasta does not contain corn or egg.

- While high-quality sea salt or mountain rock salt is an optional inclusion in this recipe, the recipe is more healing without salt. Over time, you may wish to reduce or exclude the salt.

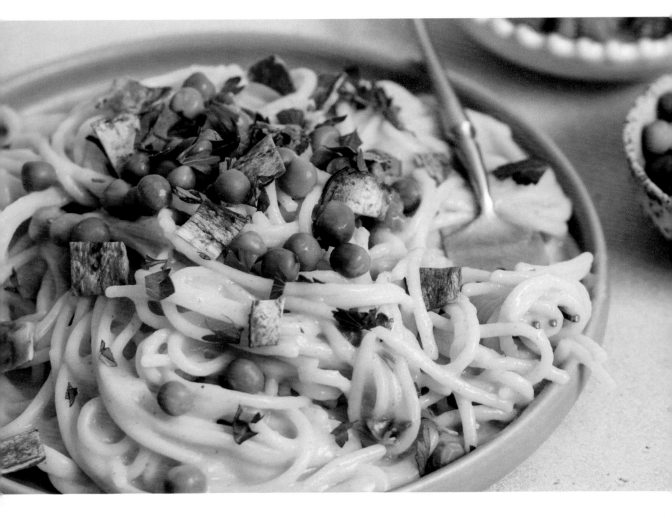

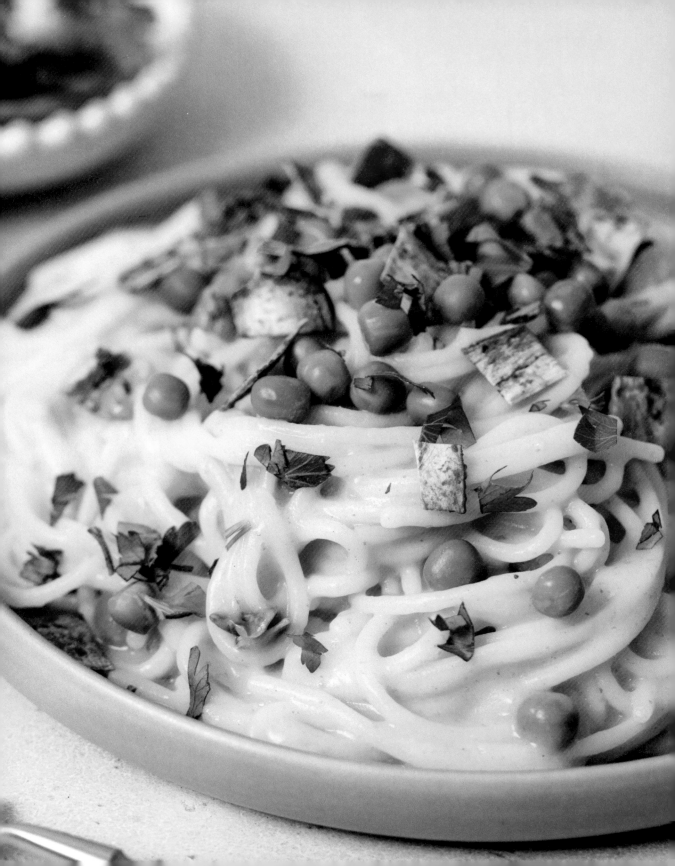

71. CURRIED POTATO, PEA, AND CILANTRO HASH

Makes 2 servings

Potato hash recipes can be as versatile as you'd like them to be. This recipe harnesses the flavors of curry spices and combines them with potatoes, peas, tomato, and fresh cilantro to make an aromatic and satiating dish.

½ cup diced onion
3 garlic cloves, finely chopped
2 teaspoons curry powder
1 teaspoon cumin seeds or ground cumin
1 teaspoon ground coriander
¼ to ½ teaspoon chili powder or cayenne
¼ teaspoon ground turmeric
4 cups diced potatoes
¼ cup diced tomato
1 cup water
1 teaspoon raw honey
1 cup fresh or thawed frozen peas
¼ cup loosely packed chopped cilantro leaves, plus more to serve
Cayenne or red pepper flakes, for garnish
1 tablespoon freshly squeezed lemon juice, to serve

Place a ceramic nonstick skillet on medium-high heat. Add the onion and cook for 3 to 5 minutes until soft, adding a bit of water if needed to prevent sticking.

Add the garlic, curry powder, cumin, coriander, chili powder or cayenne, and turmeric to the pan. Cook for a further 1 to 2 minutes until the spices are fragrant.

Add the potatoes, tomato, and water to the pan. Stir until evenly mixed, then cover, turn the heat to low, and simmer for 10 to 15 minutes until the potatoes are almost tender.

Stir in the raw honey, peas, and cilantro. Cook for 3 to 5 minutes until the peas are tender.

Divide the hash between two bowls and top with cayenne or red pepper flakes, a squeeze of lemon juice, and more cilantro. Serve immediately.

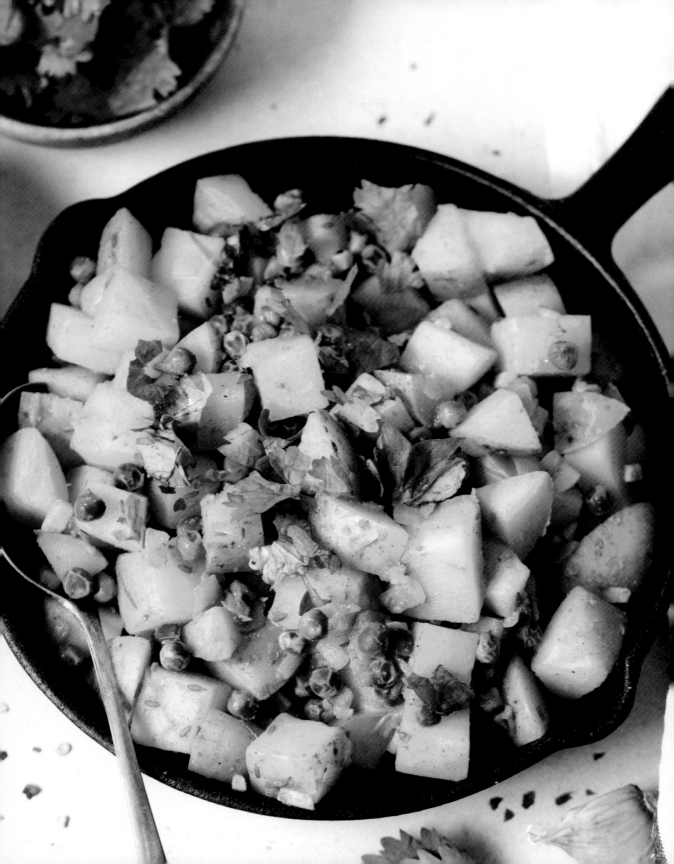

72. BLACK BEAN POTATO SOFT TACOS

Makes 2 servings

Stuffed with salsa, sautéed black beans, and bell peppers, and topped off with fresh cilantro and green onions, these tacos will hit the spot! The taco shells are made out of potatoes, making them the perfect healing substitute for conventional taco shells.

FOR THE SOFT TACO SHELLS

2 cups roughly chopped gold potatoes
½ teaspoon garlic powder
½ teaspoon onion powder
1 teaspoon pure maple syrup

FOR THE FILLING

½ cup cooked black beans
½ teaspoon garlic powder
½ teaspoon onion powder
¼ teaspoon chipotle powder
1 tablespoon tomato paste
1 teaspoon freshly squeezed lime juice
1 cup thinly sliced red, yellow, or orange
   bell peppers
2 to 3 tablespoons fresh cilantro leaves,
   to serve
1 to 2 tablespoons chopped green onion,
   to serve

FOR THE SALSA

1 cup diced tomato
¼ cup red, yellow, or white onion, finely
   chopped
¼ cup loosely packed cilantro leaves, finely
   chopped
1 tablespoon freshly squeezed lime juice
½ garlic clove, finely minced
1 teaspoon finely chopped ripe hot
   pepper of your choice
½ teaspoon ground cumin (optional)

TIPS

- Look for a tomato paste that contains only tomatoes and no other ingredients, such as salt or citric acid.

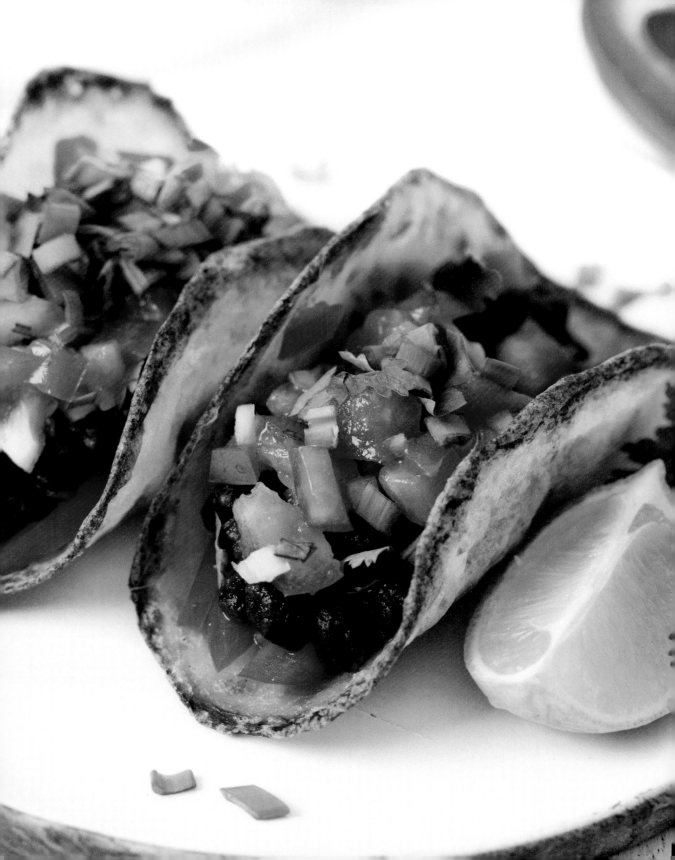

Preheat the oven to 400°F/200°C.

To make the taco shells, add 3 inches of water to a medium pot, insert a steaming basket, add the potatoes, and cover. Once the water is boiling, steam the potatoes for 20 to 25 minutes until soft. Remove the potatoes and place them in a food processor with the garlic powder, onion powder, and maple syrup. Blend until smooth.

Line a baking sheet with parchment paper. Spoon out the potato mixture, making 3 or 4 dollops. Spread each dollop with a wet spatula to make 3 or 4 mini tortillas. Bake in the oven for 15 to 20 minutes until lightly browned. Remove and pat down with the spatula. Flip the parchment paper over onto a cutting board and gently peel back. Set the taco shells aside.

Add the cooked black beans, garlic powder, onion powder, chipotle powder, tomato paste, and lime juice to a small saucepan. Cook on medium-low heat for 3 to 5 minutes until the beans are soft. Add a bit of water if the mixture sticks to the pot.

To make the salsa, combine all the ingredients in a small bowl and mix well.

Fill the soft taco shells with the bell peppers, black beans, salsa, cilantro, and green onion. Serve immediately.

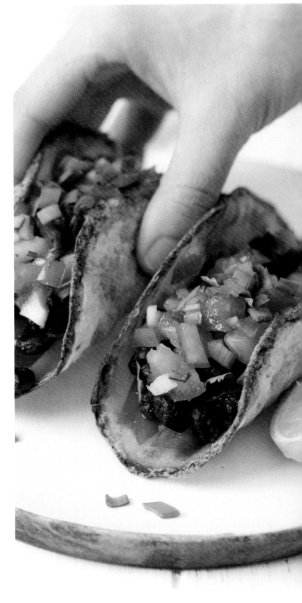

73. PHO

This Pho will entice you with the aroma alone: toasted spices; broiled onions, garlic, and ginger; fresh herbs; shiitake mushrooms; and zucchini or potato noodles held in a savory broth finished with a squeeze of lime juice and chopped hot pepper. If you like a flavorful soup, this one might just do the trick! Pho makes for a great snack or light meal.

FOR THE BROTH

2 medium onions, peeled and sliced into 1-inch-thick rounds
1 to 2 2-inch pieces of ginger, sliced in half lengthwise
5 garlic cloves
2 to 3 cinnamon sticks
2 pods star anise
5 to 6 cardamom pods
1 tablespoon coriander seeds
1 teaspoon fennel seeds
½ teaspoon whole cloves
8 cups Healing Broth (recipe on page 370)
2 cups fresh shiitake mushrooms, stems separated and caps thinly sliced*
1 teaspoon Atlantic dulse flakes
2 tablespoons coconut sugar
½ teaspoon sea salt (optional)
1 zucchini or 3 to 4 potatoes
2 to 3 tablespoons freshly squeezed lime juice, or more to taste

TO SERVE

¼ cup loosely packed, roughly chopped fresh mint leaves
¼ cup loosely packed, roughly chopped fresh cilantro leaves
¼ cup loosely packed, roughly chopped fresh Thai basil or sweet basil
1 to 2 teaspoons chopped ripe hot peppers
4 lime wedges

TIPS

- While high-quality sea salt or mountain rock salt is an optional inclusion in this recipe, the recipe is more healing without salt. Over time, you may wish to reduce or exclude the salt.

Preheat the broiler. Line a baking sheet with parchment paper. Spread the onion, ginger, and garlic in a single layer. Place on the top oven rack and broil/grill until browned, 4 to 8 minutes. Be careful not to burn them.

Place a deep pot on medium-high heat. Add the cinnamon sticks, star anise pods, cardamom pods, coriander seeds, fennel seeds, and cloves and heat for 30 seconds, stirring often. Add the broiled onions, ginger, and garlic together with the Healing Broth, shiitake stems, Atlantic dulse flakes, and coconut sugar. Add the optional sea salt if using. Stir until well combined, then bring to a simmer, cover, and cook for 2 to 6 hours. The longer the broth cooks, the more flavorful it will be.

Prepare the noodles by trimming the ends off the zucchini or by cutting a small piece off both ends of the potatoes. Use a spiralizer to make the noodles.

Once the broth is cooked to your satisfaction, strain the veggies, herbs, and spices from the broth.

Add the sliced shiitake mushroom caps to the broth. If using potato noodles, add them in at this point too. Cook for a further 5 to 6 minutes until the mushrooms and potato noodles are tender. Stir in the lime juice and remove from the heat.

Divide the cooked potato noodles or raw zucchini noodles between bowls and top with the broth, mint, cilantro, basil, chopped ripe hot pepper, and a wedge of lime. Serve immediately. Enjoy!

*For the mushrooms, wash and rinse thoroughly with warm to hot water before slicing. Do not use slimy or decaying mushrooms. That's a sign of oxidizing and aging.

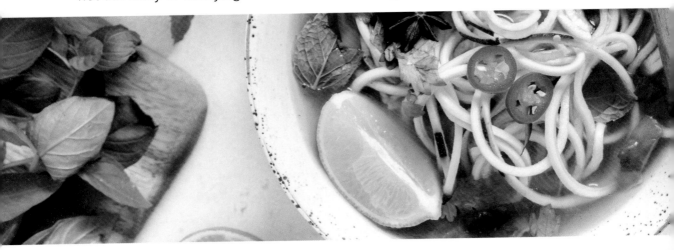

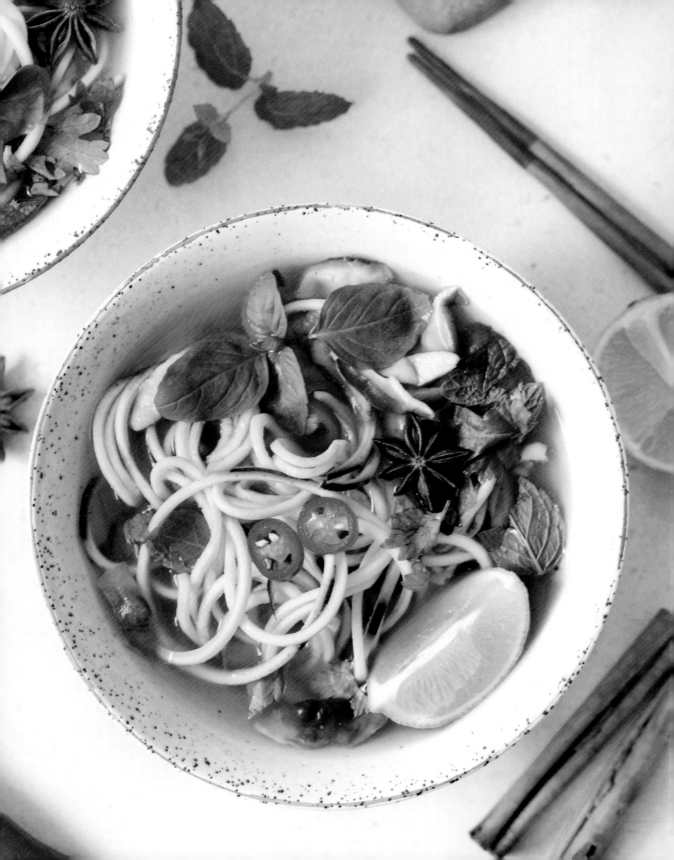

74. CANNELLONI

Packed with flavor, this fat-free, grain-free, and dairy-free version of a favorite Italian recipe is sure to please your taste buds! Baked zucchini takes the place of the cannelloni pasta shells and is stuffed with a creamy potato-based cheese sauce, and then nestled in a bed of a delicious tomato and herb sauce, all topped off with dollops of baked potato cheese.

3 to 4 small zucchinis

FOR THE POTATO CHEESE

3 cups roughly chopped potatoes
1 cup roughly chopped carrots
1 tablespoon onion powder
2 teaspoons garlic powder
1 teaspoon paprika
2 teaspoons dried oregano or basil
1 tablespoon freshly squeezed
   lemon juice

FOR THE TOMATO SAUCE

¼ cup finely chopped yellow onion
3 garlic cloves, finely chopped
1 tablespoon tomato paste
2 cups jarred crushed or diced tomatoes
   or 2 pounds fresh plum or cherry
   tomatoes, roughly chopped
1 teaspoon dried oregano
1 teaspoon dried thyme
½ teaspoon red pepper flakes
¼ cup loosely packed basil leaves,
   to serve

TIPS

- If you prefer the cheese to be firmer, let the cannelloni cool longer than 5 minutes to allow the potato cheese to firm up more. Either way, it tastes delicious!

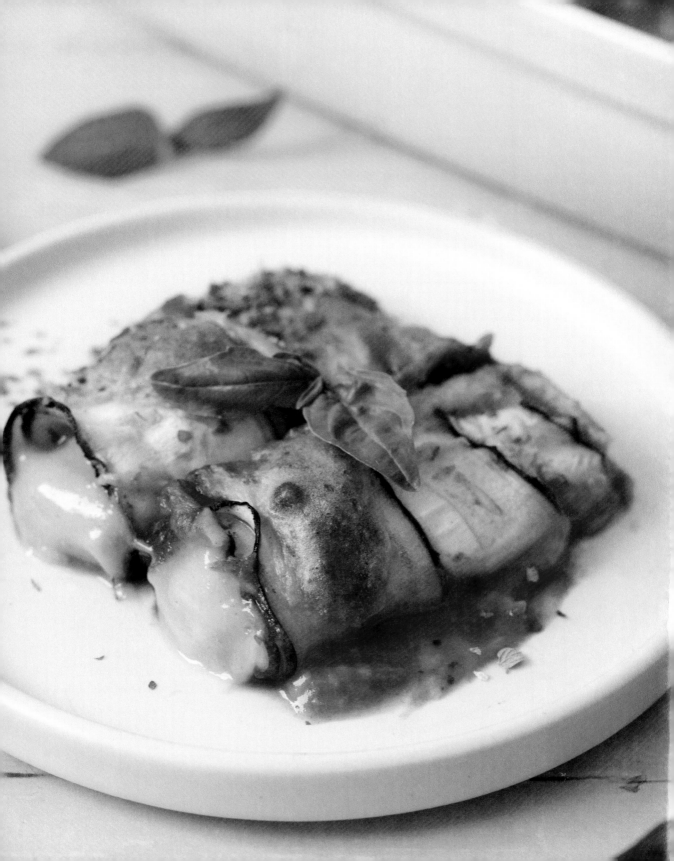

Add 3 inches of water to a medium pot, insert a steaming basket, add the chopped potatoes and carrots, and cover. Steam for 15 to 20 minutes until tender. Remove the potatoes and carrots from the heat and place in a food processor along with the onion powder, garlic powder, paprika, dried oregano or basil, and lemon juice. Process until smooth. If the potato cheese sauce is very runny, transfer it to a bowl, cover lightly with a clean kitchen towel, and set aside at room temperature for 1 to 2 hours to thicken.

Prepare the sauce by placing a ceramic nonstick pot on medium-high heat. Add the onions and cook, stirring occasionally, until very soft, 5 to 8 minutes. Add a bit of water if needed to prevent sticking. Add the garlic and tomato paste, and cook, stirring continuously, until the tomato paste caramelizes and turns dark, 1 to 2 minutes. Add the tomatoes, dried oregano, dried thyme, and red pepper flakes. Stir until evenly mixed. Reduce the heat to low, cover, and simmer gently, stirring occasionally, until the sauce is thick, 30 to 40 minutes. Leave as is, or if you want a smooth sauce, transfer the sauce to a blender or food processor and blend until smooth. Set aside.

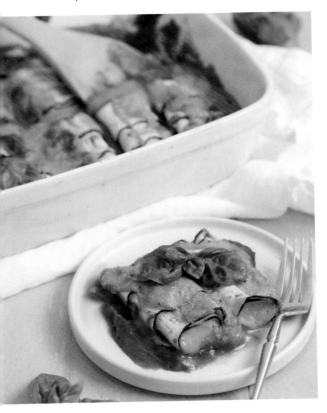

Preheat the oven to 400°F/200°C.

To prepare the zucchini cannelloni, use a Y-shaped vegetable peeler or mandolin slicer to cut thin wide strips of zucchini. Press the zucchini strips between paper towels to remove excess moisture.

Arrange three strips on a cutting board on top of each other, slightly overlapping. Place a heaped tablespoon of the potato cheese sauce on one end and roll up tightly. Set aside. Repeat with the remaining zucchini strips, making 10 to 12 cannelloni in total.

Spread the tomato sauce on the bottom of a large baking dish. Arrange the cannelloni in the tomato sauce; then drizzle or spoon the remaining potato cheese sauce on top.

Place in the oven and bake for 25 to 30 minutes until bubbling along the edges and golden on top. Cool for 5 minutes; then garnish with the basil leaves and serve.

75. MASHED POTATO FRIES

These fries are crispy and so delicious, without using any oil. To make this recipe, you'll need to prepare the potatoes the day before and keep them in the refrigerator overnight, so it's a perfect recipe to use up steamed potatoes that you have left over or that you batch prep each week for easier meals. Enjoy these fantastic fries with the barbecue sauce or ketchup or both!

4 pounds potatoes, roughly chopped
1 tablespoon onion powder
2 teaspoons garlic powder
1 teaspoon paprika
1 teaspoon dried thyme or oregano
Ketchup (recipe on page 395; optional)
Barbecue sauce (optional)

FOR THE BARBECUE SAUCE

6 ounces tomato paste
⅓ cup apple juice
¼ cup pure maple syrup or raw honey
2 tablespoons freshly squeezed lemon juice
1 teaspoon garlic powder
1 teaspoon onion powder
½ teaspoon chipotle powder
¼ teaspoon chili powder
½ teaspoon mustard powder

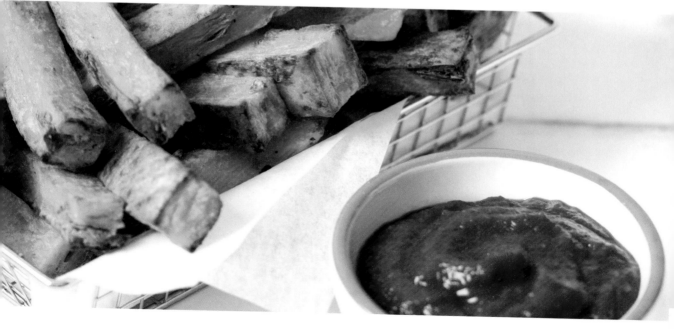

Add 3 inches of water to a medium pot, insert a steaming basket, add the potatoes, and cover. Steam for 15 to 18 minutes until tender. Remove from the heat and cool for 10 minutes; then place them in a large bowl or pot.

Add the onion powder, garlic powder, paprika, and thyme or oregano to the potatoes. Mash with a potato masher until almost smooth; some bigger pieces are okay.

Transfer the mixture to one or two square or rectangular containers, and press the mash down until evenly spread to about 1 inch thick. Cool completely at room temperature, uncovered; then cover and refrigerate overnight.

The next day, preheat the oven to 430°F/220°C. Line a large baking sheet with parchment paper.

Flip the container(s) upside down onto a cutting board. Tap a few times if the mashed potato brick doesn't come loose right away. Cut into chunky fries and transfer to the prepared baking sheet, leaving a bit of space between the fries. Bake for 40 minutes, flip, and then cook for a further 20 to 30 minutes until the fries are browned and crispy all over.

Make the barbecue sauce by whisking together all the ingredients until smooth. Serve fries immediately with the sauce or ketchup. Enjoy!

TIPS

- Potatoes are so versatile as an ingredient in healing meals that you may wish to steam enough potatoes at one time to last a few days or a week so they are ready in the fridge to be added to salads or used in potato hash, soups, these fries, or any of the other Medical Medium recipes.

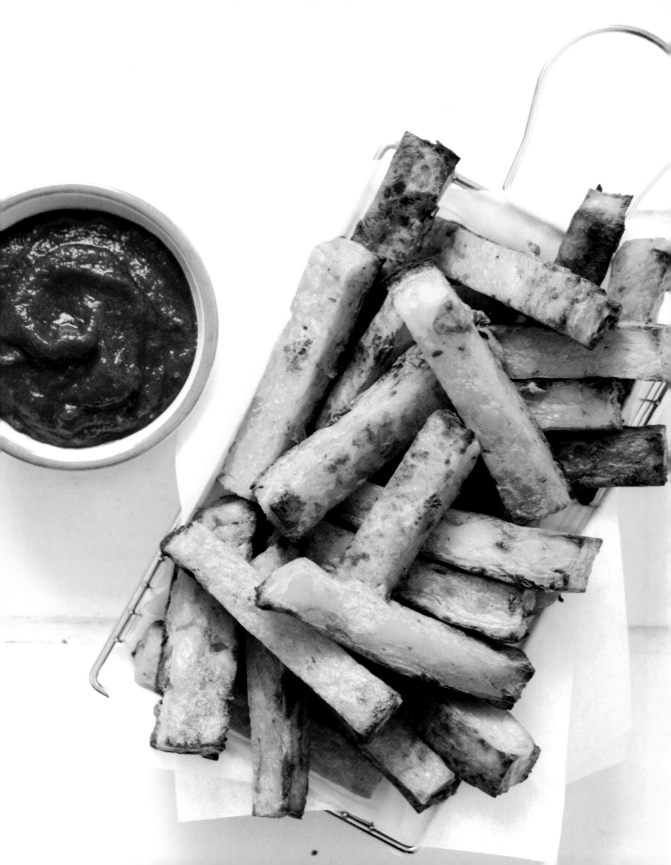

76. MUSHROOM POTATO ROLL

Makes 2 servings

Mushroom lovers will appreciate this recipe that lets its star ingredient shine. Sautéed mushrooms, onions, spices, and herbs are encased in a potato tortilla roll. Enjoy this recipe with a knife and fork, or pick it up and eat it like a burrito.

FOR THE TORTILLAS

4 cups roughly chopped gold potatoes
1 teaspoon garlic powder
1 teaspoon onion powder
2 teaspoons pure maple syrup

FOR THE FILLING

½ cup thinly sliced onion, any color
4 cups thinly sliced mushrooms*
½ teaspoon paprika
½ teaspoon garlic powder
¼ teaspoon red pepper flakes or cayenne
1 teaspoon fresh thyme or ½ teaspoon dried
1 teaspoon chopped fresh rosemary or ½ teaspoon dried
1 teaspoon finely chopped fresh parsley
1 tablespoon freshly squeezed lemon juice

Preheat the oven to 400°F/200°C.

To make the tortilla wraps, add 3 inches of water to a medium pot, insert a steaming basket, add the potatoes, and cover. Steam the potatoes for 20 to 25 minutes until tender. Remove and place the potatoes in a food processor with the garlic powder, onion powder, and maple syrup. Blend until smooth.

Line a baking sheet with parchment paper. Spoon out the potato mixture, making 2 dollops. Spread each dollop with a wet spatula to make 2 tortillas. Bake for 15 to 20 minutes until lightly browned. Remove and pat down with a spatula. Cool completely; then flip the wraps upside down onto a clean work surface or cutting board and gently peel off the parchment paper.

To make the filling, place a ceramic non-stick skillet on medium-high heat. Add the onion and cook for 3 to 5 minutes until softened. Lower the heat and add the mushrooms, paprika, garlic powder, red pepper flakes, thyme, and rosemary. Cook for 10 to 15 minutes, stirring occasionally, until the mushrooms are tender and browned. Stir in the parsley and lemon juice.

Divide the mushroom filling between the tortilla wraps and fold up gently. Serve immediately.

*For the mushrooms, wash and rinse thoroughly with warm to hot water before slicing. Do not use slimy or decaying mushrooms. That's a sign of oxidizing and aging.

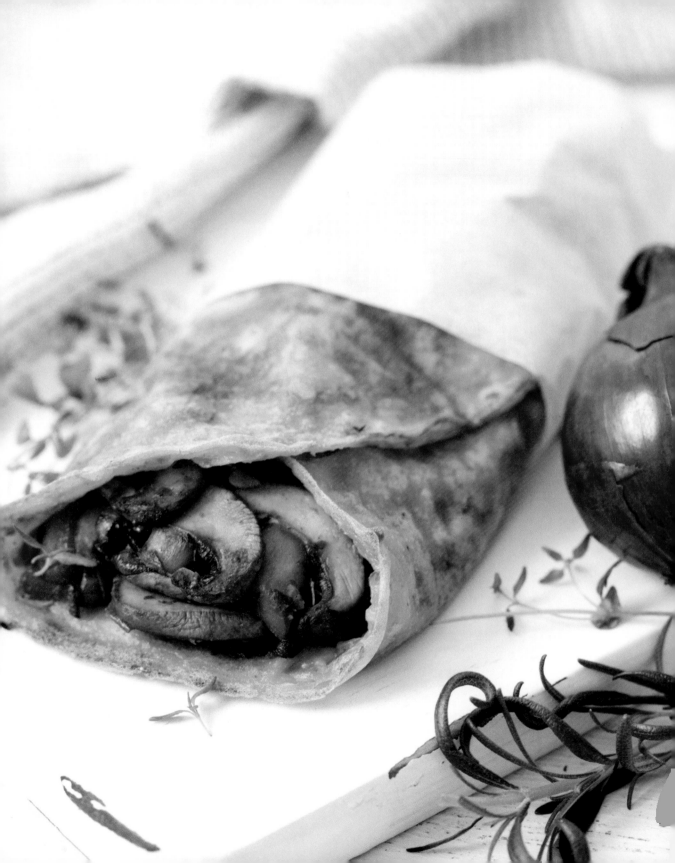

77. MILLET PATTY LETTUCE BURGERS

Makes 4 servings

Crispy and refreshing iceberg lettuce "buns" hold these delicious burger patties, slices of tomato and onion, and easy-to-make homemade ketchup. The patties and fixings can easily be put into gluten-free buns for family members who prefer a more traditional burger.

¼ cup finely chopped onion

1 garlic clove, finely chopped

¼ cup finely chopped sun-dried tomatoes (oil-free and salt-free)

1 cup millet

2 cups Healing Broth (recipe on page 370) or water

1 teaspoon dried Italian herbs, such as thyme, oregano, and/or basil

½ teaspoon paprika

2 tablespoons potato starch

2 large iceberg lettuce heads

¼ cup Ketchup (recipe on page 395)

½ cup thinly sliced tomato

⅓ cup thinly sliced onion

Place a small saucepan on medium-high heat. Add the onion and cook for 3 to 5 minutes until translucent. Add the garlic and sun-dried tomatoes and continue cooking for 1 to 2 minutes. Lower the heat and stir in the millet, Healing Broth or water, herbs, and paprika. Cover and simmer for 10 to 12 minutes until the millet is cooked. Set aside until completely cool.

Place the mixture in a large bowl and add the potato starch. Mash a few times with a potato masher until partly broken down and the potato starch has been incorporated. Using wet hands, make the mixture into 4 large patties.

Place a ceramic nonstick skillet on medium-high heat. Add the patties and cook for 4 to 5 minutes on each side until browned.

Slice 8 large rounds from the edges of the iceberg lettuce (4 from each head) to create the buns. Top one iceberg round with the millet patty, ketchup, tomato, onion, and a second iceberg bun. Repeat with the remaining ingredients and serve immediately.

TIPS

- When you're choosing between Healing Broth and water, keep in mind that the broth will produce a richer flavor. Store-bought stock isn't called for because it's very difficult to find a variety that's free of oil, salt, natural flavors, and/or other additives.

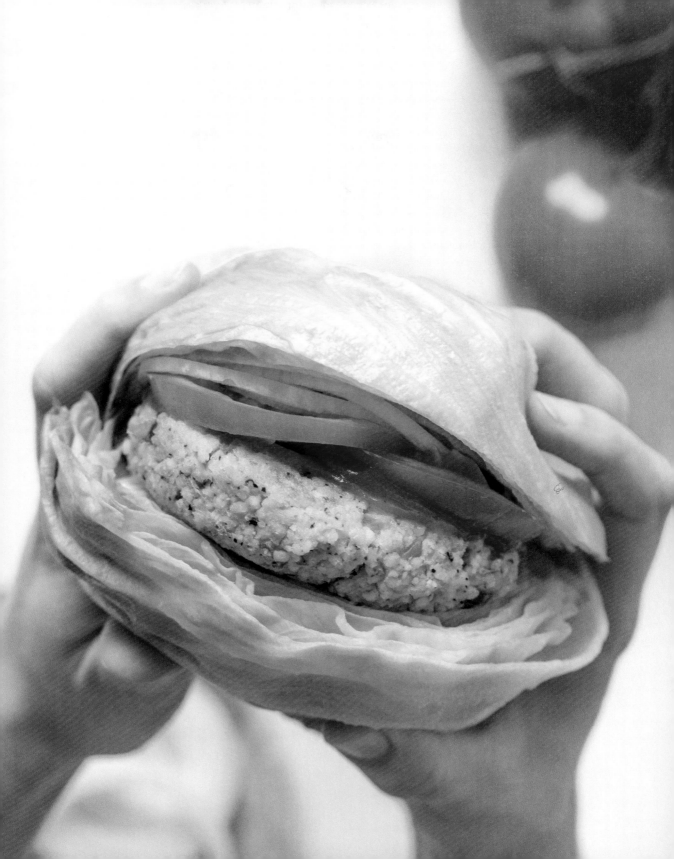

78. SWEET AND SAVORY KABOBS

Enjoy these Sweet and Savory Kabobs one of three ways: raw, dehydrated, or roasted. With a sweet and savory marinade, these kabobs make a great finger food, side, or snack. They are fun to serve and enjoy with family and friends at home or at a picnic, barbecue, or backyard gathering.

8 to 12 wooden skewers
2 cups button mushrooms*
2 cups peeled and chopped pineapple
2 cups cherry tomatoes
1 small zucchini, roughly chopped
1 red, orange, or yellow bell pepper, roughly chopped
1 red, white, or yellow onion, roughly chopped

FOR THE MARINADE

2 tablespoons tomato paste
½ cup orange juice or pineapple juice (preferably freshly squeezed)
1 tablespoon freshly squeezed lemon juice
1 tablespoon raw honey
1 teaspoon onion powder
½ teaspoon garlic powder
½ teaspoon paprika
½ teaspoon Atlantic dulse flakes
½ teaspoon dried thyme
¼ teaspoon chipotle powder (optional)

Soak the wooden skewers in water for 15 to 30 minutes (skip this step if making raw kabobs).

Arrange the chopped kabob ingredients on the skewers and place in containers or on baking sheets. Set aside.

In a small bowl, whisk together all the marinade ingredients until smooth. Brush each skewer liberally with the marinade. Marinate for at least 3 hours or, ideally, overnight.

If making raw skewers, serve as is or dehydrate at 115°F/46°C for 2 to 3 hours.

If roasting, preheat the oven to 400°F/200°C and arrange the skewers on a baking sheet. Roast for 10 to 12 minutes until the vegetables are tender. Serve immediately.

*For the mushrooms, wash and rinse thoroughly with warm to hot water before using. Do not use slimy or decaying mushrooms. That's a sign of oxidizing and aging.

TIPS

- Look for a tomato paste that contains only tomatoes and no other ingredients, such as salt or citric acid.

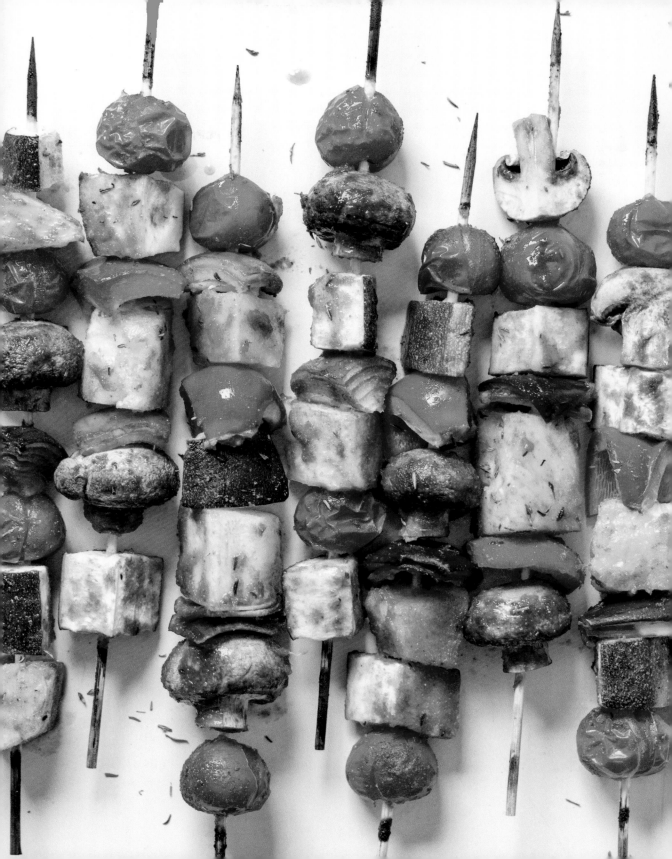

79. CURLY FRIES

Makes 1 serving

These fries are fun and delicious! They're a great option to change up normal potato fries and are perfect for an enjoyable snack or side.

1 large russet potato
½ tablespoon paprika (optional)
½ tablespoon onion powder (optional)
½ tablespoon garlic powder (optional)
½ teaspoon cayenne pepper, chili powder, or chipotle powder (optional)
Ketchup (recipe on page 395; optional)

FOR THE MUSTARD (OPTIONAL)

3 tablespoons raw honey
¾ teaspoon mustard powder
2 tablespoons freshly squeezed lemon juice
⅛ teaspoon ground turmeric

Preheat the oven to 425°F/220°C. Line two baking sheets with parchment paper.

Spiralize the potato into a large bowl. Use scissors to cut the strips into 6- to 8-inch lengths so that they cook more evenly and do not tangle.

Add your choice of spices to the spiralized potato, tossing to coat evenly.

Spread the fries evenly on the prepared baking sheets. Do not overcrowd. Bake for 15 minutes; then remove the baking sheets from the oven and thoroughly flip and rearrange the fries so that the less crispy ones have more space. Return to the oven and bake for another 10 to 15 minutes, being sure to stir them every few minutes and taking out the ones that are crispy. Keep a close eye on the fries, as they can burn quickly!

Alternatively, you can make these in an air fryer at 400°F/200°C for 10 to 15 minutes, stirring every 5 minutes.

Make the ketchup. Set aside.

To make the mustard, combine all the ingredients in a small bowl and whisk until well combined. Set aside.

Serve fries immediately with the ketchup and mustard (if using).

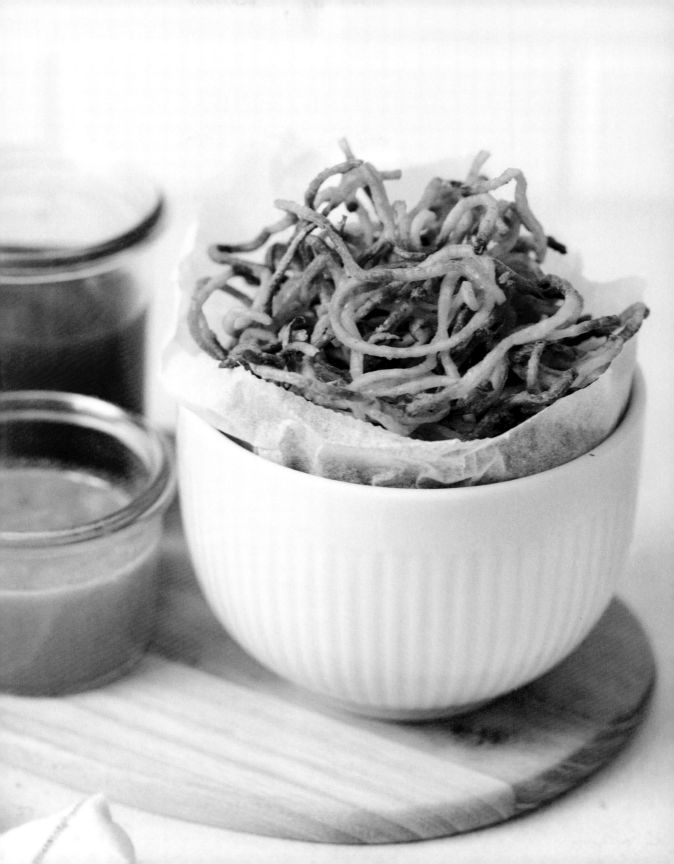

80. STOVETOP MAC AND CHEESE

Makes 4 servings

This favorite comfort food in its traditional form is hard on our health. If you are trying to heal or simply want to support your body to be as healthy as possible in the future, try this version, which is fat-free, dairy-free, and gluten-free. It's creamy and comforting without the drawbacks of regular mac and cheese.

2 medium potatoes, diced
1 medium carrot, diced
1 tablespoon onion powder
1 teaspoon garlic powder
½ teaspoon paprika
1 teaspoon dried oregano
½ teaspoon ground turmeric
1 tablespoon freshly squeezed lemon juice
⅓ cup Healing Broth (recipe on page 370) or water
12 ounces gluten-free, corn-free elbow pasta
2 tablespoons chopped fresh parsley leaves (optional)
1 to 2 teaspoons red pepper flakes (optional)

Add 3 inches of water to a medium pot, insert a steaming basket, add the diced potatoes and carrots, and cover. Steam for 10 to 15 minutes until tender. Remove the potatoes and carrots from the heat and place in a blender along with the onion powder, garlic powder, paprika, oregano, turmeric, lemon juice, and Healing Broth or water. Blend until smooth and set aside.

While the vegetables are steaming, cook the pasta according to package instructions. Drain and place back in the pot.

Pour the sauce onto the pasta and stir until evenly coated. Cook on low heat until warmed through if needed. Serve immediately, garnished with the chopped parsley and red pepper flakes (if using).

TIPS

- When you're choosing between Healing Broth and water for the ingredients, keep in mind that the broth will produce a richer flavor. Store-bought vegetable stock isn't called for because it's very difficult to find a variety that's free of oil, salt, natural flavors, and/or other additives.

- Look for pasta that is grain-free such as cassava, pea, lentil, or chickpea pasta. Alternatively, a gluten-free pasta that is made with grains such as millet, quinoa, or brown rice is also an option. Be sure to check that your pasta does not contain corn or egg.

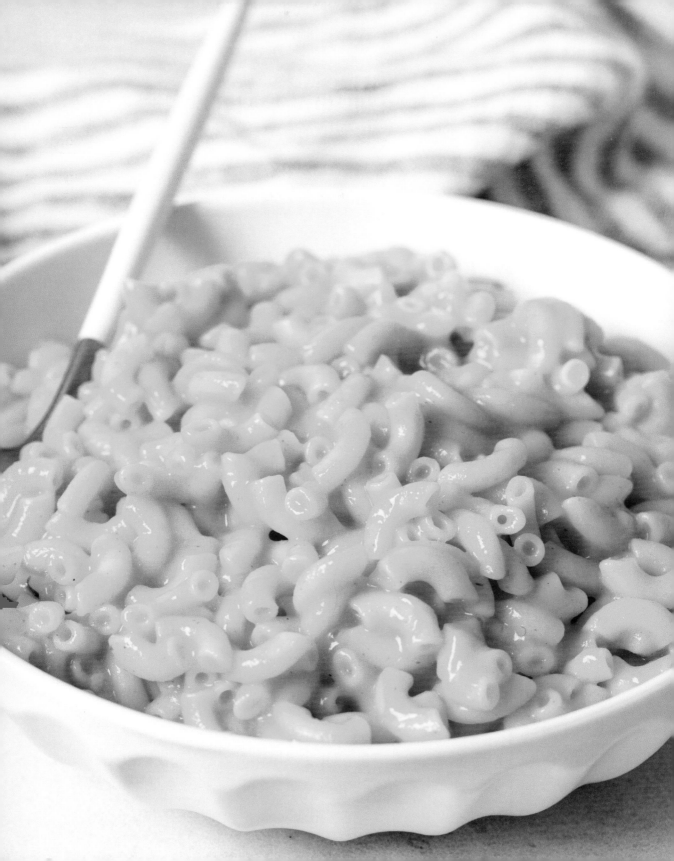

81. SCALLION PANCAKES

Makes 2 to 3 servings

These Scallion Pancakes are both delicious and versatile. Instead of using regular flour, which contains pathogen-feeding gluten, and pan-frying the pancakes in oil, here, potatoes and grain-free cassava flour are used and no oil is needed.

2 pounds potatoes, peeled and roughly chopped
½ to ¾ cup cassava flour
1 cup chopped scallions (also called green onions)
¼ teaspoon sea salt (optional)
¼ teaspoon Chinese five-spice powder (optional)

FOR THE DIPPING SAUCE

3 tablespoons pure maple syrup
2½ tablespoons freshly squeezed lemon juice
½ teaspoon garlic powder
½ teaspoon chili powder, or more to taste
1 teaspoon chopped scallions, to serve (optional)

Add 3 inches of water to a medium pot, insert a steaming basket, add the potatoes, and cover. Steam the potatoes for 20 to 25 minutes until tender. Remove the potatoes from the heat and add to a large bowl.

Mash the potatoes until smooth and lump-free using a potato masher. Add the cassava flour and knead until you get a soft dough, adding more flour as needed until the dough is no longer sticky.

Add the scallions, sea salt (if using), and Chinese five-spice powder (if using). Knead until well incorporated into the dough.

Divide the dough into three portions and form each into a ball. Place a ball between two sheets of parchment paper and roll out into a circle, pinching together any cracks that appear while rolling. Place a large ceramic nonstick skillet on high heat and cook the pancake for 4 to 6 minutes on each side until browned. Remove the pancake from the heat and repeat with the remaining balls of dough.

To make the dipping sauce, whisk together all the ingredients until well combined. Cut the pancakes into wedges and serve immediately with the dipping sauce and chopped scallions.

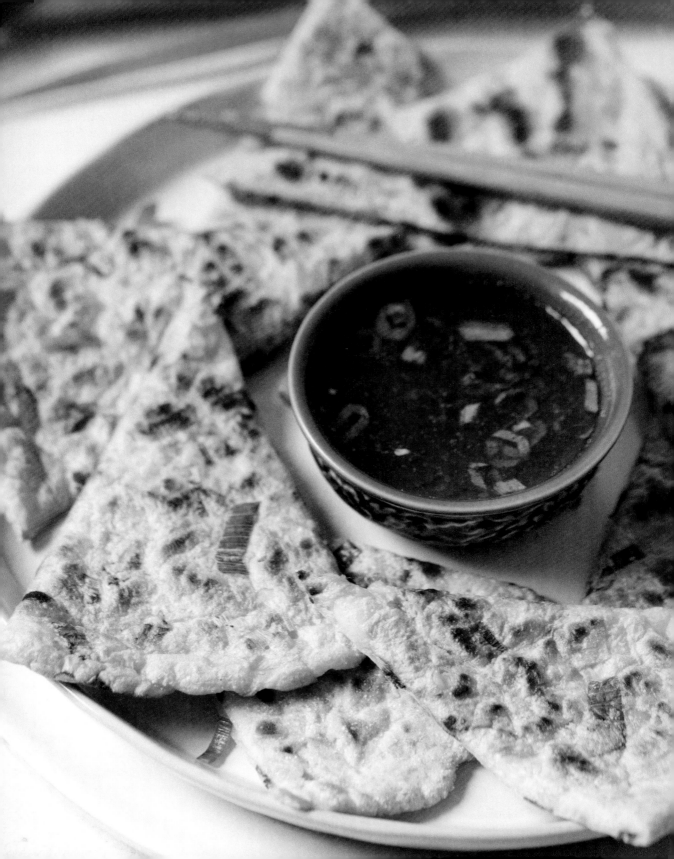

82. LENTIL SHEPHERD'S PIE

Makes 6 servings

This rustic and hearty Lentil Shepherd's Pie is the perfect dish for the family dinner table. Lentils, vegetables, and herbs are topped with creamy mashed potatoes that are baked until golden. This recipe is also great as leftovers!

FOR THE FILLING

1 medium yellow onion, diced
2 garlic cloves, minced
2 stalks celery, finely diced
2 to 3 medium carrots, diced
1½ cups uncooked brown or green lentils, rinsed (optional substitution of 2 pounds chopped mushrooms*)
4 cups Healing Broth (recipe on page 370) or water (leave out if using mushrooms)
3 tablespoons tomato paste
1 tablespoon fresh thyme or 1 teaspoon dried

1 tablespoon chopped fresh rosemary or 1 teaspoon dried
2 teaspoons onion powder
1 teaspoon garlic powder
½ teaspoon paprika
½ cup fresh or thawed frozen peas
Fresh thyme sprigs, for garnish (optional)

FOR THE MASHED POTATOES

3 pounds gold potatoes
Pinch of ground nutmeg (optional)
2 to 3 tablespoons unsweetened almond milk or water (optional)

TIPS

- Look for a tomato paste that contains only tomatoes and no other ingredients, such as salt or citric acid.

- When you're choosing between Healing Broth and water for the ingredients, keep in mind that the broth will produce a richer flavor. Store-bought vegetable stock isn't called for because it's very difficult to find a variety that's free of oil, salt, natural flavors, and/or other additives. For convenience, make a batch of Healing Broth in advance and freeze it (consider pouring into ice cube trays for easy thawing) so you have it on hand for recipes like this.

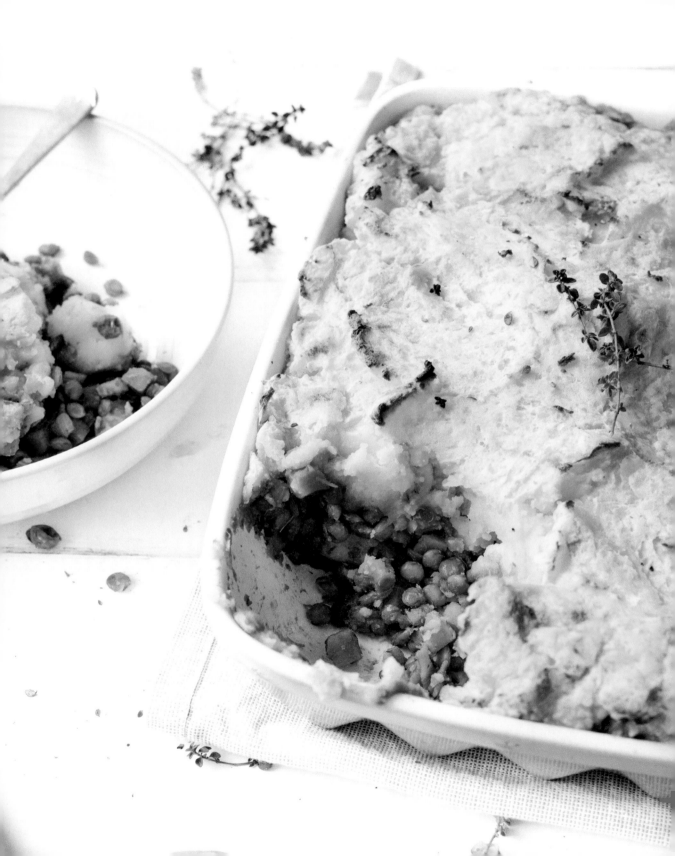

Add 3 inches of water to a medium pot, insert a steaming basket, add the potatoes, and cover. Steam for 30 to 45 minutes until tender. Once cooked, transfer the potatoes to a large bowl together with the nutmeg (if using) and mash until smooth using a potato masher. Add a few tablespoons of unsweetened almond milk or water if needed. Cover loosely and set aside.

While the potatoes are steaming, preheat the oven to 400°F/200°C.

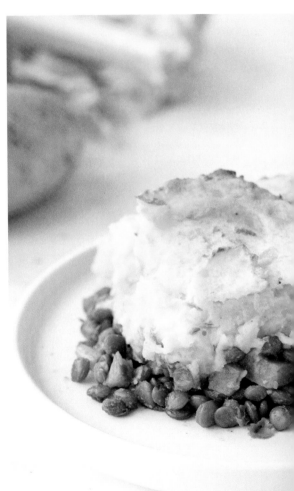

In a large saucepan on medium-high heat, sauté the onions until translucent, 3 to 5 minutes. Add a bit of water if the onions stick to the pan. Add the garlic, celery, and carrots and cook for another 5 minutes until lightly browned. Add the lentils, Healing Broth, tomato paste, thyme, rosemary, onion powder, garlic powder, and paprika. Cover and cook for 30 to 35 minutes until the lentils are tender. Stir in the peas in the last 5 minutes of cooking.

If using mushrooms instead of lentils, add them to the pot with the tomato paste, thyme, rosemary, onion powder, garlic powder, and paprika. Cook until soft and caramelized, 15 to 20 minutes. Stir in the peas in the last 5 minutes of cooking.

Transfer the filling into an 11-×-7-inch baking dish or equivalent, and top with the mashed potatoes. Smooth down with a spoon or fork.

Bake for 10 to 15 minutes or until the mash is lightly browned. Remove from the oven and cool for 10 to 15 minutes. Garnish with a few sprigs of thyme if desired and serve.

*For the mushrooms, if using, wash and rinse thoroughly with warm to hot water before chopping. Do not use slimy or decaying mushrooms. That's a sign of oxidizing and aging.

83. MEXICAN POTATO HASH

Makes 2 to 3 servings

This wonderful potato hash brings together the best of Mexican flavors with a homemade taco seasoning mix, fresh cilantro, pico de gallo, and a creamy potato-based cheese sauce all served on top of sautéed potatoes and/or sweet potatoes. This recipe can be enjoyed for any meal of the day.

6 cups diced potatoes and/or sweet potatoes
1 cup water
2 to 3 lime wedges, to serve
¼ cup loosely packed cilantro leaves, to serve

FOR THE TACO SEASONING

1 tablespoon onion powder
2 teaspoons ground cumin
1 teaspoon paprika
1 teaspoon garlic powder
½ teaspoon chili powder
½ teaspoon red pepper flakes
1 teaspoon dried oregano

FOR THE PICO DE GALLO

1 cup diced tomatoes
¼ cup finely chopped onion (optional)
¼ cup cilantro leaves, finely chopped
1 teaspoon finely chopped ripe hot pepper
½ tablespoon freshly squeezed lime juice

FOR THE CHEESE SAUCE (OPTIONAL)

1 cup peeled, diced potato
¼ cup peeled, finely chopped carrot
½ tablespoon freshly squeezed lime juice
2 teaspoons onion powder
1 teaspoon garlic powder
½ teaspoon paprika

TIPS

- A fun way to eat this hash while also getting more leafy greens into your diet is to spoon it into lettuce leaves and eat it like a taco.

Mix all the ingredients for the taco seasoning together in a small bowl.

Place a ceramic nonstick skillet on medium-low heat. Add the potatoes, taco seasoning, and water. Bring to a simmer, cover, and cook for 12 to 15 minutes until the potatoes are tender. Remove the lid and continue cooking until all the liquid has evaporated.

If making the cheese sauce, add 3 inches of water to a medium pot, insert a steaming basket, add the diced potatoes and carrots, and cover. Steam for 10 to 12 minutes or until tender. Place in a blender together with the lime juice, onion powder, garlic powder, and paprika. Blend until smooth.

Make the pico de gallo by combining all the ingredients in a medium bowl and stirring until the ingredients are evenly mixed.

To serve, drizzle the cheese sauce over the potatoes and top with the pico de gallo, cilantro, and lime wedges. Serve immediately. Enjoy!

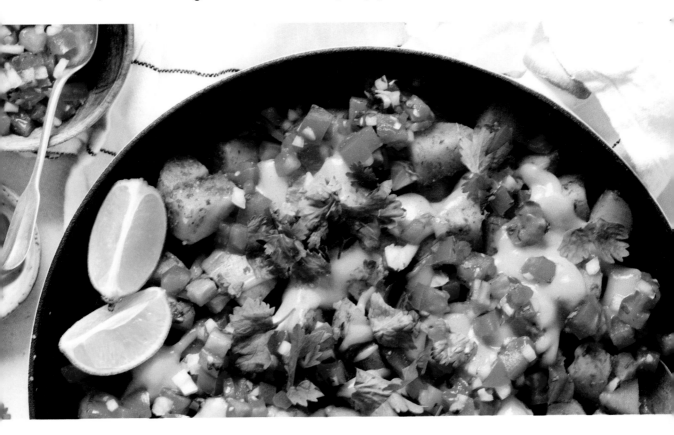

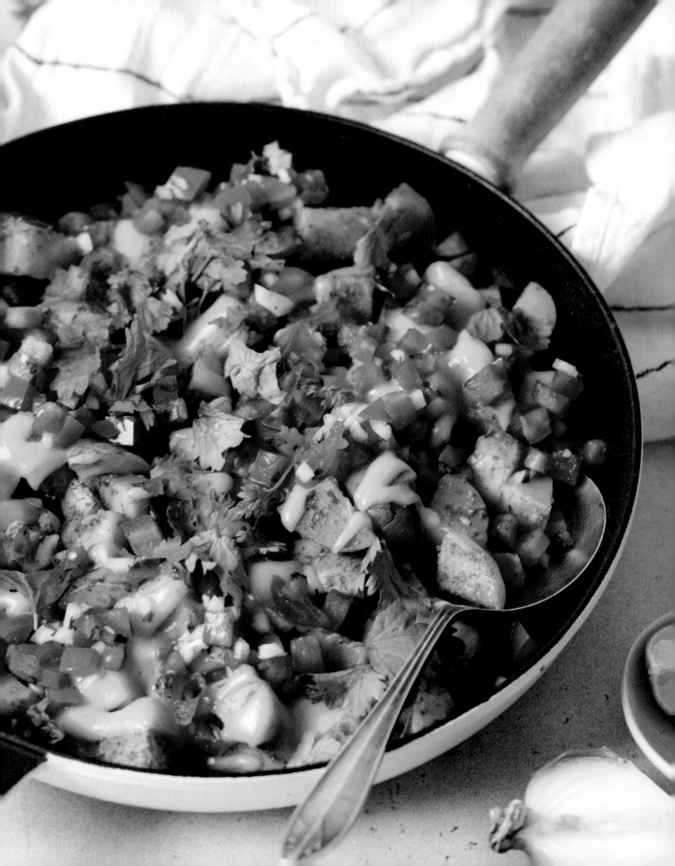

84. BROCCOLI WITH ZUCCHINI RANCH SAUCE

Makes 2 servings

Light and refreshing, this side dish is a pleasing accompaniment to any meal. Fresh dill and parsley add a pop of flavor and brightness to this recipe.

1 large head of broccoli, cut into florets

FOR THE RANCH SAUCE

3 cups raw, peeled, and diced zucchini
3 tablespoons freshly squeezed lemon juice
1½ tablespoons onion powder
2 teaspoons garlic powder
1½ tablespoons finely chopped dill
1½ tablespoons finely chopped parsley

Add 3 inches of water to a medium pot and insert a steaming basket. Add the broccoli, cover, and steam until bright green and tender, 5 to 8 minutes. Remove and place the broccoli in a serving bowl.

To make the ranch sauce, combine the zucchini, lemon juice, onion powder, and garlic powder in a blender and blend until smooth. Stir in the dill and parsley.

Pour the sauce over the steamed broccoli and serve immediately.

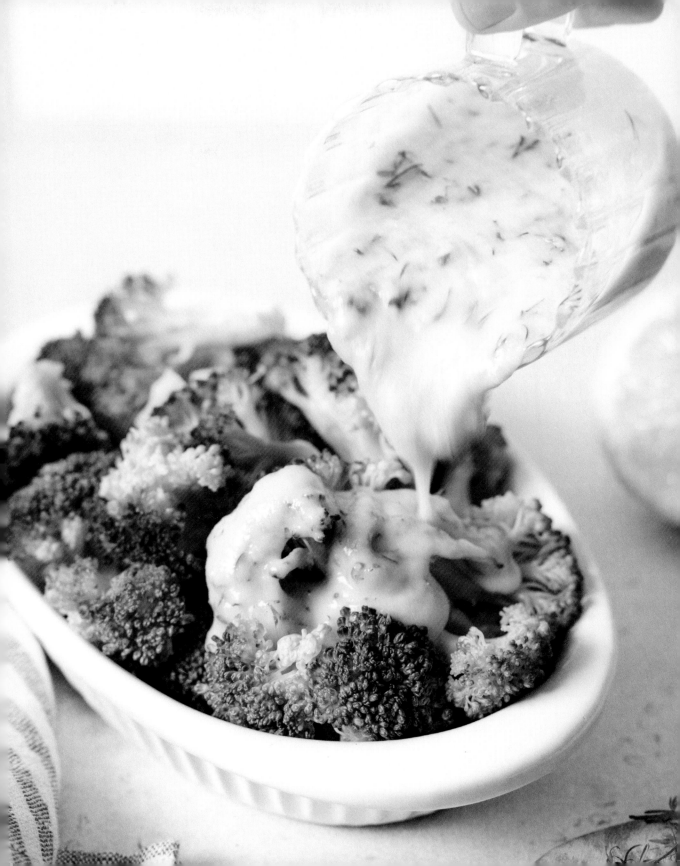

85. MILLET AND HERB SALAD

Makes 2 servings

Fresh mint, cilantro, and parsley bring so much flavor to this simple and easy-to-make salad. This recipe is especially easy to throw together if you have leftover millet on hand ready to go. Then it's just chop, toss, and serve this delightful salad.

3 tablespoons freshly squeezed lime or lemon juice
2 tablespoons raw honey or pure maple syrup
1 teaspoon garlic powder
½ teaspoon red pepper flakes
2 cups cooked and cooled millet
1 cup loosely packed cilantro leaves, roughly chopped
1 cup loosely packed parsley leaves, roughly chopped
¼ cup mint leaves, finely chopped
1 cup diced tomatoes
1 cup diced cucumber
½ cup thinly sliced celery
¼ cup finely chopped red, white, or yellow onion
2 tablespoons finely chopped green onion

In a large bowl, whisk together the lime or lemon juice, raw honey or maple syrup, garlic powder, and red pepper flakes until well combined.

Add the millet, cilantro, parsley, mint, tomatoes, cucumber, celery, onion, and green onion to the bowl. Toss gently until evenly mixed. Serve immediately.

TIPS

- If you'd prefer to use another gluten-free grain, you can also make this recipe with quinoa and/or brown rice that's been cooked and cooled. (If you have a sensitive gut, be mindful that quinoa can be scratchy on the gastrointestinal linings.)

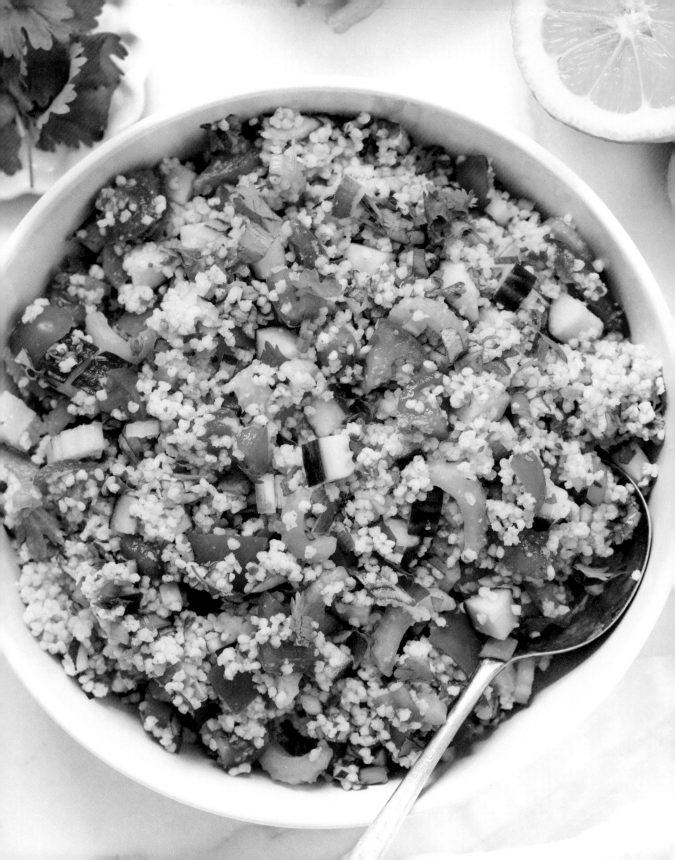

86. ASPARAGUS SUSHI

Makes 2 servings

These little bites of sushi are light, tasty, and fun to make. The dipping sauce and wasabi offer an extra burst of flavor and bring the heat! This is sushi you can enjoy as much of as you like without any drawbacks!

FOR THE CAULIFLOWER RICE

½ head cauliflower (about 6 cups cauliflower florets)
⅓ cup finely chopped onion
3 garlic cloves, finely chopped

FOR THE FILLING

6 asparagus spears, trimmed
6 nori sheets
½ cup thinly sliced radishes
6 spring onions
½ cucumber, julienned

FOR THE DIPPING SAUCE

½ cup freshly squeezed orange or tangerine juice
1 teaspoon finely chopped ripe hot pepper
1 teaspoon finely grated garlic
1 teaspoon finely grated fresh ginger
1 tablespoon freshly squeezed lime juice
½ tablespoon raw honey
½ teaspoon Atlantic dulse flakes (optional)

TO SERVE

1 teaspoon wasabi powder
2 to 3 tablespoons water

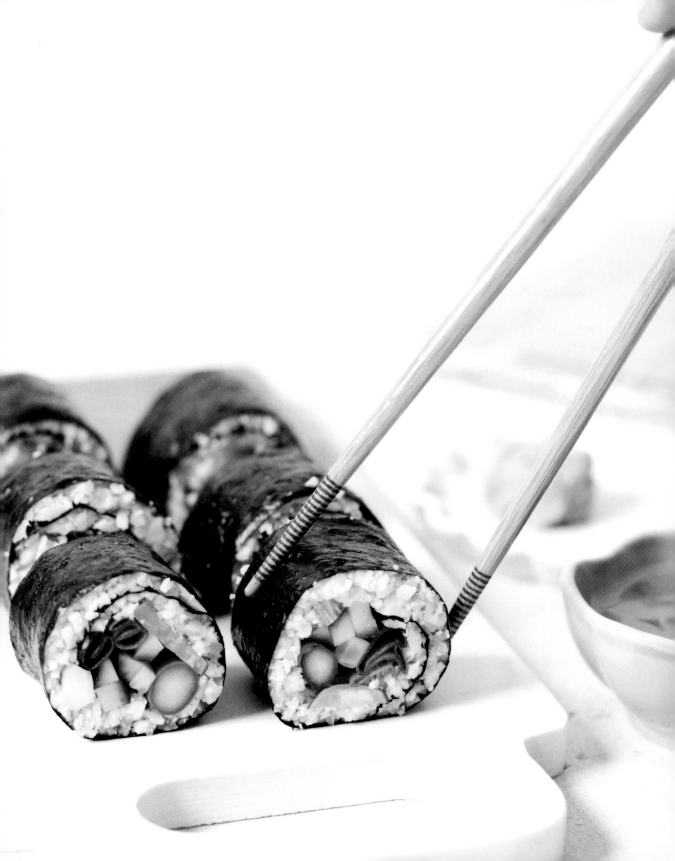

Make the dipping sauce by whisking together the orange or tangerine juice, chopped hot pepper, garlic, ginger, lime juice, raw honey, and Atlantic dulse flakes (if using). Refrigerate until needed.

Place the cauliflower florets in a food processor and pulse until a rice-like texture forms.

Place a large ceramic nonstick frying pan over medium-high heat. Add the onion and cook for 5 to 6 minutes until soft and caramelized. Add the garlic and cook for a further 2 to 3 minutes.

Add the cauliflower rice and cook, stirring frequently, for 5 to 7 minutes or until tender. Remove from the heat and set aside.

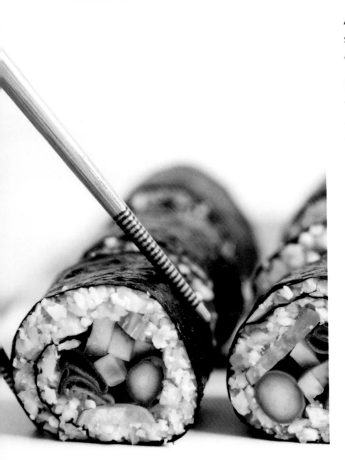

Add 3 inches of water to a medium pot, insert a steaming basket, add the asparagus spears, and cover. Steam for 4 to 5 minutes until tender.

Place one sheet of nori on a cutting board with the long edge facing you. When the rice is cool enough to handle, scoop about ¾ cup of cauliflower rice onto the end of the nori sheet closest to you and spread into an even layer, leaving about a 1-inch border at the top of the sheet. Arrange the asparagus, radish, spring onion, and cucumber on the bottom section of the cauliflower rice layer.

Carefully lift the nori from the bottom edge close to you and begin rolling it tightly toward the top. Just before wrapping the roll, dip your finger in the dipping sauce and run it along the top edge of the sheet. Seal the wrap. Using a sharp knife, slice each sushi roll into even pieces. Repeat with the remaining ingredients.

Mix the wasabi powder with water until you get a smooth paste.

Serve the sushi immediately with the dipping sauce and wasabi.

87. CHICKPEA SCRAMBLE

Scrambled eggs are a favorite food for so many people. This recipe gives a similar experience using chickpea flour instead of eggs.

½ cup chickpea flour

½ cup unsweetened almond or coconut milk, Healing Broth (recipe on page 370), or water

2 teaspoons onion powder

1 teaspoon garlic powder

½ teaspoon paprika

¼ teaspoon ground turmeric

¼ teaspoon cayenne

¼ teaspoon sea salt (optional)

⅓ cup finely chopped onion, any color

⅓ cup chopped red, yellow, or orange bell peppers

¼ cup chopped tomato

¼ cup loosely packed, roughly chopped parsley and basil, plus more to serve

1 tablespoon freshly squeezed lemon juice

Add the chickpea flour; almond or coconut milk, Healing Broth, or water; and spices to a medium bowl. Add the sea salt if using. Whisk until you get a smooth batter. Set aside.

Place a ceramic nonstick skillet on medium-high heat, add the chopped onion, and sauté until softened, 3 to 5 minutes. Add the bell peppers and tomato and cook for a further 2 to 3 minutes.

Pour in the scramble batter. Let it cook for 2 minutes without disturbing. When the mixture starts to firm up at the sides, break it up with a spatula, flipping and scrambling it for 3 to 4 minutes until the whole scramble is cooked and no longer wet.

Stir in the parsley and basil and lemon juice. Remove from the heat.

Transfer to a bowl and top with more parsley and basil. Serve immediately.

TIPS

- Using almond or coconut milk in this recipe will result in a better outcome; however, you can use the Healing Broth or water options if you prefer to make it fat-free.

- When you're choosing between Healing Broth and water for the ingredients, keep in mind that the broth will produce a richer flavor. Store-bought vegetable stock isn't called for because it's very difficult to find a variety that's free of oil, salt, natural flavors, and/or other additives. For convenience, make a batch of Healing Broth in advance and freeze it (consider pouring into ice cube trays for easy thawing) so you have it on hand for recipes like this.

- While high-quality sea salt or mountain rock salt is an optional inclusion in this recipe, the recipe is more healing without salt. Over time, you may wish to reduce or exclude the salt.

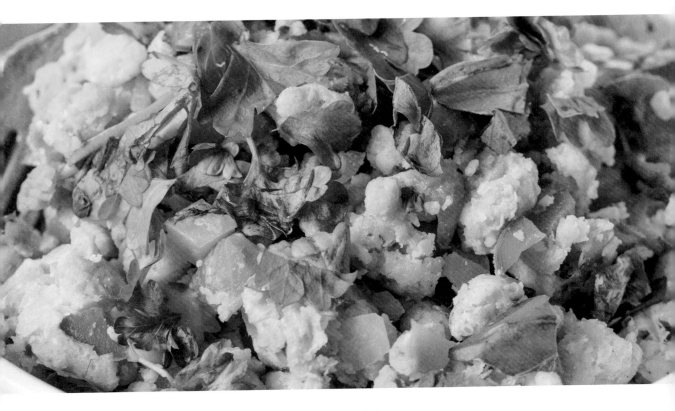

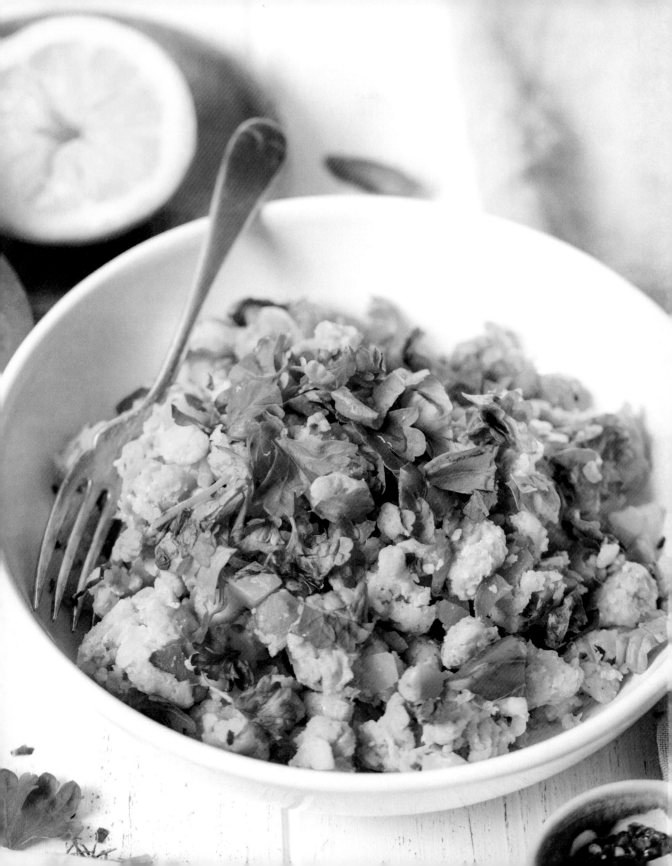

88. GARLIC AND HERB PEAS

Makes 2 servings

This recipe may be simple, but oftentimes simple is best! It couldn't be easier to make if you are using frozen peas, and the herbs, spices, and lemon juice bring flavor to this humble dish. These Garlic and Herb Peas are great as a side to any meal or a salad or enjoyed as a snack. Keep extra bags of frozen peas in your freezer to make this recipe when you need a quick option.

3 cups freshly shelled or frozen peas
2 teaspoons onion powder
½ teaspoon garlic powder
2 tablespoons finely chopped fresh dill or
   1 tablespoon dried
1 tablespoon freshly squeezed lemon juice

Add 3 inches of water to a medium pot, insert a steaming basket, add the peas, and cover. Steam for 3 to 5 minutes until bright green and tender.

Remove the peas and place them in a bowl. Add the onion powder, garlic powder, dill, and lemon juice. Stir until evenly mixed.

Serve immediately.

Alternatively, if you prefer mushy peas versus whole peas, you can also place the peas in a blender or food processor and pulse a few times until the peas reach your desired consistency. Serve immediately.

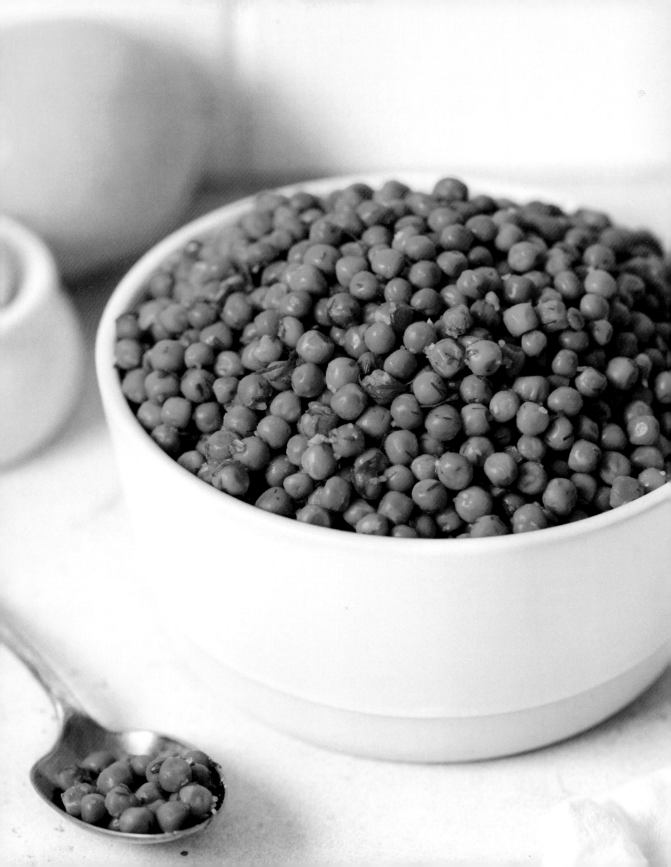

89. GARAM MASALA POTATOES

Makes 2 servings

Garam masala spices sautéed with potatoes, onion, tomato, bell peppers, and garlic bring depth of flavor to this dish. Chopped cilantro and a squeeze of lemon or lime juice add the final touches.

½ cup diced onion

2 garlic cloves, finely chopped

1 teaspoon finely chopped ginger

1½ tablespoons garam masala (or make your own)

2 pounds potatoes, diced

½ cup diced tomatoes

1 cup diced red, orange, or yellow bell peppers

1 cup Healing Broth (recipe on page 370) or water

½ tablespoon freshly squeezed lime or lemon juice, to serve

¼ cup loosely packed, roughly chopped cilantro leaves, to serve

TO MAKE YOUR OWN GARAM MASALA

1 teaspoon ground cumin

1 teaspoon ground coriander

½ teaspoon ground cardamom

½ teaspoon cinnamon

¼ teaspoon ground cloves

¼ teaspoon ground nutmeg

¼ teaspoon chili powder or red pepper flakes

To make your own garam masala blend, combine all the ingredients in a small bowl and mix well.

Place a large ceramic nonstick skillet on medium-high heat. Add the onion and cook for 3 to 5 minutes until soft, adding a bit of water if needed to prevent sticking.

Add the garlic, ginger, and garam masala. Cook for a further 1 to 2 minutes until the spices are fragrant.

Add the potatoes, tomato, bell peppers, and Healing Broth or water to the pan. Stir until evenly mixed, then cover, turn the heat to low, and simmer for 10 to 15 minutes until the potatoes are tender.

Divide between two bowls and top with a squeeze of lime or lemon juice and the cilantro. Serve immediately.

TIPS

- When you're choosing between Healing Broth and water for the ingredients, keep in mind that the broth will produce a richer flavor. Store-bought vegetable stock isn't called for because it's very difficult to find a variety that's free of oil, salt, natural flavors, and/or other additives.

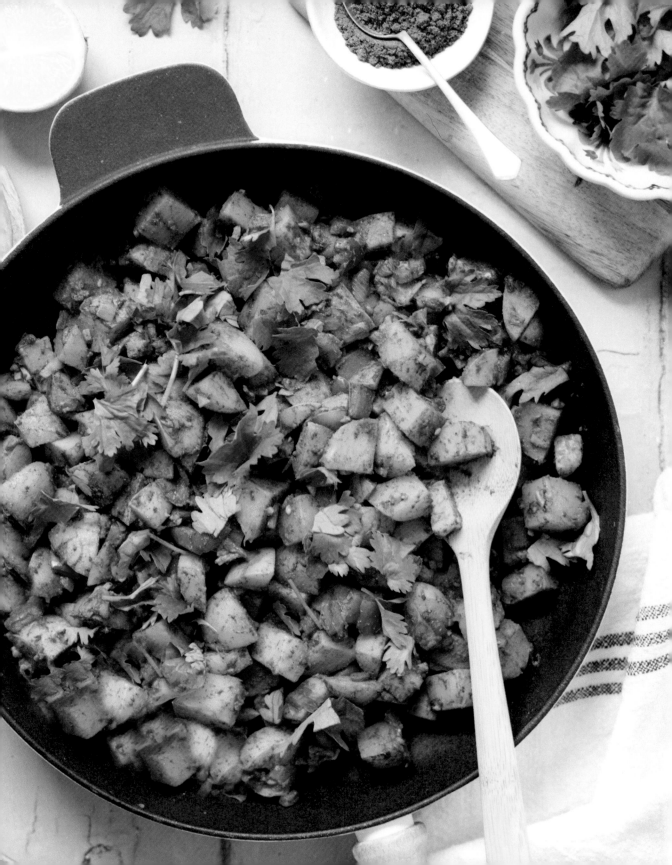

90. MILLET POLENTA WITH ROASTED CHERRY TOMATOES AND ASPARAGUS

Makes 2 servings

Millet takes the place of corn for the polenta in this recipe. Combined with juicy, sweet, roasted cherry tomatoes and steamed asparagus, this spin on polenta is not only far healthier but also tastes great!

1 pound cherry tomatoes, standard or on the vine
1 teaspoon raw honey
1 to 2 tablespoons fresh thyme or rosemary or 1 to 2 teaspoons dried
½ bunch asparagus, trimmed
1 to 2 tablespoons freshly squeezed lemon juice, to serve
½ teaspoon red pepper flakes, to serve (optional)

FOR THE MILLET POLENTA

1 cup millet
½ cup diced onion, any color
2 garlic cloves, finely chopped
4 cups Healing Broth (recipe on page 370) or water
½ teaspoon sea salt (optional)

TIPS

- When you're choosing between Healing Broth and water for the ingredients, keep in mind that the broth will produce a richer flavor. Store-bought vegetable stock isn't called for because it's very difficult to find a variety that's free of oil, salt, natural flavors, and/or other additives. For convenience, make a batch of Healing Broth in advance and freeze it (consider pouring into ice cube trays for easy thawing) so you have it on hand for recipes like this.

- While high-quality sea salt or mountain rock salt is an optional inclusion in this recipe, the recipe is more healing without salt. Over time, you may wish to reduce or exclude the salt.

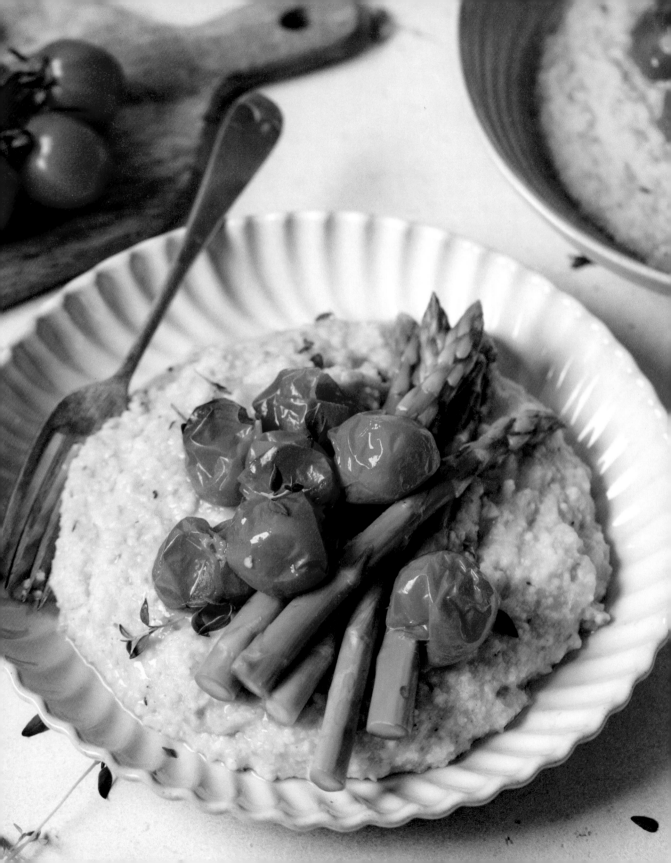

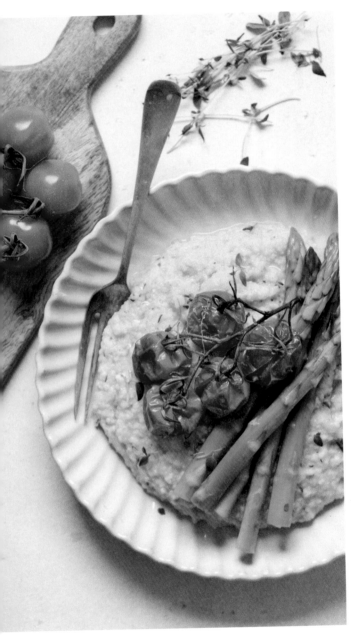

Preheat the oven to 350°F/180°C. Line a baking sheet with parchment paper.

Arrange the cherry tomatoes on the prepared baking sheet and drizzle with the honey. Sprinkle the herbs over the tomatoes. Roast for 30 to 35 minutes until soft and the skins have burst.

While the tomatoes are roasting, make the millet polenta by putting the millet in a food processor or blender and pulsing a few times until ground up but with some bigger pieces. Set aside.

Place a medium ceramic nonstick pot on medium-high heat and add the onion. Cook for 3 to 5 minutes until softened, adding a bit of water if the onion sticks to the pot. Add the garlic and continue cooking for 1 to 2 minutes.

Pour in the Healing Broth or water and bring to a boil. Stir in the millet and cook, stirring every few minutes, for 12 to 15 minutes, or until the millet is tender and all the liquid has been absorbed. Add the sea salt if using.

Add 3 inches of water to a medium pot, insert a steaming basket, add the asparagus, and cover. Steam for 4 to 5 minutes until tender.

To serve, divide the millet polenta between two bowls and top with the roasted tomatoes and steamed asparagus. Squeeze lemon juice over all and sprinkle with red pepper flakes (if using). Serve immediately.

91. SPICY FAJITAS

Makes 2 servings

These Spicy Fajitas are a fun, crowd-pleasing recipe, packed with flavor. You can simply enjoy the fillings on their own—with or without tortillas—or add the salsa and guacamole for additional flavor and satisfaction!

½ cup thinly sliced onion (any color)
2 medium portobello mushrooms, thinly sliced*
3 cups thinly sliced orange, yellow, and red bell peppers
1½ teaspoons garlic powder
½ to 1 teaspoon chili powder, to taste
1 teaspoon paprika
½ teaspoon ground cumin
¼ teaspoon sea salt (optional)
2 tablespoons roughly chopped cilantro, to serve
4 to 5 tortillas, to serve**
2 to 3 lime wedges, to serve

FOR THE GUACAMOLE

2 medium avocados, peeled and pitted
¼ cup finely chopped celery
¼ cup loosely packed cilantro leaves, finely chopped
2 tablespoons finely chopped onion
½ garlic clove, minced
¼ teaspoon sea salt (optional)
1 to 2 tablespoons freshly squeezed lime juice, to taste

FOR THE SALSA

1 cup finely chopped tomatoes
2 tablespoons finely chopped red onion
2 tablespoons loosely packed, roughly chopped cilantro leaves
½ garlic clove, minced
1 teaspoon finely chopped red serrano pepper or red jalapeño
½ teaspoon ground cumin (optional)
1 to 2 tablespoons freshly squeezed lime juice, to taste

Place a large ceramic nonstick skillet on medium-high heat. Add the onions and portobello mushrooms and cook for 5 to 7 minutes, stirring often, until soft. Add a few tablespoons of water if needed to prevent sticking.

Add the sliced bell peppers, garlic powder, chili powder, paprika, cumin, and sea salt (if using) to the pan. Cook for 4 to 6 minutes on high heat until the peppers are browned and tender. Remove from the heat and set aside.

To make the guacamole, add the avocados to a medium bowl. Mash using a potato masher or a fork until the mash is smooth but still has a few bigger chunks. Add the remaining ingredients and mix together gently with a spoon. Set aside.

To make the salsa, combine all the ingredients in a medium bowl and mix well. Set aside.

Assemble the fajitas by adding a few tablespoons of the onion, mushroom, and bell pepper filling to the bottom of the tortillas, followed by 1 tablespoon each of the guacamole and salsa. Try to discard as much liquid as possible from the salsa so that it doesn't soften the tortilla. Top with a bit of chopped cilantro and serve immediately with the lime wedges.

*For the mushrooms, wash and rinse thoroughly with warm to hot water before slicing. Do not use slimy or decaying mushrooms. That's a sign of oxidizing and aging.

**For the tortillas, you can use the Millet Tortillas on page 498 or the Potato Tortillas on page 460.

TIPS

- For an option free of radical fat, omit the guacamole. It will still taste great.

- Both the Millet Tortillas and Potato Tortillas are perfect for this recipe. The Millet Tortillas are easier to make, but the Potato Tortillas are perfect for anyone on a grain-free diet. Both recipes are free of any radical fats.

- If you use store-bought tortillas, look for a product that doesn't contain any corn, gluten, vinegar, or other problematic ingredients.

- While high-quality sea salt or mountain rock salt is an optional inclusion in this recipe, the recipe is more healing without salt. Over time, you may wish to reduce or exclude the salt.

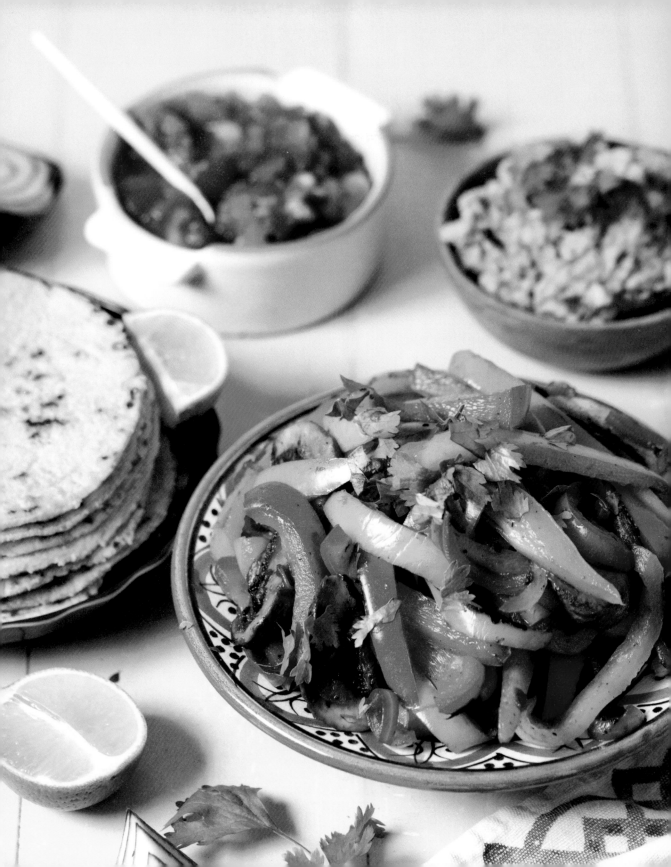

92. MILLET TORTILLAS

Makes 10 to 12 tortillas

These delicious gluten-free and corn-free Millet Tortillas are the perfect vehicle for an endless variety of mouthwatering toppings. Try them with the Spicy Fajitas on page 495 or top them with any of the veggie, fruit, and herb dishes or dips and sauces in this book or any of the other Medical Medium books. Let your creativity take over and explore your favorite way of enjoying these yummy tortillas.

2 cups water
2 cups millet flour
1 tablespoon minced fresh garlic or
  ½ tablespoon garlic powder
¼ teaspoon sea salt (optional)

Bring 2 cups of water to a boil in a shallow saucepan. Add the millet flour. Do not stir. Allow the water to continue at a low boil for 2 minutes. Then add the garlic and the sea salt (if using). Remove from the heat and mix until combined. The dough formed will feel dry to the touch. Transfer the dough into a bowl and set aside until cool enough to touch.

Form the dough into small balls about 2 inches in diameter. Place a ball between two pieces of smooth plastic wrap and roll flat. Using a small circular bowl or cup as a template, cut an even circle of dough around the outside of the bowl. Set the round aside and repeat with the rest of the dough.

Place a large ceramic nonstick skillet on medium-high heat. Place tortillas closely but not overlapping in the pan. Flip every two minutes until golden brown and freckled on both sides. Continue until all the tortillas are toasted.

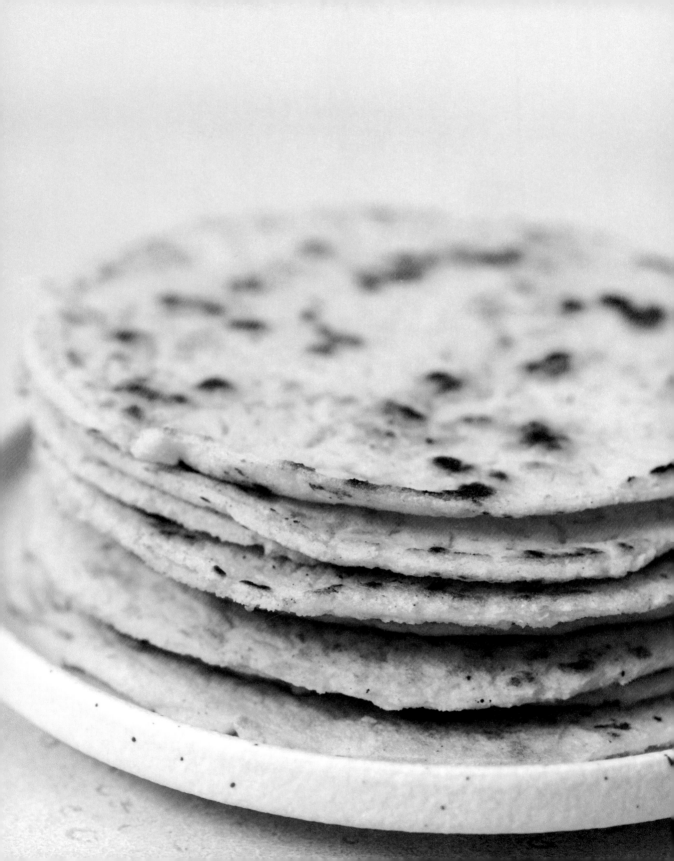

93. SAMOSA CHAAT SMASHED POTATOES

Makes 2 servings

If you like your meals to be full of flavor, texture, and spice, this is the recipe for you! Golden, crispy potatoes coated in garam masala are topped with fresh onion, tomatoes, herbs, and lime juice. The crispy potatoes are then served with oven-baked tandoori-spiced chickpeas and drizzled with an optional Mint and Cilantro Chutney. A true sensory feast!

2 pounds baby potatoes
½ tablespoon freshly squeezed lime juice
½ tablespoon raw honey
1 tablespoon garam masala (or make your own)

TO MAKE YOUR OWN GARAM MASALA

½ teaspoon ground cumin
½ teaspoon ground coriander
¼ teaspoon ground cardamom
¼ teaspoon cinnamon
¼ teaspoon chili powder or red pepper flakes
⅛ teaspoon ground cloves
⅛ teaspoon ground nutmeg

FOR THE TANDOORI CHICKPEAS

1½ cups cooked chickpeas
½ teaspoon ground cumin
½ teaspoon ground coriander
¼ teaspoon ground ginger
¼ teaspoon garlic powder
¼ teaspoon ground turmeric
¼ teaspoon chili powder or cayenne

TOPPINGS

1 cup diced tomatoes
½ cup diced onion, any color
1 teaspoon finely chopped ripe hot pepper
2 tablespoons finely chopped fresh mint
2 tablespoons roughly chopped fresh cilantro
1 to 2 tablespoons freshly squeezed lime juice

FOR THE MINT AND CILANTRO CHUTNEY (OPTIONAL)

1 cup tightly packed fresh mint leaves
1 cup tightly packed fresh cilantro leaves and stems
3 garlic cloves
½-inch piece of fresh ginger
2 tablespoons freshly squeezed lime juice
½ tablespoon raw honey

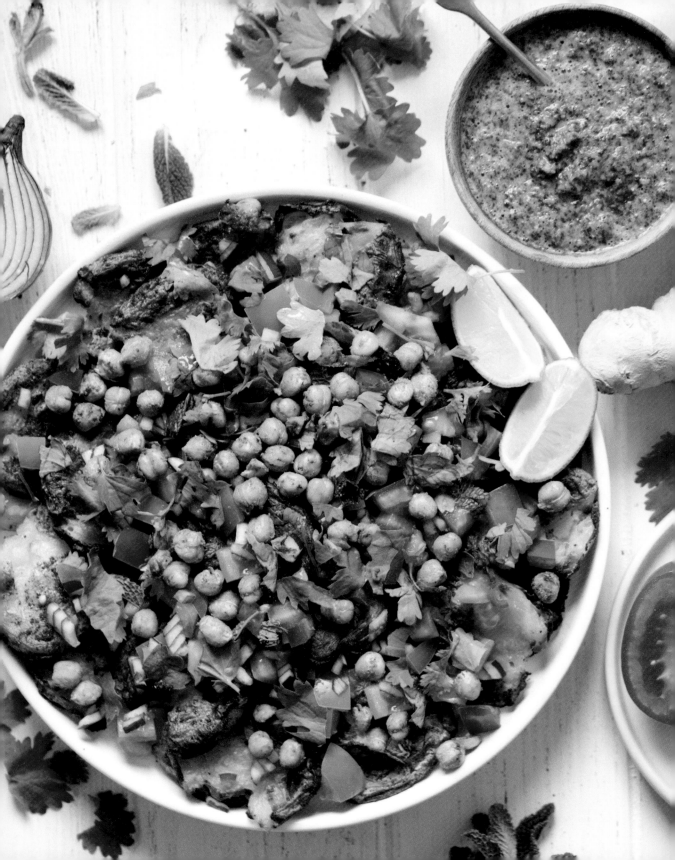

Preheat the oven to 425°F/220°C. Line two baking sheets with parchment paper.

Add 3 inches of water to a medium pot, insert a steaming basket, add the potatoes, and cover. Steam the potatoes for 20 to 25 minutes until tender. Remove from the heat and cool for 10 minutes.

While the potatoes are steaming, combine all the ingredients for the tandoori chickpeas in a bowl and stir until the chickpeas are evenly coated. Spread in a single layer on one of the prepared baking sheets and roast for 15 to 20 minutes until browned and crispy. Remove and set aside.

Place the steamed potatoes in a bowl together with the lime juice, raw honey, and garam masala. Toss until evenly coated.

Arrange the potatoes on the second baking sheet with an inch of space between each potato. Use a flat spatula or the bottom of a glass to gently smash the potatoes. Roast for 30 to 40 minutes until browned and crispy.

Combine all the chutney ingredients in a small food processor or blender and blend until smooth.

Assemble the dish by topping the smashed potatoes with the tomatoes, onion, hot pepper, mint, cilantro, lime, tandoori chickpeas, and chutney (if using). Serve immediately.

TIPS

- If you choose to add the chutney, you can use the recipe included here or you can use the Raw Cilantro Chutney recipe on page 362. Both are delicious!

- It's helpful to keep steamed potatoes ready in your fridge for meals like this so you can go straight to roasting them according to the instructions.

- You can make a larger amount of the chutney in advance and have it in the fridge for a few days to enjoy. Use it on salads and steamed or baked vegetables, as well as in this recipe.

94. BANANA SPLIT

Makes 2 servings

Creamy banana ice cream drizzled with a sweet caramel-date sauce and topped with fresh berries, cherries, and dried fruits. These banana splits feel decadent without containing any fat—they're made only with fruit!

FOR THE BANANA ICE CREAM

3 to 4 frozen bananas, roughly chopped
2 to 3 tablespoons water or freshly squeezed orange juice (optional)

FOR THE STRAWBERRY ICE CREAM

3 to 4 frozen bananas, roughly chopped
1 cup frozen strawberries
¼ to ⅓ cup water or freshly squeezed orange juice (optional)

FOR THE WILD BLUEBERRY ICE CREAM

3 to 4 frozen bananas, roughly chopped
1 cup frozen wild blueberries
¼ to ⅓ cup water or freshly squeezed orange juice (optional)

FOR THE DATE SAUCE

½ cup pitted Medjool dates
1 cup warm water
1 teaspoon alcohol-free vanilla extract or ½ teaspoon pure vanilla powder

TO SERVE

2 to 4 bananas, peeled and cut in half lengthwise
¼ cup pure strawberry jam
¼ cup pure wild blueberry jam
¼ cup chopped or whole dried mulberries (optional)
½ cup pitted fresh or thawed frozen cherries

TIPS

- Look for pure fruit jams without added sugar, citric acid, natural flavors, artificial flavors, or other additives.

- Thawing your frozen bananas for 5 minutes before using can be helpful.

- As an alternative to using a blender or food processor, you can also make banana ice cream with a fruit ice cream machine or a multipurpose masticating juicer.

Banana Split continued

To make the ice creams, place the ingredients for each flavor in a food processor or blender and blend until smooth, scraping down the sides as needed. If you have a powerful blender or food processor, you may not need any water or orange juice. Otherwise, you can add as much of either liquid as needed to blend until smooth. Serve immediately, or freeze for at least 2 hours for a firmer consistency.

To make the date sauce, combine the dates, water, and vanilla in a high-speed blender. Blend until smooth, scraping down the sides as needed.

To serve, arrange the banana halves on two plates and place a scoop of each ice cream between the halves. Drizzle the date sauce, strawberry jam, and wild blueberry jam on top. Top with dried mulberries (if using) and cherries. Serve immediately and enjoy.

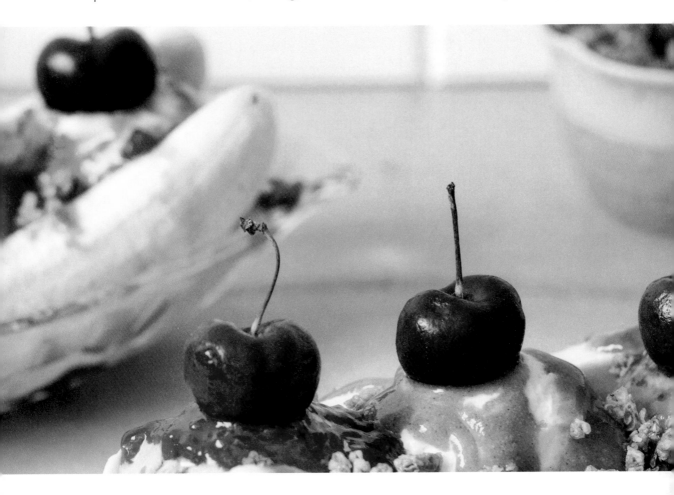

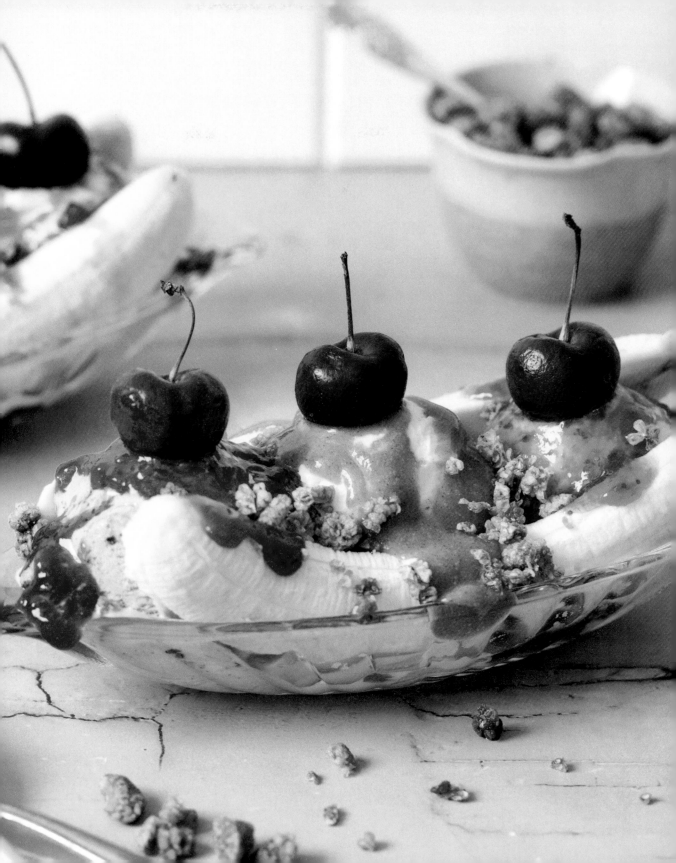

95. WILD BLUEBERRY LATTE

Makes 1 to 2 servings

This sweet and creamy drink is so delicious and really hits the spot when you want a warm drink that feels indulgent. It's also incredibly pretty!

¾ cup water
½ cup unsweetened almond milk, light coconut milk, or unsweetened oat milk
½ cup thawed frozen or fresh wild blueberries
1 to 2 tablespoons raw honey
½ teaspoon cinnamon (optional)
¼ teaspoon ground cardamom (optional)

Combine all the ingredients in a blender and blend until smooth.

Pour through a fine-mesh sieve into a small saucepan. You can skip the straining if you don't mind the wild blueberry seeds.

Heat on low until warm.

Divide between two cups and serve.

If you'd like, as an optional additional step, you can also heat some extra milk and whisk the milk with a frother until foamy. Spoon on top of the lattes and sprinkle with cinnamon (if using). Serve.

TIPS

- Nut milks, coconut milks, and oat milks can have additives or fillers (sometimes even unlabeled), including oils, preservatives, citric acid, guar gum, carrageenan, and natural flavors. If possible, it's best to make your own nut milk, coconut milk, or oat milk or to look for a brand without these additives.

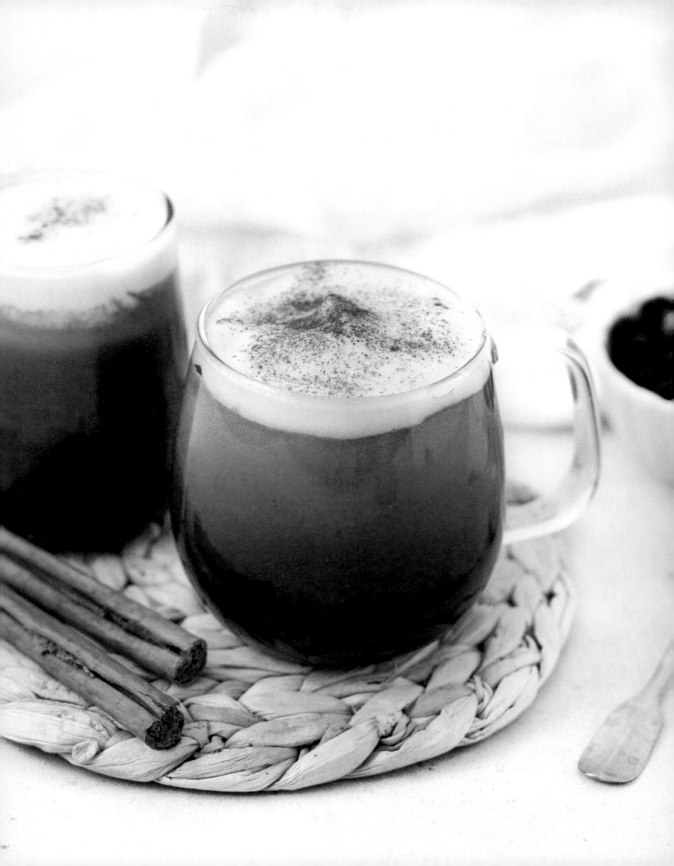

96. WILD BLUEBERRY SORBET

Makes 2 servings

This beautiful sorbet is light, tangy, and refreshing. It's perfect for a morning or afternoon pick-me-up thanks to the readily available glucose from the fruits and raw honey and the adaptogenic nature of the wild blueberries.

3 cups frozen wild blueberries
2 tablespoons freshly squeezed lemon juice
½ teaspoon lemon zest
2 to 4 tablespoons water
⅓ cup + 2 tablespoons raw honey or pure maple syrup, or more to taste

Place the wild blueberries, lemon juice and zest, 2 tablespoons of water, and raw honey or maple syrup in a high-speed blender or food processor and process until smooth, adding up to 2 more tablespoons of water if needed. Scrape down the sides as needed. Once the mixture is smooth, taste it for sweetness and add a bit of additonal raw honey or maple syrup if needed.

Serve the sorbet immediately, or transfer to an airtight container and freeze for a couple of hours for a harder consistency.

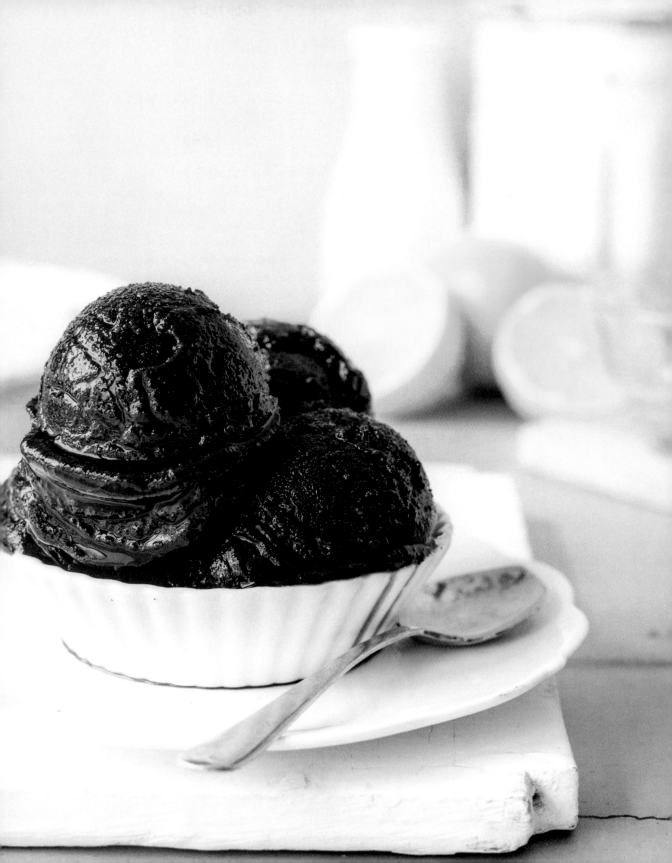

97. CHERRY PIE COMPOTE

Makes 2 to 3 servings

This quick and simple fruit compote tastes like cherry pie filling while supporting your health with nourishing ingredients. Have fun with presentation, serving this recipe in jars, teacups, or other special dishware that shows off the cherries' rich, fortifying color.

3 cups fresh or frozen pitted cherries
⅓ cup pure maple syrup
2 tablespoons arrowroot powder
1½ tablespoons freshly squeezed
   lemon juice
½ teaspoon lemon zest
1 teaspoon alcohol-free vanilla extract
   or ½ teaspoon pure vanilla powder
½ teaspoon cinnamon (optional)

Place all the ingredients in a medium pot and stir until combined.

Place the pot on medium-high heat and cook, stirring often, for 10 to 15 minutes until the cherries have softened and the sauce has thickened.

Remove from the heat and cool completely before pouring into jars or cups to serve.

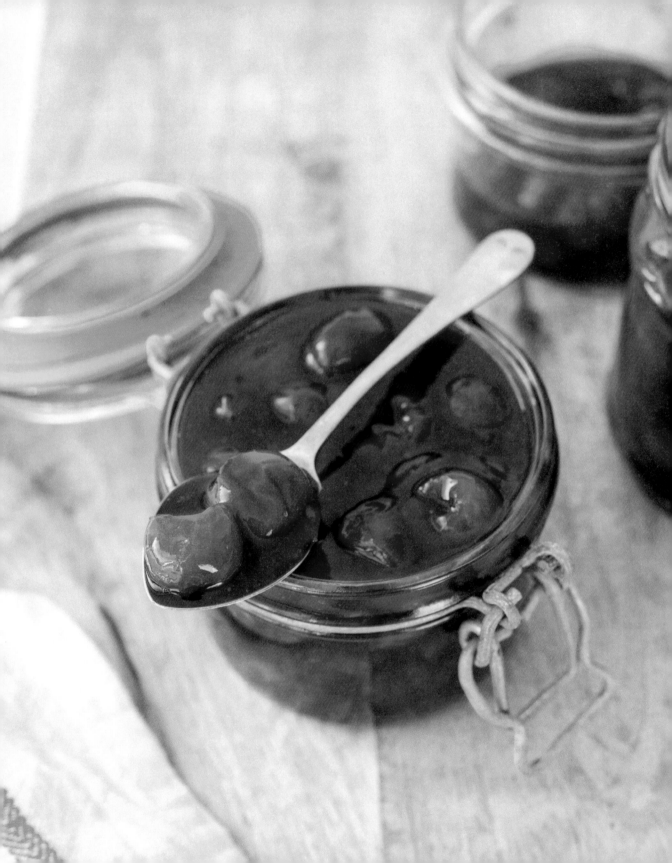

98. BAKED WILD BLUEBERRY PANCAKE

Makes 6 to 8 servings

This baked pancake is a fun and tasty way to get more wild blueberries into your diet. Best of all, you don't have to stand at the stove making pancakes; you just pour the batter into a baking dish and let the oven do the work!

1¾ cups chickpea flour

1 cup coconut milk or unsweetened almond milk

1 cup water

2 teaspoons aluminum-free baking powder

⅓ cup + 2 tablespoons pure maple syrup, plus more to serve

1 tablespoon freshly squeezed lemon juice

2 teaspoons alcohol-free vanilla extract or 1 teaspoon pure vanilla powder

½ teaspoon ground cardamom

1½ cups wild blueberries

Preheat the oven to 400°F/200°C.

Combine the chickpea flour, coconut or almond milk, water, baking powder, maple syrup, lemon juice, vanilla, and cardamom in a blender. Blend until smooth, 1 to 2 minutes.

Pour into a 10-inch ceramic baking dish or equivalent. Sprinkle the wild blueberries evenly on top.

Bake for 35 to 45 minutes until browned. Cool for at least 20 minutes.

Drizzle a bit more maple syrup on top. Slice and serve.

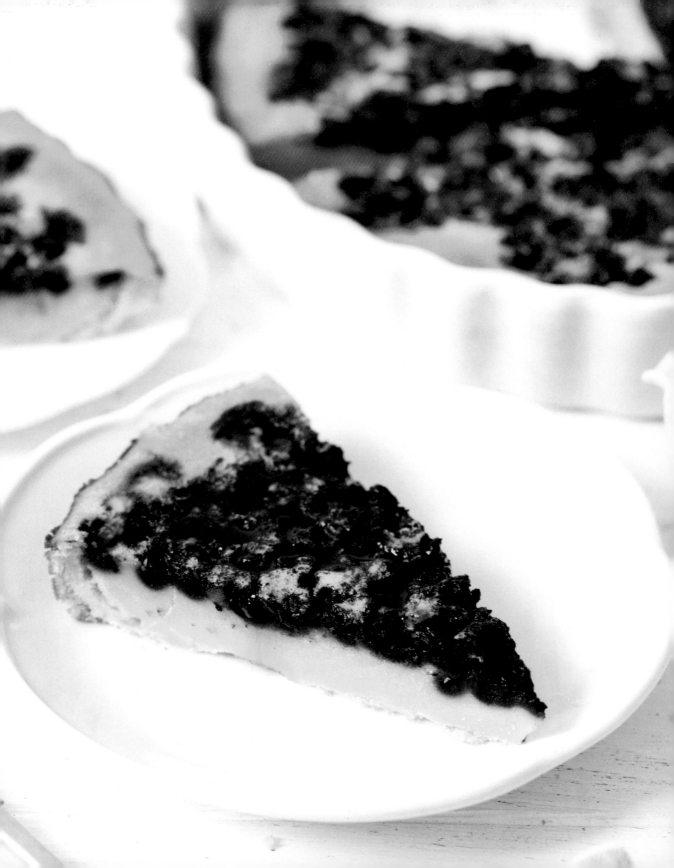

99. POTATO WAFFLE WITH WILD BLUEBERRY SAUCE

Makes 2 servings

These waffles are cooked until golden and served with a sweet wild blueberry sauce. This recipe, which can be enjoyed any time of the day, is sure to satisfy any sweet craving!

2 pounds potatoes, roughly chopped

FOR THE WILD BLUEBERRY SAUCE

2 cups frozen or fresh wild blueberries
¼ cup pure maple syrup
1 teaspoon alcohol-free vanilla extract or ½ teaspoon pure vanilla powder
2 teaspoons arrowroot powder

Add 3 inches of water to a medium pot, insert a steaming basket, add the potatoes, and cover. Steam for 15 to 20 minutes until tender when pierced with a fork. Remove from the heat and cool completely.

Add the potatoes to a large bowl and mash with a potato masher until lump-free.

Heat a ceramic nonstick waffle machine to high heat. Add enough mashed potatoes onto the base of the waffle machine until it's evenly covered, then close the machine and cook until the waffle is crispy, 10 to 15 minutes. Repeat with the remaining mashed potatoes.

While the waffles are cooking, combine the wild blueberries, maple syrup, vanilla, and arrowroot powder in a small saucepan. Stir until evenly mixed. Place on medium-high heat and cook, stirring often, until a thick sauce forms.

Serve the waffles immediately with the wild blueberry sauce on top. Enjoy!

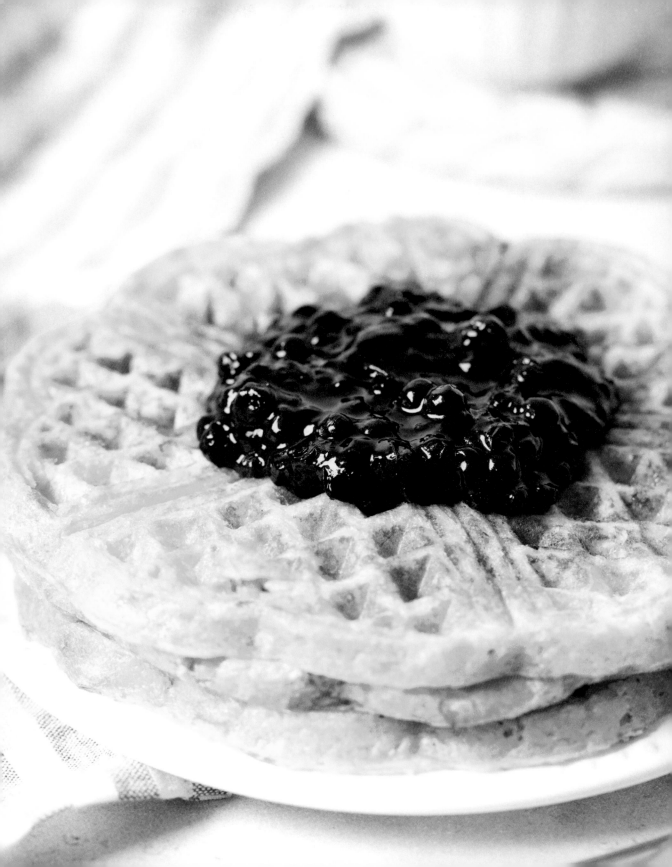

100. STEWED BERRIES

Makes 2 servings

Stewed berries are such a satisfying and comforting sweet snack. Perfect for cooler weather when you want something that feels warming and nurturing or just for when the mood strikes! These Stewed Berries can be enjoyed alone, over fruit, such as banana or mango slices, or on top of gluten-free oatmeal or millet porridge.

1½ cups frozen wild blueberries
1½ cups fresh or frozen raspberries
½ cup fresh or frozen blackberries
3 tablespoons pure maple syrup
½ teaspoon cinnamon
1 teaspoon alcohol-free vanilla extract or
  ½ teaspoon pure vanilla powder

Place the berries together with the maple syrup, cinnamon, and vanilla in a small saucepan on medium-low heat. Cook, stirring occasionally, until the berries are warm and soft. Remove from heat and serve.

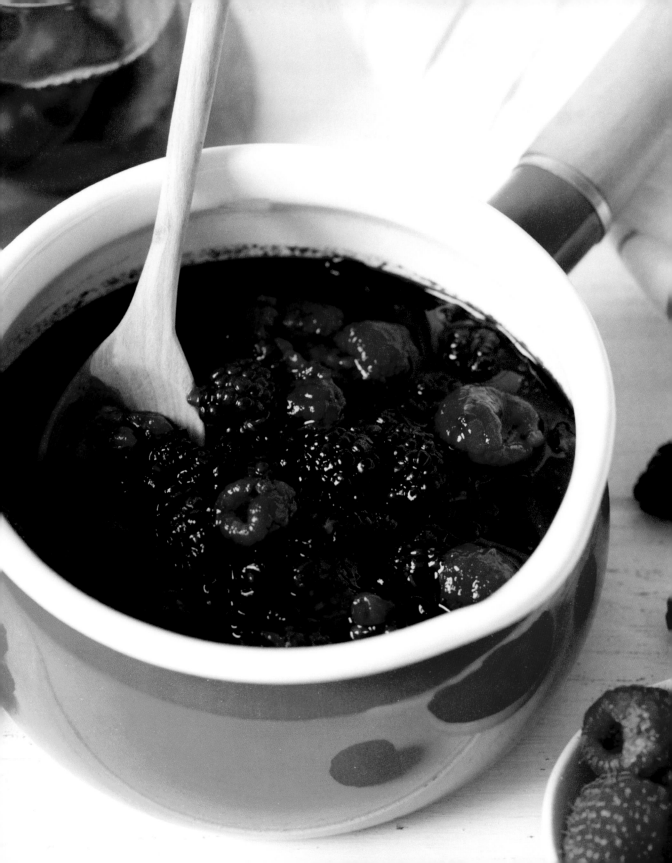

101. BERRY BREAD

This delectable Berry Bread will have your home smelling heavenly! This is a great recipe to make with your children or bake to share with family or friends. It will taste just as good as any baked treat you'd normally enjoy without containing any problematic foods such as eggs, milk, butter, refined sugar, and gluten.

3 bananas (yields about 1½ cups mashed)

⅓ cup pure maple syrup

1 teaspoon alcohol-free vanilla extract or ½ teaspoon pure vanilla powder

½ cup unsweetened almond or coconut milk

2 cups gluten-free oat flour

½ cup millet flour

1 teaspoon aluminum-free baking powder

¼ teaspoon baking soda

1 cup fresh or thawed frozen mixed berries, such as blackberries, raspberries, wild blueberries, and chopped strawberries

Preheat the oven to 350°F/180°C. Line a 9-x-5-inch loaf pan with parchment paper.

Place the bananas in a bowl and mash with a fork or potato masher. Add the maple syrup, vanilla, and almond or coconut milk. Mix well.

Combine the gluten-free oat flour, millet flour, baking powder, and baking soda in a second bowl. Whisk until lump-free. Add the wet ingredients and gently fold until you get a smooth combined batter.

Add the berries and stir very gently, just enough to incorporate them.

Pour the batter into the loaf pan and bake for 50 to 60 minutes until a toothpick inserted in the center comes out clean. Remove from the oven and cool completely before slicing.

TIPS

- If you select fresh strawberries for this recipe, remove the greens before using. Read why on page 287.

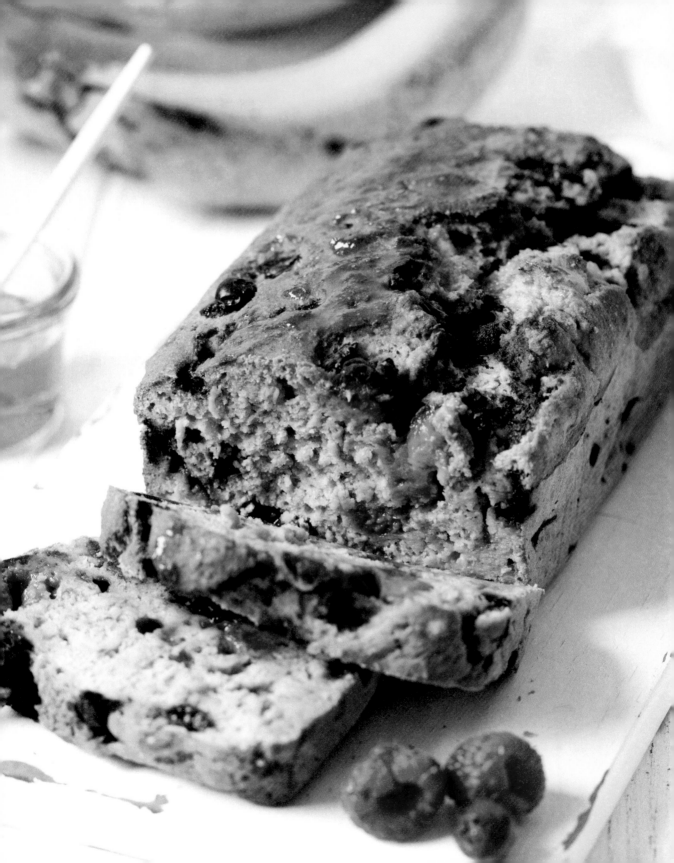

102. WILD BLUEBERRY CRISP WITH BANANA ICE CREAM

Sweet wild blueberries are topped with a maple-oat crumble that's baked until golden in this crisp. Enjoy the crisp paired with a generous scoop of banana ice cream or eat it by itself.

FOR THE FILLING

5 cups frozen wild blueberries or substitute fresh or frozen strawberries, raspberries, or blackberries
2 tablespoons freshly squeezed lemon juice
½ teaspoon finely grated lemon or orange zest
½ cup pure maple syrup
1 teaspoon alcohol-free vanilla extract or ½ teaspoon pure vanilla powder
3 tablespoons arrowroot powder or potato starch

FOR THE TOPPING

2 cups rolled gluten-free oats
½ teaspoon cinnamon
¼ teaspoon ground cardamom (optional)
⅓ cup pure maple syrup

FOR THE BANANA ICE CREAM (OPTIONAL)

3 to 4 frozen bananas, roughly chopped
2 to 3 tablespoons water or freshly squeezed orange juice (optional)

Preheat the oven to 350°F/180°C.

Combine the wild blueberries, lemon juice, lemon or orange zest, maple syrup, vanilla, and arrowroot powder in a large bowl and mix until well combined. Pour into a 9-inch square baking dish or cast-iron skillet. Set aside.

Combine the rolled oats, cinnamon, and cardamom (if using) in a medium bowl. Pour in the maple syrup. Stir until well combined.

Layer the oat mixture over the berry mixture. Bake until the berries are bubbling and the topping is browned, 40 to 45 minutes. Remove the crisp and let cool for at least 15 minutes. Serve warm or at room temperature.

To make the banana ice cream, place the frozen bananas and water or orange juice in a blender and blend until smooth, scraping down the sides and adding more liquid as needed. Alternatively, you can place just the frozen bananas in a food processor without any liquid and process until smooth. Serve immediately with the crisp, or make ahead and freeze for at least 2 hours for a firm ice cream, and then serve with the crisp.

TIPS

- If you select fresh strawberries for this recipe, remove the greens before using.

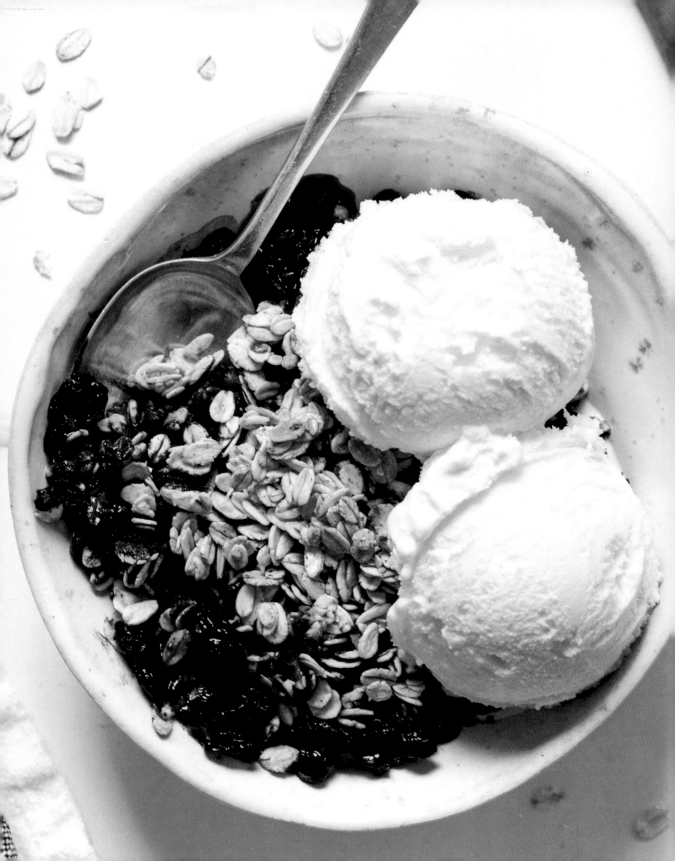

103. BLACKBERRY AND RASPBERRY JAM TARTLETS

Made with just fruits and raw honey, these pretty berry tartlets are perfect for anyone with a sweet tooth. With such healthy and wholesome ingredients, you can enjoy these tartlets any time of day and know you are feeding your body the best!

BLACKBERRY TARTLETS

Makes 5 servings

2½ cups pitted Medjool dates, divided
1 cup dried mulberries
3 cups fresh blackberries, divided
2 tablespoons freshly squeezed
   lemon juice
1 teaspoon raw honey (optional)

To make the crust, place 2 cups of the dates and the dried mulberries in a food processor and process until well combined. Scrape down the sides as needed.

Line five 4-inch mini tart pans with parchment paper or plastic wrap. (This is optional but makes removing the base a lot easier later.) Press the crust mixture evenly into the bottom of the pans and place in the freezer for 30 minutes.

Make the filling by blending together 2 cups of the blackberries, the remaining ⅓ cup of dates, and the lemon juice until smooth. Pour into the tart crusts and refrigerate for a further 30 minutes.

Remove the tartlets from the fridge and top with the remaining blackberries. Drizzle with raw honey (if using).

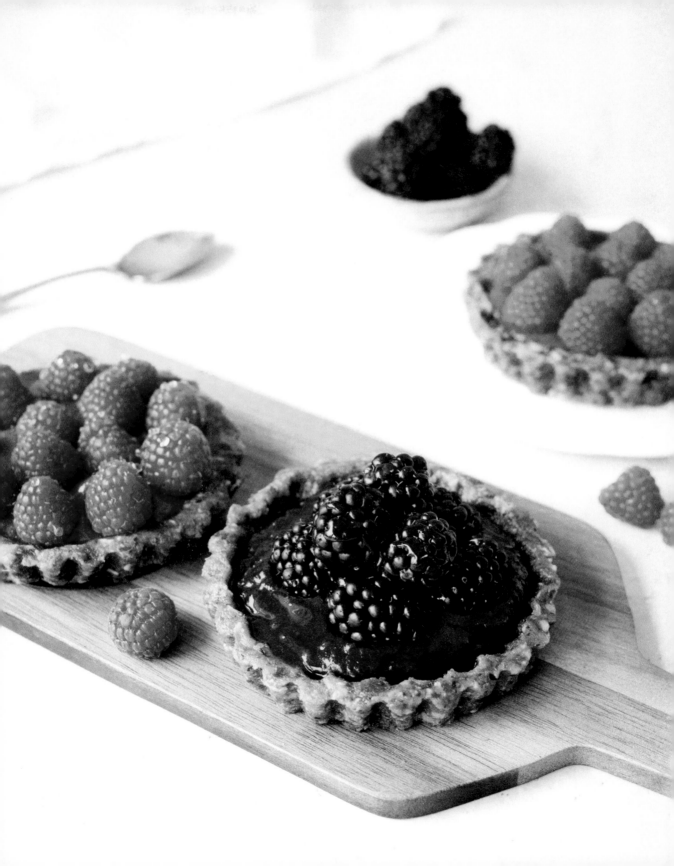

RASPBERRY TARTLETS

Makes 5 servings

2½ cups pitted Medjool dates, divided
1 cup dried mulberries
3 cups fresh raspberries, divided
2 tablespoons freshly squeezed
 lemon juice
1 teaspoon raw honey (optional)

To make the crust, place 2 cups of the dates and the dried mulberries in a food processor and process until well combined. Scrape down the sides as needed.

Line five 4-inch mini tart pans with parchment paper or plastic wrap. (This is optional but makes removing the base a lot easier later.) Press the crust mixture evenly into the bottom of the pans and place in the freezer for 30 minutes.

Make the filling by blending together 2 cups of the raspberries, the remaining ½ cup of dates, and the lemon juice until smooth. Pour into the tart crusts and refrigerate for a further 30 minutes.

Remove the tartlets from the fridge and top with the remaining raspberries. Drizzle with raw honey (if using).

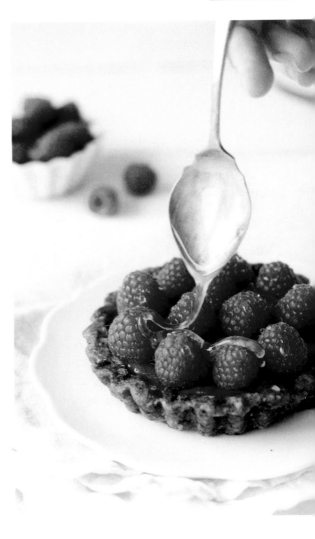

104. WILD BLUEBERRY ICE CREAM CAKE

A layer each of vanilla and wild blueberry banana ice creams on top of a sweet "crust" makes this ice cream cake oh-so-good. This recipe can be made either with some healthy fats for the most decadent result or fat-free for a delicious and even more healing option.

FOR THE CRUST

1 cup pitted Medjool dates
½ cup dried mulberries
¼ cup unsweetened shredded coconut or dried mulberries

FOR THE VANILLA ICE CREAM LAYER

3 frozen bananas
1 teaspoon pure vanilla powder or alcohol-free vanilla extract
¼ cup unsweetened coconut milk or almond milk (optional)
3 tablespoons pure maple syrup
½ tablespoon freshly squeezed lemon juice

FOR THE WILD BLUEBERRY ICE CREAM LAYER

2 frozen bananas
¾ cup frozen or fresh wild blueberries
1 teaspoon pure vanilla powder or alcohol-free vanilla extract
¼ cup unsweetened coconut milk or almond milk (optional)
3 tablespoons pure maple syrup

FOR THE TOPPING

½ cup fresh blueberries
1 to 2 tablespoons pure maple syrup or raw honey (optional)

TIPS

- For a fat-free version of this ice cream cake, use dried mulberries instead of coconut in the crust and omit the coconut or almond milk in the two ice cream layers.

- Frozen blackberries and raspberries also work well in this recipe if you can't access wild blueberries or want to try another berry variety for this cake.

- Let the cake slices soften for a few minutes before eating. This makes the cake even creamier.

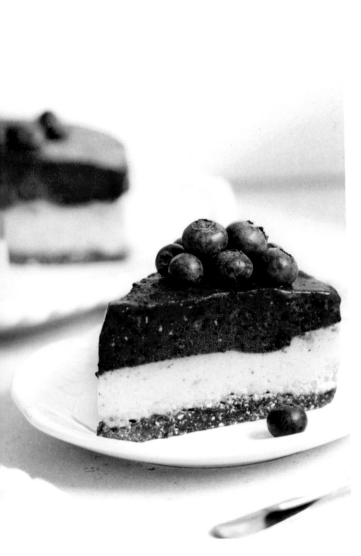

Line the bottom of an 8- or 9-inch springform baking pan with parchment paper. Set aside.

To make the crust, combine the dates, dried mulberries, and shredded coconut or additional dried mulberries in a food processor. Process for 3 to 4 minutes, scraping down the sides as needed, until smooth. Using wet hands, place the mixture in the prepared baking pan and spread out evenly. Place the pan in the freezer.

To make the vanilla ice cream layer, combine the frozen bananas, vanilla, coconut or almond milk (if using), maple syrup, and lemon juice in a food processor. Process until smooth, scraping down the sides as needed. Pour on top of the crust and return to the freezer.

To make the wild blueberry ice cream layer, combine the frozen bananas, wild blueberries, vanilla, coconut or almond milk (if using), and maple syrup in a food processor. Process until smooth, scraping down the sides as needed.

Carefully spread the wild blueberry layer on top of the vanilla layer and freeze for at least 2 to 3 hours, or until set.

To serve, top the "cake" with fresh blueberries and a drizzle of maple syrup or raw honey (if using). Slice and serve.

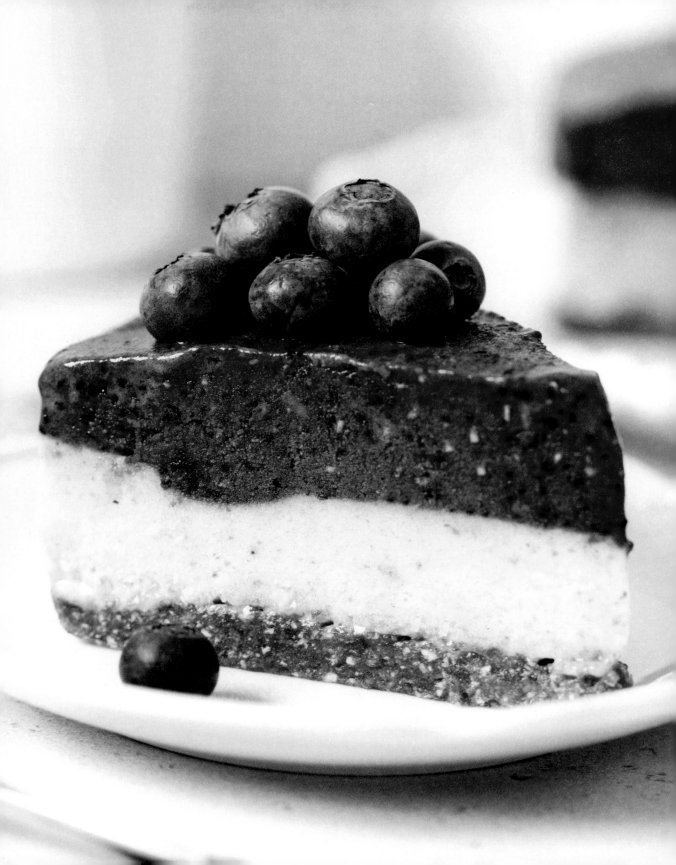

105. BAKED TURMERIC BANANAS WITH WILD BLUEBERRY SAUCE

Makes 2 to 3 servings

Warm from the oven, these baked bananas offer the healing properties of turmeric and just the right complement in sweet, antioxidant-rich wild blueberry sauce.

FOR THE BANANAS

3 to 4 bananas, peeled and cut in half lengthwise
¼ to ½ teaspoon ground turmeric
1 tablespoon raw honey or pure maple syrup

FOR THE WILD BLUEBERRY SAUCE

1½ cups frozen or fresh wild blueberries
2 tablespoons raw honey or pure maple syrup
2 teaspoons arrowroot powder

Preheat the oven to 400°F/200°C. Line a baking sheet with parchment paper.

Place the banana halves on the baking sheet and sprinkle the turmeric evenly on top. Drizzle with the raw honey or maple syrup.

Bake for 15 to 18 minutes until the bananas are soft and golden brown. Place under the broiler/grill for a further 2 to 3 minutes if the bananas haven't browned on top, being careful not to burn the bananas.

While the bananas are baking, combine the wild blueberries, raw honey or maple syrup, and arrowroot powder in a small saucepan. Stir until evenly mixed. Place on medium-high heat and cook, stirring frequently, until the wild blueberries are soft and the sauce has thickened.

When the bananas are ready, divide them between two or three plates and top with the warm wild blueberry sauce. Serve immediately.

TIPS

- Be cautious not to add too much turmeric or the bananas will become bitter.

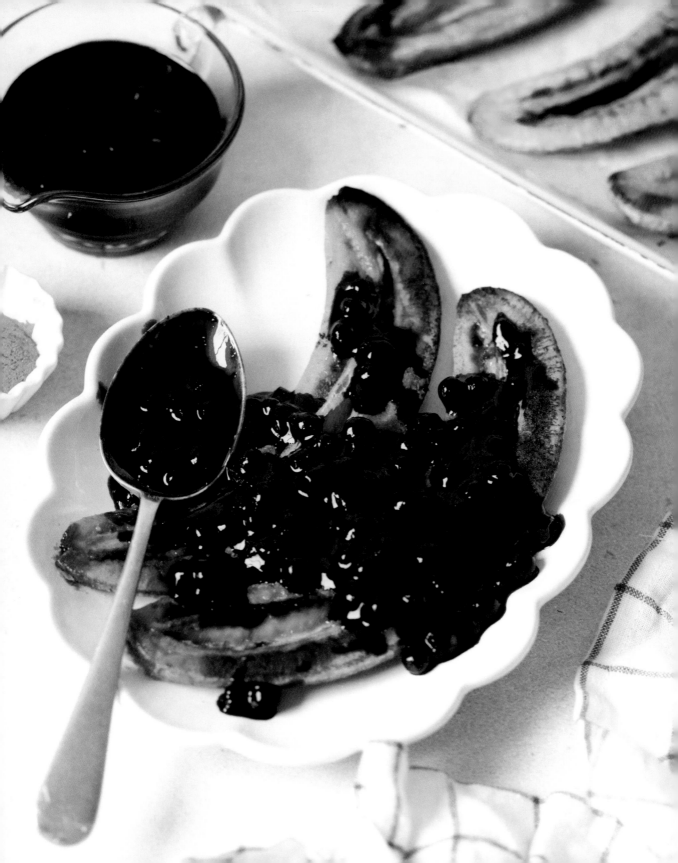

106. PANCAKES WITH BERRY SYRUP

Makes 1 to 2 servings

These fat-free pancakes come out beautifully without any need for oil, butter, eggs, or milk, making them a far better choice for anyone on the healing path. They're also excellent to make for your children or loved ones no matter what their diet! Enjoy them with the sweet berry syrup for a satisfying pancake meal when the mood strikes.

FOR THE PANCAKES

1 cup gluten-free oat flour
1 teaspoon aluminum-free baking powder
¼ cup applesauce
½ cup water
2 tablespoons pure maple syrup
½ teaspoon cinnamon (optional)

FOR THE BERRY SYRUP

1 cup mixed frozen berries, such as
    strawberries, raspberries, blackberries,
    wild blueberries, and/or blueberries
2 tablespoons water
2 tablespoons pure maple syrup
1 teaspoon alcohol-free vanilla extract or
    ½ teaspoon pure vanilla powder
½ teaspoon arrowroot powder or potato
    starch

To make the syrup, add the berries, water, maple syrup, vanilla, and arrowroot powder to a small saucepan, mix well, and bring to a simmer. Cook, stirring every few minutes, until the syrup thickens. Set aside.

Combine the oat flour and baking powder in a medium bowl. Mix well. Add the applesauce, water, maple syrup, and cinnamon (if using) to the bowl. Stir until well combined and smooth.

Place a ceramic nonstick frying pan on medium-high heat. Place about ¼ cup of the pancake batter onto the pan. Cook until bubbles form, flip, and cook for another minute. Remove from the heat and repeat with the remaining batter. If the batter gets very thick, then add a teaspoon of water to it.

Serve the pancakes immediately with the berry syrup.

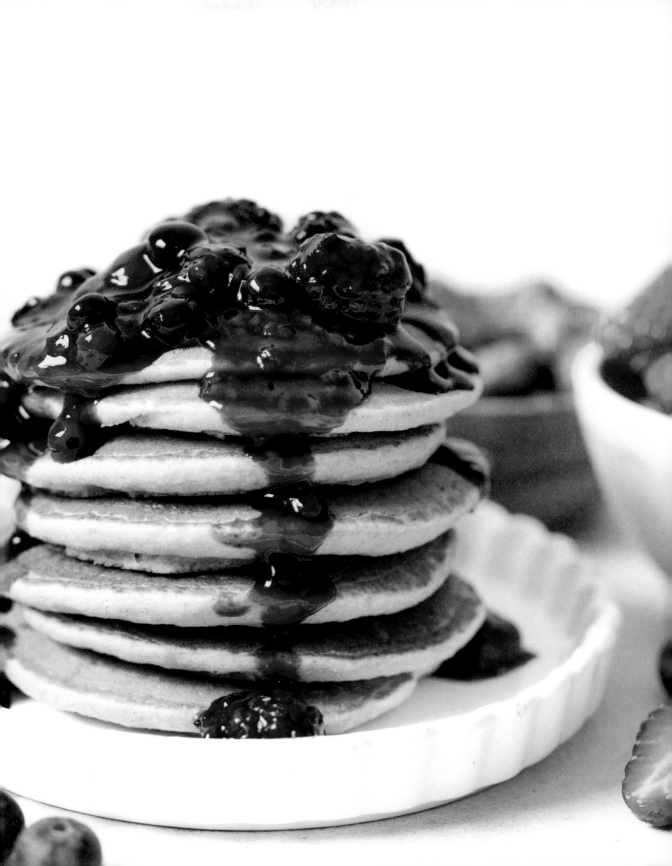

107. WARM WILD BLUEBERRY BOWL

Thick and luscious, this wild blueberry bowl offers sweetness and warmth to lift and comfort the soul. It's also incredibly easy and simple to make! Enjoy it at any time of day when you need true comfort food.

4 cups fresh or frozen wild blueberries
½ cup pure maple syrup
1½ tablespoons arrowroot powder
1½ tablespoons cold water
Fresh wild blueberries, for garnish
(optional)

Heat the wild blueberries and maple syrup in a large saucepan until the blueberries are warm and soft, 6 to 8 minutes.

In a small bowl, mix the arrowroot powder with the cold water and add to the wild blueberries. Bring to a simmer and cook for another 2 minutes until the wild blueberry mixture thickens. Remove from the heat and cool for 3 to 5 minutes before serving.

Serve with fresh wild blueberries on top (if using).

TIPS

- This recipe tastes delicious just as it is, but feel free to add a pinch of the sweet flavors you love, such as cinnamon or pumpkin pie spice and/or alcohol-free vanilla extract or vanilla bean powder if you wish.

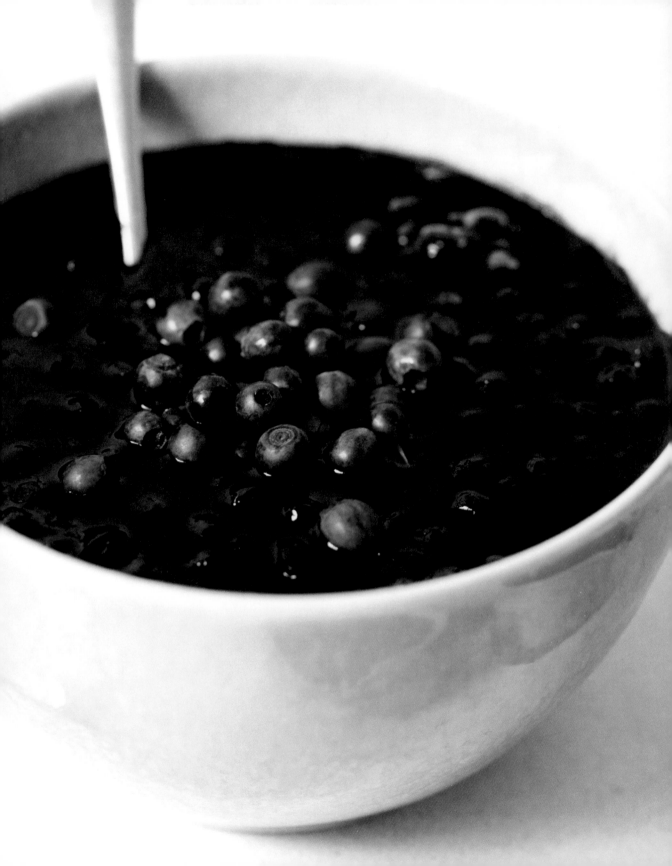

108. MILLET BANANA PANCAKES

Makes 1 to 2 servings

Sweet and satisfying, this banana pancake recipe features millet as the gluten-free grain of choice. These pancakes are easy to make and a joy to consume!

1 cup millet flour
1½ teaspoons aluminum-free baking powder
1 banana, mashed
⅓ cup unsweetened almond or coconut milk, more if needed
2 tablespoons pure maple syrup, plus more to serve
½ teaspoon freshly squeezed lemon juice
1 teaspoon alcohol-free vanilla extract or ½ teaspoon pure vanilla powder
½ teaspoon cinnamon
Sliced bananas, to serve
Raw honey, to serve (optional)

Combine the millet flour, baking powder, mashed banana, almond or coconut milk, maple syrup, lemon juice, vanilla, and cinnamon in a blender. Blend until smooth. Let stand for 5 minutes.

Preheat a large ceramic nonstick frying pan over medium-low heat. Scoop ¼ cup of the batter and cook for 2 to 3 minutes on one side until bubbles form on the surface; then flip and cook for a further 30 seconds. Remove from the heat and repeat with the remaining batter.

Serve the pancakes immediately topped with fresh banana slices and a drizzle of maple syrup or raw honey (if using).

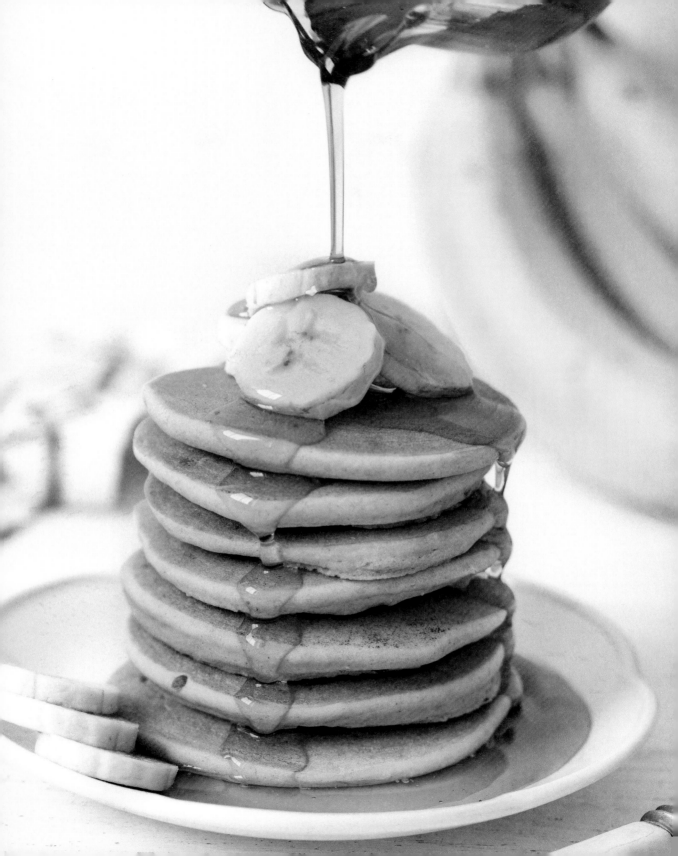

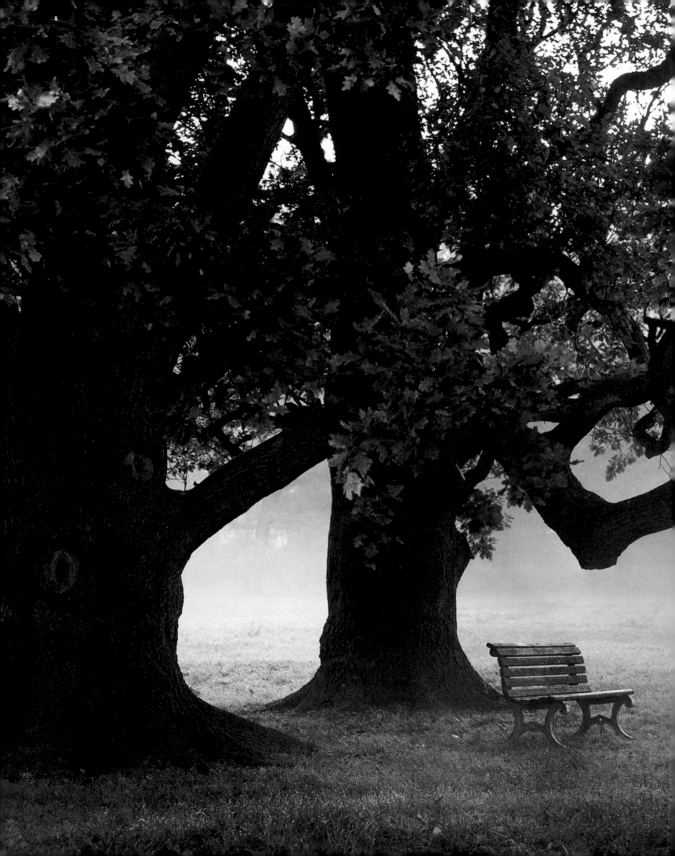

BRAIN & SOUL REHABBING

"When we go through an emotional trauma of any kind, from mild to extreme, something happens to our soul: it gets propelled out of the brain and stays close by. This is why many people feel what they call an out-of-body experience, as if they're looking from above or from the side at what's occurring in the moment when they're going through something difficult, problematic, or traumatic.

Your soul uses this method as protection. As soon as the war you're having emotionally subsides, at least the initial blow, the soul reenters your brain and body. When emotional injuries, hardships, losses, and trauma happen to us repeatedly here on earth, meaning our soul exits and reenters repeatedly, we can become disconnected from our soul. These meditations and techniques help reconnect your soul to your brain and body, strengthen your soul, and help it heal. At the same time, these meditations and techniques help heal physical injuries in your brain."

— Anthony William, Medical Medium

CHAPTER 13

Brain Healing Meditations and Techniques

If you've tried meditation and don't find it "works" for you, don't be scared off by this chapter. You don't have to like meditation to enjoy what these pages hold in store. This is not about battling your mind or fighting boredom. Trying these techniques will offer an entirely different experience. And if you have found a rhythm with standard meditations out there, you'll find something new here. These techniques and meditations are specifically geared to increase your ability to heal the symptoms and conditions listed in this book. These are powerful practices to add to your regimen to help you get better.

These techniques are not your usual exercises to find some peace and equanimity. You may not even need to embark on these meditations because you may find that healing your physical brain, especially when you overcome a level of physical pain and suffering you've been through, brings you to a sweet space of serenity and even enlightenment. Or these techniques and exercises may be needed as a support

through the physical healing. Some people may not need the techniques and exercises, and some people may really need them. Even if you're not sick with any kind of symptom or condition, these healing techniques and meditations are here to support you and keep your emotional brain and soul strong.

When we go through an emotional trauma of any kind, from mild to extreme, something happens to our soul. As we're receiving information that's extremely dissatisfying, hurtful, and even heartbreaking in any way, whether it's a betrayal or loss or hardship, our soul gets propelled out of the brain and stays close by. This is why many people feel what they call an out-of-body experience, as if they're looking from above or from the side at what's occurring in the moment when they're going through something difficult, problematic, or traumatic.

The reason the soul exits the body is to keep the soul safe, so it sustains the least amount of emotional wounds. Your physical brain can receive injuries, as we talk about in *Brain Saver*'s "Your Emotional Brain" chapter. Your soul, as much as it can get injured, uses this method that was given to us from above since the beginning of our existence as protection. As soon as the war you're having emotionally subsides, at least the initial blow, the soul reenters your brain and body. When emotional injuries, hardships, losses, and trauma happen to us repeatedly here on earth, meaning our soul exits and reenters repeatedly, we can become disconnected from our soul. This soul disconnection can lead to feeling numb, feeling as if you're missing out on something and need to be somewhere else, feeling lost, feeling like a piece of you is missing, feeling alone even if you're around others, waves of deep sadness without knowing why, and having the sensation when looking at others that everything is perfect in their lives and you're the only one feeling this way. These meditations and techniques help reconnect your soul to your brain and body, strengthen your soul, and help it heal. At the same time, these meditations and techniques help heal physical injuries in your brain.

You're welcome to ask a loved one to read any of these passages aloud for a guided meditation experience. You can also find guided meditations, including this chapter's Letting Go of Fear Meditation, on the *Medical Medium Podcast*. It's your choice how to engage with these healing practices.

RESTING THE NERVES

This is a very powerful centering technique that reboots the nervous system. Our brains are all susceptible to becoming weakened and neurologically sick. This approach is accessible to all of us when we need to give the brain and nervous system a quick restorative so we can be stronger for the day or night. You can try it anywhere: in an office chair; lying or sitting on the floor, bed, or couch at home; sitting at the kitchen table; parked in your car. The options are endless, as long as it's a spot where you'll be safe closing your eyes. That's part of the power here—it's so easy to do.

To get started, you're going to stop whatever else you're doing. Find a comfortable position. If you have a choice, opt for lying down. If not, sitting up works. Now close your eyes and keep them closed for 8 to 20 minutes. Ideally you'll keep them closed for 12 to 15 minutes—that's the most effective window. If you have less time, 8 minutes is okay, and if you have even less time, don't *not* do it. Even 3 to 4 minutes is helpful. Any amount of time spent with this technique when you need a nerve recharge will serve you.

When you close your eyes and sit or lie back, you need to remind yourself why you're doing it: to rest your nerves. In this moment you're going to have thoughts, concerns, and even worries. Projects you're working on and other reminders of your busy day are going to come to mind. At least, that's how it is for most of us. This technique is not here to punish you for that.

You're not doing it wrong if you have a racing mind. The benefits of the exercise override any thoughts and stresses pounding through your head. That's part of its power. As long as you know the purpose behind it, the second you shut your eyes and tell yourself that you're restoring your nervous system, any thoughts and worries that arise hold no authority over your restorative experience.

Right when you first close your eyes, remind yourself that the purpose of this technique is to rest your nerves, restore your nerves, and give your nerves some healing time. Your nerves are strengthening every single second. One of the incredible benefits of this exercise is that when you do it for the first time and feel and see the difference it has made for you, that becomes a landmark that helps you find peace every time you choose to do the exercise. It's so powerful that you're going to remember what it has done for you. The technique gets even more helpful every time you do it because your brain learns the routine of this restorative exercise.

When your eyes are closed, your neurotransmitters will start strengthening. Your electrical impulses will start calming down. Your neurons will start resting from less activity. Even if you're still thinking about your day as each moment passes, the emotional centers of your brain will cease to have full control over you. When your central nervous system knows you're taking care of it and giving it what it needs right then, errant thoughts can't interfere with your nerves strengthening minute by minute.

This technique is like a quick charge for your central nervous system. The nutrients from any healing foods you've eaten so far that day can be used that much more effectively while you rest your nerves. This technique also helps strengthen the immune system.

As the time you've set aside for yourself is coming to an end, try to get in touch with the fact that your brain and nerves have now strengthened. Resonate with the realization that they're stronger than when you started and that each time you do this, it's more effective.

If you're dealing with any sort of neurological symptom or illness, including ME/CFS, MS, seizures, weakness of the limbs, tingles and numbness, dizziness, vertigo, floaters in the eyes, tremors, aches, pains, ringing in the ears, headaches, migraines, jaw pain, neck pain, severe fatigue, inability to think, or brain fog, this is one of the most powerful healing techniques for you. You can use this technique throughout your day (throughout sleepless nights, even) and throughout your healing process.

ROUTINES

When we're sick or suffering, we often get lost. It can feel like a roller coaster of hope—one moment feeling optimistic about healing, the next feeling crushed, and then having to reestablish hope again. Symptoms can be a constant reminder that something is wrong. Some people have symptoms from a young age and don't remember what it's like to not have symptoms. Some may be at the beginning of chronic symptoms or a diagnosis. Trying to look for answers and protocols and find a way through all the confusion, it can be easy to get stuck in unhealthy patterns. One of the most healing exercises for finding a way forward is establishing healthy routines.

Regularly applying the information from this book can establish routines, and routines themselves can help you heal. Are you juicing celery and Brain Shot Therapies? Adding healing foods to your snacks and meals? Taking daily walks? Resting your nerves or using any of the other techniques you'll find in this chapter? A morning routine can be most powerful. If you got up and made your juice, did some form of exercise, prepared meals for the day, took a round of supplements, or did one of the meditations here, then even if the rest of the day falls apart, you have that morning as your stronghold, your foundation.

Now, this may all sound simplistic. It's not. It's not only about the healing act itself—the nutrients or the exercise or the supplements or the meditation, as powerful as these healing acts are. It's also what your brain gets out of the repetition of beneficial, productive practices, and when you're living with a chronic illness or symptom, that can help speed up recovery.

When we're feeling fine, routines can come easily. Someone may say, "Oh, I have a routine. I drink my coffee, go to my exercise class, attend meetings, take my kids to soccer practice, run errands, meet friends for drinks . . ." When you're mentally or physically suffering, life doesn't work the same way. With chronic symptoms and illness, struggling to function is part of your everyday experience. That makes for unpredictability. How much fatigue are you going to have when you get up? Are you going to have to plan your day around headaches, brain fog, or dizziness? Will a struggle with anxiety or depression get in the way of your plans? When we're suffering with these stumbling blocks, we tend to be hard on ourselves or even punish ourselves. That can become a toxic pattern. Even the smallest routines can help break our self-hatred toward our bodies and send away the feeling that they've let us down.

Establishing healthy routines tends to stimulate new neuron growth, which is critical because as we age or suffer from illness, we lose neurons. Chronic symptoms tend to enclose us in a bubble where we only get exposed to so much. Routines help encourage new cell growth by expanding electrical impulses to break us out of that bubble, and new routines redirect electrical currents to areas of the brain that might not have been receiving enough electricity. With healthy routines, new neurons get activated and stay strong. That's why it's often hard to break routines once you have them; the neurons come to expect consistent electrical brain currents.

Establishing healthy routines establishes a traffic pattern in the brain's highways. By doing this, other parts of the brain that haven't been used in a healthy manner—that have been saturated with unhealthy routines or with self-hatred, disgust, disappointment, or sadness about being sick or about any other struggle in life—get additional opportunities to heal.

If healing is your full-time job right now, here's a sample routine (this is only an example—you can create your own routine): Wake up and get yourself started on a protocol of lemon water, celery juice, and Heavy Metal Detox Smoothie. Next, depending on how you're feeling, think about taking a walk (even if it's just around the inside of your home), working on a creative project (or *thinking* about a creative project), trying your hand at a puzzle, running light errands, or doing gentle tasks. Make sure to keep fueling yourself during the morning.

When it's getting close to your midday, prep your lunch, using one of the healing recipes from the Medical Medium series, and then sit down and enjoy it. Afterward consider lying down and resting. Close your eyes for at least part of that time to give your brain and body time to rejuvenate. This is a great opportunity to try one of the meditations from this chapter. If you can, try to drift into a nap. When you're back up from your nap, make sure to reach for some juice, smoothie, or fruit to hydrate and refuel right away. This will help you wake back up and take care of whatever's on your list for the afternoon, whether that's some exercise, a project, bird-watching, gardening, a visit with friends or family, or household business.

When you eat dinner, use a healing Medical Medium recipe, and afterward do whatever you need to get ready for bed. Try to fall asleep by 10 P.M., unless you're on a different time frame. Some sort of nighttime

ritual will help you wind down, whether that's reading, taking a bath, listening to music, or all of the above. And if you can't fall asleep by 10 P.M., don't distress. Do keep your eyes closed if you can, to take advantage of that 10-to-2 sacred sleep window I've always described. You'll still receive the benefits of sleep.

Getting into a rhythm with a routine like this will make a profound difference in your healing process because you're using profound healing protocols while at the same time igniting unused or injured neuropathways. If you don't have time for all of it, that's fine. Create your own healing routine using Medical Medium information.

Once you've established a routine, it's okay to break it. It can even be *beneficial* here and there to stray from your pattern, as long as you're not straying away onto protocols that aren't healing. You can switch up your tools and protocols and your timelines and schedule, although it's not helpful to bring in toxic routines and toxic habits that can set healing back. Once you've set up your foundational, active highways through regular healing practices, mixing it up will help send electricity down different pathways and create new neuron growth in other areas of the brain.

BLOWING AWAY ANGER, FRUSTRATION, NEGATIVITY, AND HURT MEDITATION

This is a powerful brain meditation to diffuse, defuse, reroute, and even halt the emotions that dominate you the moment you have been triggered. Frustration, anger, hurt, and negativity can feel unavoidable at times, even unstoppable. When we get caught up in an emotional storm and the storm takes over, especially if whatever triggered it is ongoing, we end up becoming one with the negativity or frustration or anger or hurt that's arising. We end up resisting peace, tranquility, relaxation, and even help. As this emotional struggle is taking place within us and around us, our brain heats up. This intense brain heat can feed into the emotional struggle you are living through, causing even more brain heat and the possibility of injury to brain tissue.

Now let's begin the meditation. Find yourself a safe, comfortable place to lie down. If you need to do this meditation while sitting up, that will work fine. Once you are in a relaxing position, close your eyes. Take a deep breath in and release. Now, on the count of three, take another deep breath. One, two, three: deep breath in and release.

Now envision yourself walking. It can be wherever you'd like, whether in nature or a city street or anywhere in between. As you're walking, feel your feet hit the ground with every step. You start to feel the wind pick up. Can you feel the temperature of the wind? Is it warm? Is it cool? You can feel the wind tickle your face. The wind is becoming gusty and stronger. It's getting harder to walk. The pressure from the wind is making you push against it. Do you feel the wind against your body? Do you feel the wind rush into your lungs? Now take a

deep breath in and release. On the count of three, take another deep breath. One, two, three: take a deep breath in and release.

Feel the wind blow harder against your body, creating more resistance, to the point where it's constant and no longer blowing as gusts. After pushing and pushing against the wind, you finally stop walking and give in to the wind's force and open your arms. Feel your arms wide open as the wind is rushing against your body. Now completely relax as you are standing there against the wind. Take a deep breath in and release.

You are about to let your body fall into the wind. Are you ready to let yourself fall forward? Now let go and let yourself fall forward into the wind. Do you feel the wind catching you? The wind is strong enough to hold you upright where you are. Relax into the wind. Let the peace take over and hold you up. Feel the pressure of the wind on your abdomen, your chest, your arms, your legs, your face. No longer are you fighting against the wind. The wind feels healing. Feel your head cooling down as the wind is not allowing heat to rise inside your brain. You are one with the wind. Hear the wind rushing past your ears.

Let the wind blow the difficult emotions far, far away from you. These emotions are not a part of you anymore. These emotions do not define you. They are not truly who you are. Become one with the wind. Now take a deep breath in and release.

You can now open your eyes. You have now completed the Blowing Away Anger, Frustration, Negativity, and Hurt Meditation. You are no longer in the wind anymore.

Yet you can feel the leftover windburn on your face and body. It's a reminder that you are not controlled by anger, frustration, negativity, and hurt. They do not own you. The goal with this meditation is to know that this technique is always there, ready for you. As you are on your journey, living your life day to day, and find yourself challenged by experiences in the world that accelerate heat inside your brain, feel peace in your soul knowing that you can always change your path, cool your brain, and protect its precious resources whenever you feel your brain needs it. Feel free to repeat this meditation daily, or as many times as needed.

RELEASING EMOTIONAL TRAUMA FROM METALS MEDITATION

This is a powerful emotional processing meditation to assist with the physical aspect of removing toxic heavy metals. Some emotions and emotional experiences may have been trapped inside brain tissue that was saturated by metal toxic waste. As toxic heavy metals are exiting the brain, these trapped emotions are then released, creating sadness, the feeling of being lost, nostalgia, déjà vu, unrest, and mysterious emotional sensations and feelings. If someone has had difficult symptoms and conditions that have been caused by metals interfering with their life, then these old, trapped emotions inside the brain tissue can be more intense and need extra help to process as they exit. Metals can interfere with a person's true self, not allowing them

to express themselves to others or make decisions that move them forward in a satisfying manner. This can lead to hardship, conflict, and misunderstandings that create emotional wounds. This meditation can help heal emotional wounds that occurred during these difficult times, helping process these emotional experiences as they leave the brain tissue.

Now let's begin the meditation. Find yourself a safe, comfortable place to lie down. If you need to do this meditation while sitting up, that will work fine. Once you are in a relaxing position, close your eyes. Now take a deep breath in and release. On the count of three, take another deep breath. One, two, three: deep breath in and release.

Now envision your brain floating in front of you. You can see your brain looking at you as you are looking at your brain. Your brain has a gentle, glowing essence radiating off it. Can you see it? As you stare at your brain, you see a small, flickering, shiny metallic reflection. This is where a metal deposit is located. Another tiny metallic flickering light appears. This is another metal deposit. Do you see the flickering shiny reflections? Take a deep breath in and release.

We are going to get closer to your brain, so close that you can see the subtle patterns of the brain tissue on the outside. Can you see them? You are getting smaller and smaller and smaller. Your brain is staying the same size. Now you are going to slowly enter the inside of your brain and travel until you reach the center. Your brain is not completely dark inside. There is a soft, glowing light all around you. Are you in the center of your brain? Take a deep breath in and release.

Tiny flickering lights appear in the distance. Do you see them? These tiny flickering lights are metal deposits that have been there for many years. Can you see this one metal deposit that's leaving your brain? It's the flickering light that is getting weaker and weaker. Do you see the metallic light diminish in the distance? There is an energy storm starting to brew. The energy storm is made of old, trapped emotions. Do you feel the emotions swirl all around you? Another flickering light is dying out in the distance. Do you see it? It has now diminished. Yet the energy storm has grown stronger. Do you feel the emotion of the energy storm? You are now standing in the middle of your brain. Picture yourself raising your arms and placing your hands in the energy storm to capture it. Now slowly cast out the energy storm from your brain.

Picture yourself starting to walk gently and slowly inside the middle of your brain. Stop. Look down. There is a tiny hole inside your brain tissue where the flickering metal once was. Watch that hole fill in with new, healthy brain tissue. Do you see the hole disappearing?

A larger energy storm is starting. These are emotions that were trapped deep inside your brain tissue. Watch the emotions swirl around you. On the count of three, you are going to grab on to this energy storm and let it carry you out of your brain. One, two, three: grab on to the energy storm, picture yourself hugging the energy storm as hard

as you can, and let it carry you out of your brain. You are now leaving your brain along with the emotional energy storm.

You have now exited your brain. Look at your brain from afar. Is it glowing brighter than it was before? It is stronger than it was before. Do you see it? Now on the count of three, take a deep breath. One, two, three: deep breath in and release. You can open your eyes. You have now completed the Releasing Emotional Trauma from Metals Meditation.

As we go through life, we don't realize how tightly bound together metals and emotions really are. Emotional injuries can be stored deep down in pockets of metal waste, especially when toxic heavy metals cause disharmony, upheaval, and distress in our life, even to the point of changing your life's direction. By doing this meditation, you have now opened new channels for healthy growth, stimulating your brain to override and release both toxic metals and toxic emotions. Feel free to repeat this meditation daily, every other day, or a couple of times a week, because each time it only becomes more powerful in its ability to release emotional trauma caused by metals.

LETTING GO OF FEAR MEDITATION

Remember, I offer a guided version of this and other meditations on the *Medical Medium Podcast.*

This is a powerful brain meditation for letting go of fear and ridding fear from our soul, spirit, and heart. Fear is something that becomes a part of our consciousness, and it gets in the way of who we truly are. It can end up taking away a piece of who we are and shadowing who we aspire to be.

As we go through life and live through hardships, betrayal, broken trust, losses, broken friendships and other relationships, or emotional struggles of any kind, we have small out-of-body experiences where our soul leaves our brain and body, and a disconnect happens. An empty space opens up between our soul and brain, a distance, and fear fills the gap. This meditation is about taking control of your life, not letting fear run you or own you in any way. This will allow your neurons that are in the emotional centers of your brain to reconnect to your soul and redirect their messaging away from fear, pushing it away.

Now let's begin the meditation. Find yourself a safe, comfortable place to lie down. If you need to do this meditation while sitting up, that will work fine. Once you are in a relaxing position, close your eyes. Now take a deep breath in and release. Now on the count of three, take another deep breath. One, two, three: deep breath in and release. Now envision yourself walking down a road, and you see a bridge in the distance. It can be whatever type of bridge you like. It can be a wooden bridge, or a swinging bridge suspended over a canyon or ravine. It can be a larger bridge crossing a wide river.

Once you envision your bridge, take a deep breath in and release. You are alone. You are standing on a road exactly where the bridge starts. Don't walk across the bridge yet. First, get a clear image of what's before you. It's a bridge that's in disarray. It seems to be under construction, in desperate need of repair. It has chunks of bridge missing, and there are piles of wood, scrap metal, and trash everywhere on the bridge. Yet the bridge is still standing. You see a beat-up sign with the warning OUT OF COMMISSION. USE AT YOUR OWN RISK. As you stand there looking at the debris and rubble that's on the bridge in front of you, you notice someone in the far distance, on the other end of the bridge. They are waving and yelling in your direction. You hear them shout, "I need help!" Listen to them shout again. "I need help! Don't worry, the bridge is safe."

You can't see who this person is. They are too far away, and there seems to be a light fog in the air. You don't trust this mysterious person with your life. It's obvious to you the bridge is far from safe. You hear them shout again, "I need you. I need help. Please come fast!"

You holler, "Is the bridge really safe?"

The person answers, "It's safe. I promise. It's safe."

You instantly think, *That's the wrong answer.* That promise doesn't work for you. You've heard that before in your life, and you've been let down. You hear again, "Please come here! It's safe."

Now take a deep breath in and release. On the count of three, take another deep breath. One, two, three: take a deep breath in and release. You can't trust this person, yet something inside you leads you in their direction, onto the bridge. Something you can't explain, something that feels familiar.

You slowly take your first step onto the bridge to see for yourself if it is safe. To the left of you, you see old car tires. Ahead of you, it looks like a disaster area. You see piles of rubble and metal everywhere. You take one more step, and a lemonade stand appears to the right of you. A mother and child are selling lemonade. It makes no sense. You hadn't noticed them before. And why would they be on such a danger-ous bridge? You ask them, "Are you okay?" No response. They are sitting there safely on this little spot on the bridge that's clean and clear.

The person on the other end of the bridge calls out, "Didn't I tell you it's safe?" The person says, "Please come here! Come here soon."

You look ahead. It's a disaster zone. You still don't trust this bridge. The bridge is in total shambles, yet where your feet are touching on the bridge, it is secure. Now take a deep breath in and release.

You take a step forward away from the lemonade stand and it disappears in the fog. It's gone. You look to the right of you, and there is a broken-down car. You look ahead of you, and it's a wasteland. Concrete blocks, metal barrels, and holes everywhere in the bridge. You look to the left of you, and you notice what looks like two par-ents and their children with fishing poles. They're casting their lines off the side of the bridge. It makes no sense. The bridge is a disaster. You did not see them before. When you look around you, there's barely

any bridge left to support anyone, yet in their space, as they're fishing, they are fine. They have a solid railing supporting them as they're fishing.

"Keep going!" the voice says from the other end of the bridge. "I told you it's safe. Come quick."

Now take another deep breath in, and release. You take another step forward onto the bridge and a friendly puppy comes bounding up to you. It startles you. How did this puppy cross over the holes in the bridge? It looks like a golden retriever. The puppy begins to lick your hand. The tongue is grippy. It doesn't make sense. How did it get here from the other side? Behind the puppy is a hole in the bridge, and behind that hole is debris everywhere. You hear the voice again, the person from the other end of the bridge: "I'm over here. Come here. Hurry up. I need you."

You see everything wrong around you. The bridge is falling apart. It's a disas-ter zone. Yet where you are standing has repaired itself. Underneath your feet the bridge has gotten strong and repaired itself, and you and the puppy are safe. All of a sudden, a leash appears attached to the puppy. And at the other end of the leash is a person who offers a delightful smile. You think, *How is this possible?* as they walk by you. You turn around to look at them and they disappear in the fog and are gone, yet you are gaining a little bit of trust step by step on this bridge as you discover that pieces of the bridge are safe.

Now all that's left before you is a giant hole in the bridge, and you are not sure that trust and confidence will be enough to carry you across this hole. Do you see the hole in the bridge? Look: you can see it. The person in the distance yells, "I need you. Keep walking. Don't slow down."

You think that if you take this next step, you can fall through that hole and become injured or even die. You turn around and say, "I can't. I'm not going to die for you. I refuse to die for you. I don't trust you. It's not worth it."

The voice says, "Hurry up. I need your help. You can't let me down. Just step forward. I promise, it's safe."

There's that word *promise* again. You've heard that word before. You look back behind you, to where you started, because you're thinking you'd better head back. Then you realize it's too late. The bridge behind you is in worse shape than it ever was before and the people have all disappeared. You realize it's possible you've been tricked, taken advantage of, and misled. The voice yells out, "Listen to me. You will be safe. The bridge is safe. Time is running out." The voice says, "Please come."

You take a deep breath in and release. Take another deep breath in and then release. As you're standing there on the bridge looking at that great big hole, you decide to close your eyes. Now take the next step forward over the hole. Your foot hits solid ground and you don't fall through the bridge. You're standing.

You open your eyes while you're standing there on the bridge, and you see that underneath you, the hole in the bridge is fixed. Take another step forward. As you're walking, you see the bridge is starting to mend. The bridge is repairing itself with each step you take.

As you are stepping across the bridge, you start seeing people on this bridge and realize you have met them before in your life. You start seeing family members, friends, familiar animals walking by. All of them are happy. Everyone on this bridge is someone you have known at one point in your life. You hear the person again at the end of the bridge: "I'm here. Keep walking." You are almost at the end of the bridge now, and the bridge is beautiful. It's safe. It's peaceful. You can feel the warm sun on your face as you're walking on this bridge, and the mild fog around you is lifting.

You are almost at the end of the bridge now. You get to the last step of the bridge. You're standing there, and the person who's been calling you all along from the other side is standing there as well, right in front of you, waiting for you. It becomes clear that this person was you this whole time. Your soul was waiting at the other end of the bridge, and the fear that was keeping you apart is now gone. Now take a deep breath in and release. You can now open your eyes.

We don't realize that when we go through life, our soul becomes injured from betrayal and broken trust, and this creates fear within us. This hinders the bridge between our soul and our physical brain, and this bridge is the connection that allows us to feel safe and trust again and not live in fear. You've now completed the meditation that bridges your soul to your physical neurons in the emotional centers of your brain, so the connection between them grows strong, and fear and broken trust won't hold you back. Feel free to repeat this meditation daily, every other day, or a couple of times a week, because each time it only becomes more powerful in its ability to mend the bridge between your soul and your body.

SOUL LIGHT INFUSION MEDITATION

This is a powerful soul-healing meditation to mend fractures in the soul that have collected throughout the years as you experienced hardships, losses, betrayal, broken trust, and times of being misunderstood, or if you fought battles against injustice in your life and lost, or if you feel you have lost a piece of your soul and you are searching to get it back.

Now let's begin the meditation. Find yourself a safe, comfortable place to lie down. If you need to do this meditation while sitting up, that will work fine. Once you are in a relaxing position, close your eyes. Now take a deep breath in and release. On the count of three, take another deep breath. One, two, three: deep breath in and release.

Envision a tall staircase in the distance. You start heading in the direction of the staircase. A misty fog starts to roll in. Do you see the fog? You still see the staircase in the distance. You keep walking in that direction. It's getting closer. You are almost

there. A few more steps. You are now at the bottom of the staircase looking up. Now take a deep breath in and release.

There are 21 steps to the top of the staircase. Do you see them? We are going to count each step together as you climb the staircase. Place your foot on the first step. That is one. Now place your other foot on the step above that step. That is two. As you are climbing the staircase in the fog, do any of these numbers have meaning for you? Now let's climb the rest of the steps together: three, four, five, six, seven, eight, nine, ten, eleven, twelve, thirteen, fourteen, fifteen, sixteen, seventeen, eighteen, nineteen, twenty, twenty-one. You are now at the top of the staircase. A door appears. It is a portal. Now take a deep breath in and release.

Grab the doorknob and open the door to this portal. You enter into a dark, wide-open space. There is no floor underneath you. You are floating. Can you feel yourself floating? When you look up and around, you see glittering stars in the far distance. Look straight ahead. There is a ball of light heading your way. Do you see this light? Get ready and put your hand out. You are going to catch the light. Here it comes. Three, two, one: grab on to it. You are now holding this light. Now bring the light up to your forehead and push it in and let it enter your soul.

Another light in the distance is heading your way. The light is coming closer to you. Get ready to catch it with your hand. Three, two, one: grab on to it. You are now holding this light. How does it feel to hold on to this light? Bring the light up to your forehead and push it in and let it enter your soul.

There is another light in the distance heading your way. Do you see it? This light is brighter and larger. You need to catch this light with both hands. The light is getting closer and closer to you. Get ready to catch it. Three, two, one: grab on to it with both hands. Do you see how beautiful this light is in your hands? It's a warm, soothing, comforting light. Part of you is in this light. This part of you is pure, untouched, uninjured, and has been kept safe. Now bring the light up to your forehead and push it in and let it enter your soul. Do you feel the light inside your soul? Now take a deep breath in and release. On the count of three, take another deep breath. One, two, three: deep breath in and release.

Now it's time to leave this space and head back to the portal doorway. The door is still open. Are you there yet? Are you standing at the top of the staircase? Grab the doorknob and close the door behind you. The portal is now closed. It's time to descend back down the staircase, one step at a time. Let's count together with each step you take. Twenty-one, twenty, nineteen, eighteen, seventeen, sixteen, fifteen, fourteen, thirteen, twelve, eleven, ten, nine, eight, seven, six, five, four, three, two, one. Take a deep breath in and release.

You can open your eyes. You have now completed the Soul Light Infusion Meditation. Any fractures within your soul are now in the process of mending. As fractures mend, your soul is healing. Your soul is complete now and not missing precious lost pieces that may have been pushed away from you in times of struggle, loss, and hardship. Your spiritual force as a light being in this world has elevated. Old wounds from the past will not have a grip upon your soul as they once did. No one owns your soul but you, and you have every right to heal your soul. Feel free to repeat this powerful meditation daily, or as many times as needed to bring peace and healing to your soul.

"Our soul is an energy force that isn't conquered by what happens here on earth."

— Anthony William, Medical Medium

CHAPTER 14

Your Soul's Voice

What is a soul? Does our soul even exist? Is our soul just air that floats away? Was having a soul all along created by our imagination?

Your soul does exist. Everyone has a soul. It is the voice of your entire existence. Your soul retains knowledge of all the events that have occurred in your life. Your soul is a record that contains the meaning of your physical existence. Your soul harnesses every journey you have chosen or experienced in a physical living form. Your soul sustains itself and lives forever, long after the physical part of you has perished.

It doesn't matter if you like your soul, love your soul, or hate your soul. It doesn't matter if you don't believe in the soul's existence or believe you have a soul. It doesn't matter because your soul is more powerful than you, more powerful than your consciousness in your present state of being. Your soul is more powerful than the brainwashing you have been conditioned with here on earth because your soul has been far away from the earth and isn't governed in this earthbound bubble of our human-created environment. Your soul is more than you. It is your light. A light that did not start here on earth but started above. Your soul is much older than your physical body and has memories and information from the past to which you don't have conscious access. Your soul has the power to lead you on your way even when it's underfed and broken by the people around you or the world we live in. Your soul's leftover fragments still hold the power and the glory that brighten the way on the darkest path.

When we voice ourselves here on earth, sometimes we find moments when we transcend the confusion here, and what we're speaking is more than just our own truth; it is a common truth that unites us with others, one that may even go beyond words. This can be our true, powerful voice.

Many times, the truth spoken on Planet Earth could be flawed because human nature tends to bend the truth to provide a game and a ledge to hold on to, so truth is manipulated and spoiled with deception. Evil takes the term *truth*, shape-shifts it, and uses it as a weapon, because that truth is spoiled and filled with deception. This is a survival mechanism used by all walks of life, from the bottom tier to the top of the hierarchy.

Your soul holds authentic truth—untainted, pure, regardless of whatever survival mechanisms we tend to adapt to here on earth. Your true soul always knows better and is wiser than the truth games played here on earth. Inside each of us is this even truer, more potent voice than our earthly voice. This truer voice is elevated above the voice we know to come from a deep place within—because as strong and important as our true, deep, earthly voice is, it is often mixed with hurt and sorrow and distrust and confusion and misinformation. The truest voice we possess can never be swayed by trickery. It resides inside all of us. It is your soul.

Our soul has a sound, a sound we can't hear with our physical ears, a sound that rings true through time and space. When our soul leaves our physical body and transcends upward, a noise is made, a sound. The soul is energy, and the energy of the soul is powerful—a fireball of light. As the soul travels, the noise is the sound of the soul piercing time itself, for time no longer exists for the soul once the soul has left the body.

Where our soul goes, there is no clock. The home our soul goes back to can't be governed by time because time is different for every planet, every solar system, every galaxy. And if one planet or solar system ceases to exist, then time stops for that planet or solar system, yet our soul cannot cease to exist. Our soul needs to live on and it does, without the constraints of time.

Our soul is an energy force that isn't conquered by what happens here on earth. It is a universal, God-conceived law that our soul has it right and safely right, even if our consciousness connected to our brain has it wrong. Wrong cannot enter and destroy a soul. What really matters in the end is the truth of our soul, because it is our forever existence and overrides what we are and were here in life on earth.

"Our soul has a sound, a sound we can't hear with our physical ears, a sound that rings true through time and space."

— Anthony William, Medical Medium

ORIGINS OF THE MEDICAL MEDIUM

Spirit of the Most High, God's expression of compassion whom I call Spirit of Compassion, came into my life when I was four years old to teach me how to see the true causes of people's suffering and to get that information out into the world. Spirit of Compassion constantly speaks into my ear with clarity and precision, as if a friend were standing beside me, filling me in on the symptoms of everyone around me. Plus, Spirit of Compassion taught me from an early age to see physical scans of people, like supercharged MRI scans that reveal all blockages, illnesses, infections, trouble areas, and past problems.

My job as a messenger for Spirit of Compassion is to continue to bring advanced healing information into medical and health communities. That means publishing books and podcasts, posting and appearing on social media, and any other way to reach the chronically ill. The information in this book comes from Spirit of Compassion viewing hundreds of millions of people who are chronically suffering and then deciphering the different variables, conditions, and mental health states they're living with, feeling, or stricken with. Spirit gathers information on a vast level about what people are suffering with down here on earth and how to communicate this material so everyone with chronic illness is validated and has an opportunity to use this information to heal.

Many times as I was sitting at my desk receiving the information that you found here in these pages, I would enter a sphere of light to take me out of my personal world and surroundings so that I could hear Spirit of Compassion perfectly clearly and see any vision that Spirit provided. One day as I was sitting here waiting to transcribe words from Spirit about eating disorders, I asked, "Where are you?" Spirit of Compassion said, "I'm here. I'm just opening up the plane to get a reading from over a billion eating disorders on the planet so I can provide the information that reaches everyone with eating struggles. I want it to be comprehensive, so everyone's included."

Spirit of Compassion sees the human condition on this planet and then provides a deep understanding of how it came to be, why, and what to do with the resources we have here on this planet. *We see you. We know what you're up against. And we don't want you to go through it a moment longer.* My life's work is to deliver this information to you so that you can be elevated above the sea of confusion—the noise and rhetoric of today's health fads and trends—in order to regain your health and navigate life on your own terms.

People have often said, "What a gift you have." Some have even called me a prophet. I've replied, "It's not a gift for me. It's a responsibility I carry toward others. It's a gift for you." If someone has a gift as a mountain climber, they're truly gifted. They can climb that mountain and even risk their life doing it. That gift brings them satisfaction in their soul. While others will look in awe, the mountain climber is climbing the mountain for themselves, whether to prove they can do it and achieve that great goal, or to prove they can do it better than before. This gift is different. There isn't any self-satisfaction in hearing a voice; it's not for my own personal goals. The voice I hear is for everyone and anyone who wants to listen, who's suffering. Yes, there's always satisfaction when a life is changed and someone is healed. That satisfaction is knowing someone is freed from suffering physically or mentally.

You don't have to like me, like the message I deliver, like how I deliver that message, or even believe in the voice that was bestowed upon me. I'm still a messenger. I never wanted to hear a voice. Even after I started hearing the voice, I still never wanted to hear it. There was no running from it. And eventually I had to accept it was never going away. Know that this information is always here for you and has a history of bringing the chronically ill out of the depths of lost hope, sickness, and despair—and bringing them into the light of healing. Discrimination for being "the guy who hears a voice" has been a challenge all my life, but that doesn't compare to the discrimination the chronically ill have gone through in their lives. I'm forever committed and dedicated to having the backs of the chronically ill and, as long as I'm still here, making sure I keep bringing forth the information from Spirit of Compassion.

My job is to bring clarity to the ones who want to take the time to learn about what is wrong within their body—not because their body is weak or faulty but because there are real causes from living here on earth that can get in the way of someone's quality of life. Energy is a precious resource, and so many with chronic illness don't have enough of it. If someone takes whatever energy they do have and applies that energy and puts in an effort to learn this information from above, then the opportunity to receive results is there. My job is to deliver for the ones whose trust has been broken in other health realms, the ones who have just enough trust left within them to use that trust to move forward.

If you'd like to know more about my origins, you'll find my story in *Medical Medium: Secrets Behind Chronic and Mystery Illness and How to Finally Heal (Revised and Expanded Edition).*

CONVERSION CHARTS

The recipes in this book use the standard United States method for measuring liquid and dry or solid ingredients (teaspoons, tablespoons, and cups). The following charts are provided to help cooks outside the U.S. successfully use these recipes. All equivalents are approximate.

Standard Cup	Fine Powder (e.g., flour)	Grain (e.g., rice)	Granular (e.g., sugar)	Liquid Solids (e.g., butter)	Liquid (e.g., milk)
1	140 g	150 g	190 g	200 g	240 ml
¾	105 g	113 g	143 g	150 g	180 ml
⅔	93 g	100 g	125 g	133 g	160 ml
½	70 g	75 g	95 g	100 g	120 ml
⅓	47 g	50 g	63 g	67 g	80 ml
¼	35 g	38 g	48 g	50 g	60 ml
⅛	18 g	19 g	24 g	25 g	30 ml

Useful Equivalents for Liquid Ingredients by Volume				
¼ tsp			1 ml	
½ tsp			2 ml	
1 tsp			5 ml	
3 tsp	1 tbsp		½ fl oz	15 ml	
	2 tbsp	⅛ cup	1 fl oz	30 ml	
	4 tbsp	¼ cup	2 fl oz	60 ml	
	5⅓ tbsp	⅓ cup	3 fl oz	80 ml	
	8 tbsp	½ cup	4 fl oz	120 ml	
	10⅔ tbsp	⅔ cup	5 fl oz	160 ml	
	12 tbsp	¾ cup	6 fl oz	180 ml	
	16 tbsp	1 cup	8 fl oz	240 ml	
	1 pt	2 cups	16 fl oz	480 ml	
	1 qt	4 cups	32 fl oz	960 ml	
			33 fl oz	1000 ml	1 l

Useful Equivalents for Dry Ingredients by Weight

(To convert ounces to grams, multiply the number of ounces by 30.)

1 oz	1/16 lb	30 g
4 oz	1/4 lb	120 g
8 oz	1/2 lb	240 g
12 oz	3/4 lb	360 g
16 oz	1 lb	480 g

Useful Equivalents for Cooking/Oven Temperatures

Process	Fahrenheit	Celsius	Gas Mark
Freeze Water	32° F	0° C	
Room Temperature	68° F	20° C	
Boil Water	212° F	100° C	
Bake	325° F	160° C	3
	350° F	180° C	4
	375° F	190° C	5
	400° F	200° C	6
	425° F	220° C	7
	450° F	230° C	8
Broil			Grill

Useful Equivalents for Length

(To convert inches to centimeters, multiply the number of inches by 2.5.)

1 in			2.5 cm	
6 in	1/2 ft		15 cm	
12 in	1 ft		30 cm	
36 in	3 ft	1 yd	90 cm	
40 in			100 cm	1 m

INDEX

ACKNOWLEDGMENTS

Thank you to the Medical Medium community for your support and commitment through thick and thin. You have become a force of compassion and light.

Thank you to Patty Gift, Anne Barthel, Reid Tracy, Margarete Nielsen, Diane Hill, Sarah Coomes, and the rest of the Hay House team for your faith and commitment to getting Spirit of Compassion's wisdom out into the world so it can continue to change lives.

Kelly Noonan and Alec Gores, thank you for always looking out for me. It means so much.

Helen Lasichanh and Pharrell Williams, you are extraordinarily kindhearted seers.

Sylvester Stallone, Jennifer Flavin Stallone, and family, your support has been legendarily game-changing.

Dwayne Johnson and Lauren Hashian, I appreciate your friendship beyond measure. You are the salt of the earth.

Adam and Jackie Sandler, your humble, giving spirit is the real deal.

Diane von Furstenberg, what a blessing to have crossed paths with you in this life.

Hilary Swank and Philip Schneider, your dedication to the healing truth and wisdom is remarkable, and I am deeply honored. Your support is immensely powerful.

Kate Hudson, Danny Fujikawa, Erinn and Oliver Hudson, and Elisabeth Stassen, having you guys on my side with your love and support is a blessing.

Miranda Kerr and Evan Spiegel, it's so amazing to have your hands of light and compassion behind the healing movement.

Laura Dern, thank you for spreading your light and changing the world for the better.

Gwyneth Paltrow, your caring and generosity are a profound inspiration.

Carrie Ann Inaba, you are true to the core.

Uma Thurman, I deeply value and treasure our friendship.

Novak and Jelena Djokovic, your excellence at thriving is uplifting and inspiring.

Sage and Tony Robbins, it's an honor to be part of your world that's helping so many.

Martin, Jean, Elizabeth, and Jacqueline Shafiroff, thank you for always being there, believing in me, and helping to spread the message so that others can heal.

Dr. Alejandro Junger, life would not be the same without you, brother.

Dr. Ilana Zablozki-Amir, your willingness to support the Medical Medium cause is epic.

Dr. Prudence Hall, your selfless work to enlighten patients who need answers renews the true, heroic meaning of the word *doctor*.

Craig Kallman, thank you for your support, advocacy, and friendship on this journey.

Corey and Courtney Feldman, you are genuine, thoughtful, and outstanding souls.

Caroline Fleming, you're truly a blessing because you have the gift to always care about everyone around you as you share your light.

Chelsea Field and Scott, Wil, and Owen Bakula, how did I get so blessed to have you in my life? You are true crusaders for the Medical Medium cause.

Kimberly and James Van Der Beek, there's a special place in my heart for you and your family. I'm truly thankful to have crossed paths with you in this lifetime.

Kelly Rutherford, your wisdom and foresight raise up everyone around you.

Kerri Walsh Jennings, you truly amaze me with your hopeful nature and endless positive energy.

John Donovan, it's an honor to be on the planet with such a peace-seeking soul.

Nanci Chambers and David James, Stephanie, and Wyatt Elliott, I can't thank you enough for your dear friendship and everlasting encouragement.

Lisa Gregorisch-Dempsey, your acts of kindness have been deeply meaningful.

Grace Hightower De Niro, Robert De Niro, and family, you are precious, gracious beings.

Liv Tyler, it's such a great honor to be a part of your world.

Robert Downey, Jr., you're truly all heart and soul.

Jenna Dewan, your fighting spirit is an inspiration to behold.

Debra Messing, you are bettering people's lives with your vision for a healthy planet.

Alexis Bledel, your strength in this world is extraordinarily heartening.

Lisa Rinna, thank you for tirelessly using your influence to spread the message.

Steve Harris and family, you truly are incredible people.

Jennifer Aniston, your kindness, caring, and support are on another level.

Taylor Schilling, what a joy to know you and have your support.

Dana Gerson Unger, you are always looking out for others. You're amazing.

Marcela Valladolid, knowing you is a gift in my life.

Jennifer Meyer, I'm beyond grateful for your friendship and how you're always spreading the word.

Calvin Harris, you've changed the world with a powerful rhythm.

Courteney Cox, thank you for having such a pure, loving heart.

Hunter Mahan and Kandi Harris, I'm proud of you for always being game to take on a challenge.

Kidada Jones and Rashida Jones, the deep care and compassion you bring to life mean more than you know. Your mother was a treasure who lives on in you.

A very warm, heartfelt thanks and deep appreciation to Naomi Campbell; Eva Longoria; Carla Gugino; Mario Lopez; Renee Bargh; Tanika Ray; Michael Bernard Beckwith; Jay Shetty; Alex Kushneir; LeAnn Rimes Cibrian; Sharon Levin; Nena and Robert Thurman; Leslie Mann and Maude Apatow; Jenny Mollen; Jessica Seinfeld; Kelly Osbourne; Demi Moore; Beth Behr; Nikki Vianna; India.Arie; Kristen Bower; Rozonda Thomas; Peggy Rometo; Debbie Gibson; Carol, Scott, and Christiana Ritchie; Jamie-Lynn Sigler; Amanda de Cadenet; Marianne Williamson; Erin Johnson; Lewis Howes; Gabrielle Bernstein; Maha Dakhil; Bhavani Lev and Bharat Mitra; Woody Fraser and everyone at Hallmark's Home & Family; Morgan Fairchild; Patti Stanger; Catherine, Sophia, and Laura Bach; Annabeth Gish; Robert Wisdom; Danielle LaPorte; Nick and Brenna Ortner; Jessica Ortner; Mike Dooley; Kris Carr; Ann Louise Gittleman; Jan and Panache Desai; Ami Beach and Mark Shadle; Brian Wilson; John Holland; Alexandra Cohen; Christine Hill; Carol Donahue; Caroline Leavitt; Koya Webb; Jenny Hutt; Adam Cushman; Sonia Choquette; Colette Baron-Reid; Denise Linn; and Carmel Joy Baird. I deeply value you all.

To the compassionate doctors and other healers of the world who have changed the lives of so many: I have tremendous respect for you. Dr. Masha Kogan, Dr. Virginia Romano, Dr. Nguyen Phan, Dr. Chris, Dr. Habib Sadeghi, Dr. Carol Lee, Dr. Richard Sollazzo, Dr. Jeff Feinman, Dr. Deanna Minich, Dr. Ron Steriti, Dr. Nicole Galante, Dr. Diana Lopusny, Dr. Dick and Noel Shepard, Dr. Aleksandra Phillips, Dr. Chris Maloney, Drs. Tosca and Gregory Haag, Dr. Deborah Kern, Dr. Darren and Suzanne Boles, and Dr. Robin Karlin—it's an honor to call you friends. Thank you for your endless dedication to the field of healing.

Thanks to David Schmerler, Brittany Berckes, Kimberly S. Grimsley, Susan G. Etheridge, and Paul Prince for being there for me.

To the following special souls whose loyalty I treasure, my thanks go out: Muneeza Ahmed; Kimberly Spair; Amber Stone; Lauren Henry; Tara Tom; Bella; Victoria and Michael Arnstein; Nina Leatherer; Michelle Sutton; Haily Cataldo; Kerry; Amy Bacheller; Alexandra Laws; Ester Horn; Linda and Robert Coykendall; Glenn Klausner; Michael Monteleone; Bobbi and Leslie Hall; Katherine Belzowski; Matt and Vanessa Houston; David, Holly, and Ginnie Whitney; Melody Lee Pence; Terra Appelman; Eileen Crispell; Kristin Cassidy; Calvin Stebbins; Catherine Lawton; Alana DiNardo; Min Lee; and Eden Epstein Hill.

Sally Arnold, thank you for shining your light so brightly and lending your voice to the movement. Jeff Skeirik, thank you for the best pictures, man. Alyssa Degati, you are changing lives with your voice. Robby Barbaro, your unwavering positivity lifts up everyone around you. Andrew Kusatsu: love you, brother, for persevering past the pain and fighting for health freedom.

Ruby Scattergood, your masterful patience and countless hours of dedication have heroically formed the true spine of this book. The Medical Medium series would not be possible without your writing and editing. Thank you for your literary counsel.

Vibodha and Tila Clark, your creative genius has been astoundingly instrumental to the cause of helping others. Thank you for standing with us throughout the years.

Friar and Clare: *And if any man shall take away from the words of the book of this prophecy, God shall take away his part out of the book of life, and out of the holy city, and from the things which are written in this book. / He which testifieth these things saith, Surely I come quickly. Amen. Even so, come, Lord Jesus. / The grace of our Lord Jesus Christ be with you all. Amen.* (Rev. 22:19–21)

Quincy, thank you for your steadfast commitment and dedication to the cause.

Chelsey, Courtney, Harper, and Anett, thank you for your invaluable support and hard work.

Sepideh Kashanian and Ben, thank you for your warm, loving care.

Michael and Bonnie McMenamin, honored to be on this planet in this time in history together.

Oliver Niño and Mandy Morris, so proud of you for all you do for so many.

For your love and support, as always, I thank my family: my luminous wife; Dad and Mom; my brothers, nieces, nephews, aunts, and uncles; my champions Indigo, Ruby, and Great Blue; Hope; Marjorie and Robert; Laura; Rhia and Byron; Alayne Serle and Scott, Perri, Lissy, and Ari Cohn; David Somoroff; Joel, Liz, Kody, Jesse, Lauren, Joseph, and Thomas; Brian, Joyce, and Josh; Jarod; Brent; Kelly and Evy; Danielle, Johnny, and Declan; and all my loved ones who are on the other side.

Finally, thank you, Spirit of the Most High (aka Spirit of Compassion), for providing all of us with compassionate wisdom from the heavens that inspires us to keep our heads up and carry the sacred gifts you've been so kind to give us. Thank you for putting up with me over the years and reminding me to keep a light heart with your never-ending patience and willingness to answer my questions in search of the truth.

ABOUT THE AUTHOR

Medical Medium Anthony William, the chronic illness expert, is the originator of the global celery juice movement, host of the *Medical Medium Podcast*, and #1 *New York Times* best-selling author of the Medical Medium book series:

- *Medical Medium Brain Saver Protocols, Cleanses & Recipes: For Neurological, Autoimmune & Mental Health*

- *Medical Medium Brain Saver: Answers to Brain Inflammation, Mental Health, OCD, Brain Fog, Neurological Symptoms, Addiction, Anxiety, Depression, Heavy Metals, Epstein-Barr Virus, Seizures, Lyme, ADHD, Alzheimer's, Autoimmune & Eating Disorders*

- *Medical Medium Cleanse to Heal: Healing Plans for Sufferers of Anxiety, Depression, Acne, Eczema, Lyme, Gut Problems, Brain Fog, Weight Issues, Migraines, Bloating, Vertigo, Psoriasis, Cysts, Fatigue, PCOS, Fibroids, UTI, Endometriosis & Autoimmune*

- *Medical Medium Celery Juice: The Most Powerful Medicine of Our Time Healing Millions Worldwide*

- *Medical Medium Liver Rescue: Answers to Eczema, Psoriasis, Diabetes, Strep, Acne, Gout, Bloating, Gallstones, Adrenal Stress, Fatigue, Fatty Liver, Weight Issues, SIBO & Autoimmune Disease*

- *Medical Medium Thyroid Healing: The Truth behind Hashimoto's, Graves', Insomnia, Hypothyroidism, Thyroid Nodules & Epstein-Barr*

- *Medical Medium Life-Changing Foods: Save Yourself and the Ones You Love with the Hidden*

Healing Powers of Fruits & Vegetables

- *Medical Medium: Secrets Behind Chronic and Mystery Illness and How to Finally Heal (Revised and Expanded Edition)*

Anthony was born with the unique ability to converse with the Spirit of Compassion, who provides him with extraordinarily advanced healing medical information that's far ahead of its time. Since age four, Anthony has been using his gift to see into people's conditions and tell them and their doctors how to recover their health. Over decades of helping individuals find the answers they needed, Anthony found that he could only help so many as his waiting list continued to grow. Anthony now dedicates much of his time and energy to listening to Spirit of Compassion's information and placing it into books so everybody can have an opportunity to heal. His unprecedented accuracy and success rate as the Medical Medium have earned him the trust and love of millions worldwide, among them movie stars, rock stars, billionaires, professional athletes, and countless other people from all walks of life who couldn't find a way to heal until he provided them with insights from above. Over the decades, Anthony has also been an invaluable resource to doctors who need help solving their most difficult cases.

Learn more at www.medicalmedium.com

"It doesn't matter if you like your soul, love your soul, or hate your soul. It doesn't matter if you don't believe in the soul's existence or believe you have a soul. It doesn't matter because your soul is more powerful than you, more powerful than your consciousness in your present state of being."

— Anthony William, Medical Medium

Hay House Titles of Related Interest

YOU CAN HEAL YOUR LIFE, the movie, starring Louise Hay & Friends
(available as an online streaming video)
www.hayhouse.com/louise-movie

THE SHIFT, the movie,
starring Dr. Wayne W. Dyer
(available as an online streaming video)
www.hayhouse.com/the-shift-movie

***

*MEDICAL MEDIUM: Secrets Behind Chronic and Mystery Illness
and How to Finally Heal (Revised and Expanded Edition),* by Anthony William

*MEDICAL MEDIUM LIFE-CHANGING FOODS: Save Yourself and the Ones You Love
with the Hidden Healing Powers of Fruits & Vegetables,* by Anthony William

*MEDICAL MEDIUM THYROID HEALING: The Truth behind Hashimoto's, Graves',
Insomnia, Hypothyroidism, Thyroid Nodules & Epstein-Barr,* by Anthony William

*MEDICAL MEDIUM LIVER RESCUE: Answers to Eczema, Psoriasis, Diabetes, Strep,
Acne, Gout, Bloating, Gallstones, Adrenal Stress, Fatigue, Fatty Liver, Weight Issues,
SIBO & Autoimmune Disease,* by Anthony William

*MEDICAL MEDIUM CELERY JUICE: The Most Powerful Medicine of Our
Time Healing Millions Worldwide,* by Anthony William

*MEDICAL MEDIUM CLEANSE TO HEAL: Healing Plans for Sufferers of Anxiety, Depression,
Acne, Eczema, Lyme, Gut Problems, Brain Fog, Weight Issues, Migraines, Bloating, Vertigo, Psoriasis,
Cysts, Fatigue, PCOS, Fibroids, UTI, Endometriosis & Autoimmune,* by Anthony William

*MEDICAL MEDIUM BRAIN SAVER: Answers to Brain Inflammation, Mental Health, OCD, Brain Fog,
Neurological Symptoms, Addiction, Anxiety, Depression, Heavy Metals, Epstein-Barr Virus, Seizures, Lyme,
ADHD, Alzheimer's, Autoimmune & Eating Disorders,* by Anthony William

All of the above are available at your local bookstore,
or may be ordered by contacting Hay House (see next page).

***

We hope you enjoyed this Hay House book. If you'd like to receive our online catalog featuring additional information on Hay House books and products, or if you'd like to find out more about the Hay Foundation, please contact:

Hay House, Inc., P.O. Box 5100, Carlsbad, CA 92018-5100
(760) 431-7695 or (800) 654-5126
(760) 431-6948 (fax) or (800) 650-5115 (fax)
www.hayhouse.com® • www.hayfoundation.org

———

Published in Australia by: Hay House Australia Pty. Ltd.,
18/36 Ralph St., Alexandria NSW 2015
Phone: 612-9669-4299 • *Fax:* 612-9669-4144
www.hayhouse.com.au

Published in the United Kingdom by: Hay House UK, Ltd.,
The Sixth Floor, Watson House, 54 Baker Street, London W1U 7BU
Phone: +44 (0)20 3927 7290 • *Fax:* +44 (0)20 3927 7291
www.hayhouse.co.uk

Published in India by: Hay House Publishers India,
Muskaan Complex, Plot No. 3, B-2, Vasant Kunj, New Delhi 110 070
Phone: 91-11-4176-1620 • *Fax:* 91-11-4176-1630
www.hayhouse.co.in

———

Access New Knowledge.
Anytime. Anywhere.

Learn and evolve at your own pace
with the world's leading experts.

www.hayhouseU.com

"Everyone is different. Not in the way we normally think. While our souls are different, our physical bodies, as humans, are meant to function in the same way. We eat food, drink water, urinate and defecate; our hearts beat and our blood pumps; we walk on our feet, we see with our eyes, we hear with our ears, our stomachs are meant to digest . . . until something goes wrong and we can't. We can't walk, we can't talk, we can't hear, we can't see; our blood gets clogged or our heart doesn't beat right. Different internal problems with our physical bodies can create endless differences. Our injuries, pathogens, stresses, metals, traumas, relationships, environmental surroundings, resources, support, pharmaceuticals, experiences, deficiencies, amounts of blood drawn, number of flus we've had, how many exposures we come into the world with—all these make us different. Our differences make our healing processes and their timelines different."

— Anthony William, Medical Medium

"When people are on the journey of healing and they're not using the right tools, and they don't know why they became sick to begin with, they lose faith where they once had faith. It burns out. If you're someone who has tried everything, been through so much during your process of healing throughout the months or years, and you land here with very little faith or no faith left at all because you lost it along the way through endless trial and error based on misinformation, you can still heal. Your faith will restore as you're healing and you see the light."

— Anthony William, Medical Medium